Primary Care of Adult Women

Editors

JAMES N. WOODRUFF
ANITA K. BLANCHARD

OBSTETRICS AND GYNECOLOGY CLINICS OF NORTH AMERICA

www.obgyn.theclinics.com

Consulting Editor
WILLIAM F. RAYBURN

June 2016 • Volume 43 • Number 2

ELSEVIER

1600 John F. Kennedy Boulevard • Suite 1800 • Philadelphia, Pennsylvania, 19103-2899

http://www.theclinics.com

OBSTETRICS AND GYNECOLOGY CLINICS OF NORTH AMERICA Volume 43, Number 2
June 2016 ISSN 0889-8545, ISBN-13: 978-0-323-44622-8

Editor: Kerry Holland
Developmental Editor: Kristen Helm

Obstetrics and Gynecology Clinics (ISSN 0889-8545) is published quarterly by Elsevier Inc., 360 Park Avenue South, New York, NY 10010-1710. Months of issue are March, June, September, and December. Periodicals postage paid at New York, NY, and additional mailing offices. Subscription price per year is $295.00 (US individuals), $597.00 (US institutions), $100.00 (US students), $370.00 (Canadian individuals), $754.00 (Canadian institutions), $225.00 (Canadian students), $450.00 (international individuals), $754.00 (international institutions), and $225.00 (international students). To receive student/resident rate, orders must be accompanied by name of affiliated institution, date of term, and the signature of program/residency coordinator on institution letterhead. Orders will be billed at individual rate until proof of status is received. Foreign air speed delivery is included in all *Clinics* subscription prices. All prices are subject to change without notice. POSTMASTER: Send address changes to *Obstetrics and Gynecology Clinics*, Elsevier Health Sciences Division, Subscription Customer Service, 3251 Riverport Lane, Maryland Heights, MO 63043. **Customer Service: Telephone: 1-800-654-2452 (U.S. and Canada); 314-447-8871 (outside U.S. and Canada). Fax: 314-447-8029. E-mail: journalscustomerservice-usa@elsevier.com (for print support); journalsonlinesupport-usa@elsevier.com (for online support).**

Reprints. For copies of 100 or more of articles in this publication, please contact the Commercial Reprints Department, Elsevier Inc., 360 Park Avenue South, New York, New York 10010-1710. Tel.: 212-633-3874; Fax: 212-633-3820; E-mail: reprints@elsevier.com.

Obstetrics and Gynecology Clinics of North America is also published in Spanish by McGraw-Hill Interamericana Editores S.A., P.O. Box 5-237, 06500, Mexico; in Portuguese by Reichmann and Affonso Editores, Rio de Janeiro, Brazil; and in Greek by Paschalidis Medical Publications, Athens, Greece.

Obstetrics and Gynecology Clinics of North America is covered in MEDLINE/PubMed (Index Medicus), Excerpta Medica, Current Concepts/Clinical Medicine, Science Citation Index, BIOSIS, CINAHL, and ISI/BIOMED.

Contributors

CONSULTING EDITOR

WILLIAM F. RAYBURN, MD, MBA
Associate Dean, Continuing Medical Education and Professional Development; Distinguished Professor and Emeritus Chair, Obstetrics and Gynecology, University of New Mexico School of Medicine, Albuquerque, New Mexico

EDITORS

JAMES N. WOODRUFF, MD
Professor of Medicine, Department of Medicine, Associate Dean of Students, Pritzker School of Medicine, The University of Chicago Medicine and Biological Sciences, Chicago, Illinois

ANITA K. BLANCHARD, MD
Professor, Residency Program Director, Department of Obstetrics and Gynecology, The University of Chicago Medicine and Biological Sciences, Chicago, Illinois

AUTHORS

NADIA N. AHMAD, MD, MPH
Director, Obesity Medicine Institute; Armada Medical Center, Dubai, United Arab Emirates

SABINA AIDAROUS, MBBS
Clinical and Research Fellow, Obesity Medicine Institute, Dubai, United Arab Emirates

ANITA K. BLANCHARD, MD
Professor, Residency Program Director, Department of Obstetrics and Gynecology, The University of Chicago Medicine and Biological Sciences, Chicago, Illinois

WINFIELD SCOTT BUTSCH, MD, MSc
Instructor in Medicine, MGH Weight Center, Massachusetts General Hospital, Harvard Medical School, Boston, Massachusetts

BETH DUNLAP, MD
Assistant Professor of Family and Community Medicine, Northwestern University, Chicago, Illinois

ELIZABETH FITELSON, MD
Director, The Women's Program, Assistant Professor of Psychiatry at the Columbia University Medical Center, Columbia University Department of Psychiatry, New York, New York

PERPETUA GOODALL, MD
Assistant Professor, Department of Obstetrics and Gynecology, University of Chicago, Chicago, Illinois

MARTHA GULATI, MD, MS, FACC, FAHA
Division Chief of Cardiology, University of Arizona-Phoenix; Professor of Medicine, Physician Executive Director for the Banner University Medicine Cardiovascular Institute, Phoenix, Arizona

ANNA R. HEMNES, MD
Assistant Professor, Division of Allergy, Pulmonary and Critical Care Medicine, Vanderbilt University Medical Center, Nashville, Tennessee

KAREN E. KIM, MD
Professor of Medicine, Section of Gastroenterology, Hepatology and Nutrition, The University of Chicago Medical Center, Chicago, Illinois

CARMELA KIRALY, MD
Department of Medicine, University of Chicago, Chicago, Illinois

EMILY G. KOCUREK, MD
Fellow, Division of Allergy, Pulmonary and Critical Care Medicine, Vanderbilt University Medical Center, Nashville, Tennessee

JODY L. KUJOVICH, MD
Assistant Professor, Department of Pediatric Hematology/Oncology, The Hemophilia Center, Oregon Health and Science University, Portland, Oregon

CHERYL McGIBBON, MD
Fellow in Women's Mental Health, Instructor in Psychiatry at the Columbia University Medical Center, Columbia University Department of Psychiatry, New York, New York

JULIE MHLABA, BS
Pritzker School of Medicine, University of Chicago, Chicago, Illinois

DEJAN MICIC, MD
Gastroenterology Fellow, Section of Gastroenterology, Hepatology and Nutrition, The University of Chicago Medical Center, Chicago, Illinois

VIJAYA L. RAO, MD
Gastroenterology Fellow, Section of Gastroenterology, Hepatology and Nutrition, The University of Chicago Medical Center, Chicago, Illinois

CARLY ROMAN, MD
Section of Dermatology, University of Chicago, Chicago, Illinois

ARLENE M. RUIZ DE LUZURIAGA, MD, MPH
Assistant Professor, Section of Dermatology, University of Chicago, Chicago, Illinois

MONIKA SANGHAVI, MD
Cardiology, Department of Medicine, University of Texas Southwestern Medical Center, Dallas, Texas

SACHIN D. SHAH, MD
Assistant Professor of Medicine and Pediatrics, University of Chicago, Chicago, Illinois

SANDRA SHI, MD
Department of Medicine, University of Chicago, Chicago, Illinois

CELESTE C. THOMAS, MD, MS
Assistant Professor of Medicine, Section of Adult and Pediatric Endocrinology, Diabetes, and Metabolism, Department of Medicine, University of Chicago, Chicago, Illinois

KATHERINE THOMPSON, MD
Assistant Professor of Medicine, Section of Geriatrics and Palliative Medicine,
Department of Medicine, University of Chicago, Chicago, Illinois

GEORGE W. WEYER, MD
Assistant Professor of Medicine, University of Chicago, Chicago, Illinois

MELTEM ZEYTINOGLU, MD, MBA
Assistant Professor of Medicine, Section of Adult and Pediatric Endocrinology, Diabetes,
and Metabolism, Department of Medicine, University of Chicago, Chicago, Illinois

Contents

Specialists in general obstetrics and gynecology are key providers of primary care in women. They diagnose and provide the initial management of many medical conditions unrelated to reproductive health. Most importantly they can impact the overall health of patients through incorporating preventive approaches in the annual well-woman visit. This article defines preventive care and identifies leading causes of mortality in women. A framework for identifying key elements of the well-woman examination is summarized. Examples of prevention are provided, which focus on major health care issues that affect adult women.

Dermatologic disease often presents in the primary care setting. Therefore, it is important for the primary care provider to be familiar with the presentation, diagnosis, and treatment of common skin conditions. This article provides an overview of acne, rosacea, melasma, vitiligo, alopecia, nonmelanoma and melanoma skin cancer, dermatitis, and lichen sclerosus.

The World Health Organization estimates that nearly 2 billion people worldwide are overweight, 600 million of whom are obese. The increasing prevalence of this condition in women is of particular concern given its impact on reproductive health and mortality. Burgeoning data implicating maternal obesity in fetal programming and the metabolic health of future generations further suggest that obesity in women is one of the most pressing public health concerns of the twenty-first century. However, health care professionals are infrequently engaged in obesity management. This article provides a conceptual understanding of obesity and a rational approach to treatment.

Providers of obstetric and gynecologic care are often the most commonly seen medical providers for adult women, providing primary and reproductive care. Even where psychiatric care is readily available, obstetricians/gynecologists are frequently the front line for recognition, education, and initial management of many mental health problems. In settings where psychiatric treatment is a more scarce resource, obstetricians/gynecologists often are responsible for ongoing treatment of these disorders. This review focuses on the impact of the female reproductive life cycle on the presentation and management of some of the most common behavioral health problems in women: major depression, bipolar disorder, anxiety disorders, and primary sleep disorders.

Anemia is a common problem in primary care. Classification based on mean cell volume narrows the differential diagnosis and directs testing. A marked macrocytosis is characteristic of vitamin B_{12} and folate deficiencies, certain medications, and primary bone marrow disorders. The three most common causes of microcytic anemia are iron deficiency, thalassemia trait, and anemia of inflammation. Additional laboratory testing is required for diagnosis. Determination of the rate of development of anemia and examination of a blood smear may provide diagnostic clues to guide more specialized testing. Diagnosis of iron, vitamin B_{12}, or folate deficiency mandates determination of the underlying cause.

Cardiovascular disease remains the leading cause of death in the United States. Primary prevention of cardiovascular disease requires involvement of an extended health care team. Obstetricians and gynecologists are uniquely positioned within the health care system because they are often the primary or only contact women have with the system. This review article discusses initial assessment, treatment recommendations, and practical tips regarding primary and secondary prevention of cardiovascular disease in women with a focus on coronary heart disease; discussion includes peripheral and cerebrovascular disease.

Hypertension is the most commonly encountered chronic medical condition in primary care and one of the most significant modifiable cardiovascular risk factors for women and men. Timely diagnosis and evidence-based management offer an important opportunity to reduce the risk of hypertension-related morbidity and mortality, including cardiovascular events, end-stage renal disease, and heart failure. Clinical trials have shown significant improvements in patient-oriented outcomes when hypertension is well-controlled, yet many hypertensive patients remain undiagnosed, uncontrolled, or managed with inappropriate pharmacotherapy. This article discusses the initial diagnosis, evaluation, and management of hypertension in nonpregnant women, with topics for obstetrician-gynecologists and women's health providers.

Although the lung is not traditionally thought of as an organ affected by sex-based differences, emerging literature elucidates major differences between men and women in the development, physiology, and predilection to and outcomes in lung diseases. These differences are driven by both differences in sex hormones and differences in environmental exposures. However, in many cases the underlying etiology of these sex- and gender-based differences is unknown. This article outlines the state-of-the-art knowledge on the etiology of sex differences in lung disease, including differences in lung development and physiology, and reviews therapy recommendations that are sex-based.

Diabetes mellitus, thyroid disorders, and osteoporosis are endocrine conditions affecting a significant proportion of women presenting to the obstetrician-gynecologist. Obstetrician-gynecologists are often the first health-care providers that young women see in adulthood, and thus, have a critical opportunity to identify women at risk for gestational and overt diabetes and manage the condition in those who have developed it. The obstetrician-gynecologist should be aware of the appropriate therapeutic options and treatment goals (eg, hemoglobin A1c) for women with diabetes. Thyroid disorders often present with menstrual irregularities or infertility, can affect pregnancy outcomes, and contribute to cardiovascular and bone disorders as women age. Finally, osteoporosis and low bone mineral density affect a substantial proportion of older women and some younger women with risk factors for secondary osteoporosis. The morbidity and mortality of osteoporotic fractures is substantial. There are many lifestyle interventions and therapeutic options available for these conditions, and the gynecologist plays a key role in optimizing risk factor assessment, screening, and providing treatment when appropriate.

Gastrointestinal disorders often present to the primary care setting where initial preventive, diagnostic, and treatment strategies are implemented. This article reviews the presentation and diagnosis of common gastrointestinal disorders, including colorectal cancer, irritable bowel syndrome, peptic ulcer disease, gallbladder disorders, inflammatory bowel disease, gastroesophageal reflux, and Barrett's esophagus. We focus on the evaluation and management of these diseases in women.

Older adults are the fastest growing segment of the US population and the majority of older adults are women. Primary care for the older adult patient requires a wide variety of skills, reflecting the complexity and heterogeneity of this patient population. Individualizing care through consideration of patients' goals, medical conditions, and prognosis is paramount. Quality care for the older adult patient requires familiarity with common geriatric syndromes, such as dementia, falls, and polypharmacy. In addition, developing the knowledge and communication skills necessary for complex care and end-of-life care planning is essential.

OBSTETRICS AND GYNECOLOGY CLINICS

FORTHCOMING ISSUES

September 2016
Hysterectomy and the Alternatives
John A. Occhino and
Emanuel C. Trabuco, *Editors*

December 2016
**Critical Care Obstetrics for the Obstetrician
and Gynecologist**
Carolyn M. Zelop and Stephanie R. Martin,
Editors

March 2017
Health Care for Underserved Women
Wanda Kay Nicholson, *Editor*

RECENT ISSUES

March 2016
**Medical and Advanced Surgical
Management of Pelvic Floor Disorders**
Cheryl B. Iglesia, *Editor*

December 2015
Contraception
Pamela S. Lotke and Bliss Kaneshiro,
Editors

September 2015
**Obstetric and Gynecologic Hospitalists and
Laborists**
Brigid McCue and
Jennifer A. Tessmer-Tuck, *Editors*

Foreword

Are Obstetrician-Gynecologists Primary Care Physicians?

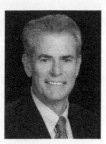

William F. Rayburn, MD, MBA
Consulting Editor

This issue of *Obstetrics and Gynecology Clinics of North America* is a concise reference that encompasses a broad spectrum of management issues relating to the primary care of women. It was developed and edited very capably under the direction of Dr Jim Woodruff and Dr Anita Blanchard from the University of Chicago. Past issues were edited by obstetrician-gynecologists (OB-GYNs) who were accomplished in their specialty. Instead, this issue is mostly authored by experts in internal medicine who represent diversity among women's health care providers from academic and private practices, as well as from general and subspecialty medicine.

Primary care can be viewed as the day-to-day health care given by a health care provider. Typically, the provider acts as the first contact and principal point of continuing care and coordinates other specialty care that the patient may need. Although information contained in this issue is intended for the OB-GYN, much is applicable to others in women's health care, such as nursing staff, physician assistants and other allied health providers, health care administrators, and health plan decision-makers.

This issue provides a digest of clinical information that is not easily found in most OB-GYN textbooks. The overall issue is not intended to be comprehensive; instead, it consolidates useful information from a variety of relevant medical topics that encompass primary care. The authors draw on recommendations from many professional organizations, especially those from the American College of Obstetricians and Gynecologists' practice bulletins, committee opinions, and policy statements.

The issue begins with health care of women that focuses on routine screening and prevention. New information is provided in separate articles that pertain to cardiovascular disease, hypertension, lung development and disease, endocrinology, and gastroenterological disorders. Obesity, anemia, and many dermatologic conditions commonly faced by OB-GYNs in their offices are nicely covered. In addition, one article addresses primary care of older women, who constitute the most rapidly growing group of patients in the United States.

Obstet Gynecol Clin N Am 43 (2016) xiii–xiv
http://dx.doi.org/10.1016/j.ogc.2016.03.002
0889-8545/16/$ – see front matter © 2016 Published by Elsevier Inc.

obgyn.theclinics.com

Are OB-GYNs primary care physicians? In order to provide primary care, a physician must offer a broad spectrum of care directed to many aspects of a woman's health. During the reproductive years, many women turn to an OB-GYN's office as a point of entry into the health care system. It is here where continuity of care begins with encouragement of routine screening and preventive care. Routine visits are opportunities for OB-GYNs to educate and counsel their patients about risk factors and lifestyle issues, as identified from the screening history or physical examination.

Whether an OB-GYN is a primary care physician depends on the scope of services provided predominantly in the ambulatory setting. For example, a practitioner may feel very comfortable in providing preventive screening for healthy asymptomatic women and care for those with acute uncomplicated illness, but not necessarily in treating worse or chronic diseases. Therefore, it is important to clarify with the patient whether the OB-GYN's office is the site for medical care delivery and for specialty referrals for issues that are outside the OB-GYN's purview. The scope of services at inpatient settings also varies depending on the OB-GYN's training and experience. Hospitalists in internal medicine and in obstetrics and gynecology are more common in urban settings to serve primary care physicians.

Without question, obstetrics is a medical field in which primary care is provided. Following a delivery and at the first postpartum visit, the obstetrician or other obstetric provider should identify interval care recommendations for general health promotion. Regardless of whether the woman's subsequent care is provided by that same practitioner or by a family physician, internist, or other health care provider, it is important to clearly identify needed follow-up care, such as blood pressure monitoring and repeat anemia or diabetes screening. Patient handoffs are a necessary component of current medical care. Accurate and timely communication of information about a patient from one member of the health care team to another is essential for patient care and safety.

I wish to thank Dr Woodruff and Dr Blanchard for enlisting the cooperation of several clinician authors who are experts in a broad range of women's health care needs. Addressed in the articles are also issues involving access to health care and an awareness of women with diverse needs. Clinical recommendations presented here are based on the best available evidence and factor in age group and risk factors. Assessments, whether annually or as appropriate, vary according to that specific patient's needs and any high-risk conditions that require targeted screening or treatment.

William F. Rayburn, MD, MBA
Continuing Medical Education
and Professional Development
Obstetrics and Gynecology
University of New Mexico School of Medicine
MSC 10 5580
1 University of New Mexico
Albuquerque, NM 87131-0001, USA

E-mail address:
Wrayburn@salud.unm.edu

Preface

Primary Care of Adult Women

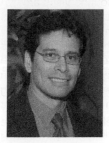
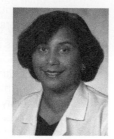

James N. Woodruff, MD   Anita K. Blanchard, MD
Editors

Access to high-quality primary care enhances the health of populations.[1] The focus on prevention, early detection of disease, and successful management of commonly encountered diseases enables primary care practitioners to promote health.[2]

Obstetrician-Gynecologists are frequently responsible for management of the primary care needs of their patients. A survey performed in 2005 found an estimated 37% of private, nonpregnant patients rely on gynecologists for routine primary care. The same study found that almost a quarter of gynecologists reported they would benefit from additional primary care updates in training.[3] In response to language in the Affordable Care Act, the Institute of Medicine (IOM) developed a report on clinical preventive services necessary for women.[4] The US Department of Health and Human Services has adopted these IOM recommendations and, as a result, health plans are required to include these services. As a result, the impetus for enhanced training of gynecologists in primary care skills is increasing. While ACOG's Well-Woman Task Force recommendations and recent cross-specialty ACOG educational collaborations address many primary care educational needs, additional ongoing efforts inspire in-depth handling of key primary care topics.

The *Obstetrics and Gynecology Clinics of North America* series is an ideal means for accomplishing this important goal. In this issue, commonly encountered medical conditions are reviewed through the lens of primary care for women. Selected topics are reviewed by experts in their respective fields. These authors take an evidence-based approach to practical office-based decision-making. In several areas, authors also provide contemporary insights into the modulation of specific diseases by female physiology.

The collaborative nature of this issue with contributions from a variety of specialists in many fields will hopefully enhance the delivery of high-quality primary

Obstet Gynecol Clin N Am 43 (2016) xv–xvi
http://dx.doi.org/10.1016/j.ogc.2016.03.001
0889-8545/16/$ – see front matter © 2016 Published by Elsevier Inc.

obgyn.theclinics.com

care, support interprofessional teamwork, and promote the overall health of our patients.

James N. Woodruff, MD
Department of Medicine
Pritzker School of Medicine
The University of Chicago Medicine
& Biological Sciences
924 East 50th Street
Chicago, IL 60637, USA

Anita K. Blanchard, MD
Department of Obstetrics and Gynecology
The University of Chicago Medicine
& Biological Sciences
5841 South Maryland Avenue
Room L235, MC 2050
Chicago, IL 60637, USA

E-mail addresses:
jwoodruf@medicine.bsd.uchicago.edu (J.N. Woodruff)
ablancha@bsd.uchicago.edu (A.K. Blanchard)

REFERENCES

1. Macinko J, Starfield B, Shi L. Systems to health outcomes within Organization for Economic Cooperation and Development (OECD) countries, 1970–1998. Health Serv Res 2003;38(3):831–65.
2. Starfield B, Shi L, Macinko J. Contribution of primary care to health systems and health. Milbank Q 2005;83(3):457–502.
3. Coleman V, Laube D, Hale R, et al. Obstetrician–gynecologists and primary care: training during obstetrics–gynecology residency and current practice patterns. Acad Med 2007;82:602–7.
4. Gee R, Brindis C, Diaz A, et al. Recommendations of the IOM Clinical Preventive Services for Women Committee: implications for obstetricians and gynecologists. Curr Opin Obstetr Gynecol 2011;23:471–80.

Preventive Care in Women's Health

Anita K. Blanchard, MD*, Perpetua Goodall, MD

KEYWORDS

- Women's health • Preventive care • Health maintenance • Screening tests

KEY POINTS

- Reproductive aged women often receive primary care from specialists in general obstetrics and gynecology.
- Prevention is the mainstay of health care. There are primary, secondary, and tertiary forms of prevention.
- Preventive measures may include immunizations, behavioral counseling, screening tests, and chemoprevention.
- Leading causes of death vary by age group.
- Leading causes of death can be mitigated by promoting healthy practices that focus on primary, secondary, and tertiary prevention.

INTRODUCTION

Preventive care is a major cornerstone of clinical medicine. The focus of health care is shifting from problem-based medicine toward preemptive care, seeking to intervene before harmful problems develop. Obstetric and gynecologic physicians provide approximately half of all preventive care visits in reproductive-aged women.[1] There is great opportunity to expand the focus of these visits beyond reproductive health issues. Given the wide reach of the specialty, it is important to promote disease prevention through detailed history taking, assessing risk, and coordinating the appropriate interventions in all aspects of health. Eliminating inequity and advancing health literacy among patients are also complex but important aspects of preventive medicine. This article provides an overview of preventive care, leading causes of mortality in adult women, and examples of prevention focused on these major health care issues.

Preventive care includes primary prevention, secondary prevention, and tertiary prevention. Primary prevention controls risk factors that contribute to disease with

Disclosure Statement: The authors have nothing to disclose.
Department of Obstetrics and Gynecology, University of Chicago, Chicago, IL, USA
* Corresponding author. 5841 South Maryland Avenue, Room L235, MC 2050, Chicago, IL 60637.
E-mail address: ablancha@uchicago.edu

Obstet Gynecol Clin N Am 43 (2016) 165–180
http://dx.doi.org/10.1016/j.ogc.2016.01.008
0889-8545/16/$ – see front matter © 2016 Elsevier Inc. All rights reserved.

the goal of preventing disease onset. Secondary prevention targets early staged disease to decrease morbidity or death by eradicating or slowing disease progression. Tertiary prevention limits sequelae once a disease is fully manifested to reduce further complications. Distinctions between the three types of clinical prevention may be blurred and interventions may fulfill more than one type of prevention.

Clinical interventions supporting preventive care fall into several categories: immunizations, behavioral counseling, screening tests, and chemopreventive measures. Procedural interventions may also contribute to preventive care. Examples include bariatric surgery for obese women and prophylactic oophorectomy in patients with hereditary cancer syndromes. Deciding which interventions are appropriate for individual patients is a challenge. Evidence of overall clinical benefit as outlined by professional and scientific organizations supports decision-making.

Counseling and patient education are important components of the preventive care model. Materials supporting these efforts should be obtained from credible sources and be designed to effectively promote patient understanding.

Risk stratification is important in any preventive care program. Examples of variables contributing to risk include age, genetic, and environmental factors. Mitigation of risk is accomplished by interventions tailored to the individual's personal and hereditary attributes. For example, screening should be targeted to populations demonstrating the highest prevalence of disease to enhance cost effectiveness and test reliability. Epidemiologic data including disease prevalence and death rates help identify target groups. Leading causes of death by age in women are summarized in **Table 1**.[2] The goals of preventive interventions may evolve as patients age and risks change. In younger women, health maintenance may consist of only primary prevention including healthy habits and immunizations designed to minimize morbidity from common disorders. As women age and chronic illness becomes more frequent, care shifts to secondary prevention to include preservation of quality of life and preventing mortality. In the elderly, tertiary prevention may become the main focus.

Preventive measures should target disorders that demonstrate a burden of impairment, that have common prevalence, and that are treatable in the precursor state. Screening should be safe, accessible, and cost effective with analytical validity and clinical utility to alter the natural course of the disease. Screening tests can be evidence based, evidence informed, and based on expert opinion. Several governing bodies dictate these recommendations including US Preventive Services Task Force (USPSTF), National Institutes of Health, World Health Organization, Institute of Medicine, and Centers for Disease Control and Prevention (CDC). Other data-gathering analytical resources include the Cochrane library, and specialty-based medical societies, such as the American Congress of Obstetrics and Gynecology (ACOG) and the American College of Physicians.

Recently ACOG published the Well-Woman Task Force Report highlighting evidence that supports components of a well-woman examination with consensus from experts from 15 major organizations in women's health.[3] The task force compiled and reviewed the major recommendations of many societies and surveillance organizations, then made joint recommendations. Their completed extensive report to the US Department of Health and Human Services is based on three levels of consensus including the following categories: evidence based, evidence informed, or uniform expert agreement. Strength of the recommendation was further scored as strong or qualified. Although this document does not attempt to duplicate the recommendations of other agencies, it creates a convenient resource compiling elements of the well-woman examination. It also fills the gaps between data-driven care and practical decision making in areas with limited data. As recommendations continue to be revised,

Table 1
Leading causes of death in US women by age group 2013

Age	20–24	25–34	35–44	45–54	55–64	65–84	85+
Leading cause of death	Unintentional injuries	Unintentional injuries	Cancer	Cancer	Cancer	Cancer	Heart disease
Second leading cause of death	Suicide	Cancer	Unintentional injuries	Heart disease	Heart disease	Heart disease	Cancer
Third leading cause of death	Homicide	Suicide	Heart disease	Unintentional injuries	Chronic lower respiratory disease	Chronic lower respiratory disease	Alzheimer disease

Adapted from Centers for Disease Control and Prevention (CDC). Available at: http://www.cdc.gov/women/lcod/2013/WomenAll_2013.pdf. Accessed October 10, 2015.

it also gives the references needed for health care providers to continue to update their practices.

The Well-Woman Task Force recommendations identify key components of the health care maintenance examination varied by age group. Of the approximately 40 elements reviewed by the Task Force, **Box 1** lists the components that were recommended in average-risk, reproductive-aged adult, nonpregnant women. Screening for anemia, bacteriuria, glaucoma, hearing, hypothyroidism, kidney disease, and ovarian cancer was not routinely recommended in the asymptomatic nonpregnant adult woman.

A complete review of preventive measures is beyond the scope of this article. Important screening measures including those focused on hypertension, atherosclerotic cardiovascular disease, and colon cancer are reviewed in other articles in this issue. The focus of this article is directed toward the components of adult preventive care that target the leading causes of morbidity and mortality in women and highlight examples of the four types of clinical prevention: (1) behavioral counseling, (2) immunizations, (3) screening interventions, and (4) chemoprevention.

BEHAVIORAL COUNSELING: UNINTENTIONAL INJURIES, SUICIDE, AND HOMICIDE
Incidence and Mortality

Unintentional injuries, suicides, and homicides are three leading causes of death in young adult women less than 44 years of age. In 2013, unintentional injuries accounted for 130,557 deaths among US women.[4] In women age 20 to 24 unintentional injuries accounted for 40% of deaths and in age 25 to 34 approximately 30% of deaths. Motor vehicle accidents are the leading cause of death in this age range.

Suicide is the second most common cause of death in these age groups. In 2013 there were 41,149 deaths from suicide and 16,121 deaths from homicide.[4] Suicide and homicide are much more common in males than females. High-risk behaviors are important contributors to unintentional injuries, homicide, and suicide. Drug and alcohol abuse impact all three causes of mortality. Depression impacts suicide and homicide incidence. These causes of death are also influenced by socioeconomic and environmental stressors. These behaviors may be modified with early identification and counseling in individuals at risk.

Screening Modalities and Recommendations

Motor vehicle accidents
The two leading primary preventive interventions to reduce fatalities from motor vehicle accidents are correct use of occupant restraint devices and decreasing alcohol-related driving.[5] It is proposed that many accidents can be averted or injuries limited by educational interventions to increase seat belt use and other driving safety precautions. In addition to avoidance of alcohol and seat belt use, adherence to speed limitation while driving and helmet use while biking can impact accident prevention. Mitigating such hazards as distracted driving includes avoidance of cell phone use or other technology use while driving. Physicians should advise patients of medical conditions and medications that can prohibit driving because of delayed reaction time, syncope, seizure, or somnolence. Vision examination, hearing testing, and early identification of cognitive decline in elderly drivers can also impact motor vehicle safety. Counseling on accident prevention is an important component of health care maintenance.

Suicide
Reported suicide fatalities do not capture the full scope of the problem because many people have suicidal thoughts or have unsuccessful attempts. Young adults are more

---

Box 1
Screening elements recommended by the well woman task force for healthy, reproductive-aged nonpregnant adult women

Abdominal examination

Alcohol misuse

Blood pressure

Breast awareness

Breast cancer chemoprevention

Breast cancer screening

Cardiovascular disease/dyslipidemia

Cervical cancer

Colorectal

Contraception, sexually transmitted infections, and reproductive health

Depression

Diabetes

Diet, fitness, nutrition

Domestic and intimate partner violence

Drug use

Genetic screening

Hepatitis B screening

Hepatitis C screening

Immunizations

Injury prevention

Mental health

Metabolic syndrome

Obesity

Oral cavity examination

Oral hygiene

Pelvic examination

Sexual health

Skin health

Tobacco use

Data from Conry JA, Brown H. Well-Woman Task Force: components of the well-woman visit. Obstet Gynecol 2015;126(4):697–701.

---

likely to commit suicide than older adults. Women are more likely than men to have suicidal ideation and have nonfatal suicide attempts. Firearm use is the most common mode of suicide in men, whereas poisoning is the most common method used by women.

Most individuals who attempt or commit suicide have a diagnosable psychiatric disorder. Risk factors for suicide include prior personal history or family history of a suicide attempt, depression or other mental illness, alcohol misuse, drug abuse, physical illness, and feeling of isolation. Suicide risk may be altered if treatable psychiatric disorders are identified and addressed. It is estimated that 50% of individuals who commit suicide have sought professional care within approximately 1 month of suicide.[6] Physician education in depression recognition with subsequent treatment can have an impact. Usual health care maintenance may miss up to 50% of patients with depressed mood. Detecting overt and subtle signs including changes in mood, diet, and sleep patterns with feedback and intervention may reduce the risk of persistent depression.[7] Somatic symptoms that sometimes present with depression may include headache, sexual dysfunction, appetite changes, menstrual-related symptoms, chronic pain, chronic medical conditions, digestive problems, fatigue, and sleep disturbances.[8] Depression rating scales may be used to identify at-risk individuals who need further evaluation. Many screening instruments are available. Beck Depression Inventory, Beck Hopelessness Scale, Beck Scale for Suicide Ideation, Suicide Intent Scale, and SAD PERSONS scale, are some commonly used risk scales.[9] These tools help identify individuals who need further evaluation. The concept of increased connectedness has been advocated by the CDC and the Surgeon General as a measure toward reducing suicide through enhanced social connections. Improved engagement may contribute to increased well-being.[10] Health care providers are important sources of information to make supportive services available through counseling and enhanced relationships with mental health care providers.

Homicide

According to the Federal Bureau of Investigation's Uniform Crime Reports, in 2014, of the female murder victims for whom the relationships to their offenders were known, 35.5% were murdered by their husbands or partners.[11] Most murders are committed by firearm use. Characteristics of perpetrators of female intimate partner homicide include access to guns, unemployment, low education, drug use, leaving the home of the abuser, and having a nonbiologic child as major risk factors.[12] One study controlling for education level, marital status, and year demonstrated significantly greater adjusted odds ratio for homicide mortality among Hispanics (2.6) and blacks persons (2.1) compared with whites persons (1.0).[13]

Physicians should assess their patients for modifiable circumstances including screening for intimate partner violence. **Table 2** identifies common modifiable risks and screening recommendations.[3,14] Screening women for intimate partner violence in the hospital setting may identify those at risk for further violence and other mental and physical health problems. Physicians can play a vital role in providing education and resources of police, community, and public health organizations for intervention and prevention against further harm.[15]

IMMUNIZATIONS
Impact of Immunizations on Disease Incidence and Mortality

An important part of providing primary preventive health care to women is immunization against vaccine-preventable disease. Studies have shown that recommendation from a health care provider is one of the strongest influences on patient acceptance.[16] Annual health maintenance visits offer excellent opportunities to discuss vaccination history and to provide age-appropriate counseling and risk-based immunization.

Table 2
Screening recommendations for modifiable behaviors contributing to unintentional injuries, suicide, and homicide (compiled from Well-Woman Task Force and USPTF)

Modifiable Behaviors	Well-Woman Task Force Recommendation	USPSTF
Alcohol misuse	Annual screening of adults for alcohol misuse by questionnaire, history, or both, but not by testing, is recommended. Provide or refer persons engaged in risky or hazardous drinking to brief behavioral counseling interventions to reduce alcohol misuse (Level of evidence: Strong).	Recommends that clinicians screen adults aged 18 y or older for alcohol misuse and provide persons engaged in risky or hazardous drinking with brief behavioral counseling interventions to reduce alcohol misuse (2013 Guideline, Grade of recommendation: B)
Depression	Annual screening for depression, using a validated tool, is recommended (Qualified). Screening postpartum women for depression, using a validated tool, is recommended (Qualified).	Recommends screening for depression in the general adult population, including pregnant and postpartum women. Screening should be implemented with adequate systems in place to ensure accurate diagnosis, effective treatment, and appropriate follow-up (2015 Draft Guideline, Grade of recommendation B).
Intimate partner violence	Screening is recommended at least annually for intimate partner violence, such as domestic violence or reproductive or sexual coercion. Provide or refer women who screen positive to intervention services (Strong).	Recommends that clinicians screen women of childbearing age for intimate partner violence, such as domestic violence, and provide or refer women who screen positive to intervention services (2013 Guideline, Grade of recommendation B).
Drug use	At least annual screening for substance abuse by history (not laboratory testing) is recommended. Provide or refer patients to counseling as needed (Strong).	Concludes that the current evidence is insufficient to assess the balance of benefits and harms of screening adolescents, adults, and pregnant women for illicit drug use (2008 Guideline, Grade of Recommendation I)
Mental health and psychosocial issues/suicide/behavioral assessment	Evaluation of psychosocial aspects of health (interpersonal and family relationships, intimate partner violence, work satisfaction, lifestyle and stress, sleep disorders [all women]; acquaintance rape prevention [women aged 19–39 y]; advance directives [women 40 y and older]; neglect and abuse; depression [all women]) is recommended as part of routine health assessment (Strong). Routine screening for suicide risk in asymptomatic general populations is not recommended (Strong).	Concludes that the current evidence is insufficient to assess the balance of benefits and harms of screening for suicide risk in adolescents, adults, and older adults in primary care (2014 Guideline, Grade of Recommendation I)

Data from Conry JA, Brown H. Well-Woman Task Force: components of the well-woman visit. Obstet Gynecol 2015;126(4):697–701; and U.S. Preventive Services Task Force. Recommendations for primary care practice: published recommendations. 2016. Available at: http://www.uspreventiveservicestaskforce.org/BrowseRec/Index/browse-recommendations. Accessed October 15, 2015.

Recommendations

The CDC currently recommends routine vaccination to prevent 17 vaccine-preventable diseases that occur in the lifespan from infancy through adulthood. The 2015 Adult Immunization Schedule was approved by the CDC Advisory Committee on Immunization Practices, American Academy of Family Physicians, the American College of Physicians, ACOG, and the American College of Nurse-Midwives. In February 2015, the adult immunization schedule and a summary of changes from 2014 were published in the *Annals of Internal Medicine*.[17] A full review of adult immunizations is found at www.cdc.gov/vaccines/hcp/acip-recs/index.html. Commonly recommended vaccines in adulthood include influenza vaccine, human papilloma virus (HPV) vaccine, hepatitis B vaccine, meningococcal vaccine, pneumococcal vaccine, tetanus-diphtheria-pertussis vaccine, and zoster vaccine. Additional adult vaccines include hepatitis A, varicella, *Haemophilus influenzae* type b, measles, mumps, and rubella. Special consideration in immunization should include pregnancy, individuals with severe allergic reactions, and those who are immunocompromised.

A comprehensive review of immunization is beyond the scope of this article. Instead, this article includes one example of vaccination, HPV immunization, and its impact on cervical cancer.

Human Papilloma Virus Vaccine and Cervical Cancer Prevention

Incidence and mortality of cervical cancer

Screening for cervical cancer and treatment of its precursor lesions is an important example of how primary and secondary prevention can greatly impact disease. Since the advent of screening with the Papanicolaou test the incidence of cervical cancer has drastically decreased in the United States with a 2012 incidence of at 12,042 cases.[18] About half of the cases of invasive cervical cancer are found in women who have never been screened.[19] Current consensus screening guidelines are listed in **Table 3**.[3,8,20] Age, immune status, history of abnormal pap smear, presence of an intact cervix, and diethylstilbestrol exposure affect surveillance frequency. Worldwide cervical cancer remains prevalent representing the third most common cancer in women, most frequently occurring in underresourced countries without widespread screening and immunization.

Immunization and primary prevention

In addition to cytology screening, cervical cancer prevention has been further enhanced by the linkage of cervical cancer to high-risk HPV virus types. HPV testing combined with cytology improves sensitivity over cytology alone. HPV plays an important role in the pathogenesis of cervical cancer and also is associated with other cancers including vulvar, vaginal, oropharyngeal, and anal cancer in women. Prophylactic HPV vaccine in adolescent and young women and men is predicted to have significant clinical impact on several diseases including cervical cancer and genital warts. The implementation of the HPV vaccine is gaining acceptance as a primary prevention strategy and can greatly impact the incidence of cervical cancer in future decades. Bivalent, quadravalent, and nine-valent vaccines are available. The Advisory Committee on Immunization Practices recommends immunization of adolescents at age 11 to 12. The vaccine can be administered as early as age 9 with catch-up vaccination recommended from age 13 to 26.[17] Vaccine effectiveness in reducing the incidence of genital warts has already been demonstrated in population-based studies with greatest effect seen with early age of immunization.[21]

Table 3
Guidelines for cervical cancer prevention in average-risk individuals with a cervix but with no diagnosis of high-grade cervical lesion/cancer, DES in utero exposure, or immunocompromise

Age	USPSTF	ACS/ASCCP/ASCP	WWTF
Less than 21	Screening is not recommended.	Screening is not recommended.	Screening is not recommended.
21–29	Recommend cytology alone every 3 y. HPV testing should not be used for screening in this age group.	Recommends cytology every 3 y. Recommends against screening for cervical cancer with HPV testing, alone or in combination with cytology.	Screening for cervical cancer is recommended with cytology alone every 3 y. Screening with HPV testing is not recommended.
30–65	Recommends cytology every 3 y. For women who want to lengthen the screening interval, screening with a combination of cytology and HPV testing every 5 y.	HPV and cytology cotesting every 5 y is the preferred approach. Cytology alone every 3 y is acceptable. Screening by HPV testing alone is not recommended for most clinical settings.	Screening for cervical cancer with a combination of cytology and HPV testing (cotesting) is recommended every 5 y. Screening with cytology alone every 3 y is acceptable.

Abbreviations: ACS, American Cancer Society; ASCCP, American Society for Colposcopy and Cervical Pathology; ASCP, American Society for Clinical Pathology; DES, diethylstilbestrol; WWTF, Well-Woman Task Force.
Data from Refs.[3,14,20]

CANCER SCREENING

According to National Institutes of Health estimates, there will be approximately 1,658,370 new cases of cancer diagnosed in 2015.[22] Cancer is the leading cause of death in women aged 35 to 84. An estimated 589,430 people will die from cancer but the number of people who live beyond a cancer diagnosis is steadily increasing. This trend is largely related to earlier detection and improved success of intervention through secondary and tertiary prevention. In average-risk individuals, in addition to age-specific screening tests, general preventive measures include physical activity, maintaining normal weight, and a healthy diet high in fruits and vegetables and whole grains with low saturated and trans fats. Excessive sun exposure and tobacco use should be avoided. Alcohol consumption should be limited. Heredity plays an important role in cancer but there are modifiable factors based on early identification of risk. Women at risk for hereditary cancer syndromes should be identified by careful history and referred for genetic assessment. Individualized surveillance plans can be offered including heightened imaging and testing, chemoprevention, and prophylactic surgery.

Breast Cancer

Incidence and mortality
Breast cancer is the most commonly diagnosed cancer in US women excluding skin cancer. In 2015, the American Cancer Society estimated there will be 60,290 cases of in situ breast cancer, 231,840 new cases of invasive breast cancer, and 40,290 disease-related deaths.[23] Based on current incidence rates, a woman has an approximately one in eight (12.08%) lifetime risk of developing breast cancer.[24] Incidence

rates dropped significantly (7%) between 2002 and 2003 in large part because of the decline in the use of postmenopausal hormone-replacement therapy.[24] In more recent years, incidence has remained stable for white women but has slightly increased for African American women. As a result of increased early detection and improved therapy, breast cancer mortality has had a steady decline in the past two decades.[23]

Screening modalities and recommendations

Screening and intervention in breast cancer demonstrate important concepts of primary, secondary, and tertiary prevention. The goal of breast cancer screening includes identification of preinvasive lesions, and early detection of invasive neoplasms. Differentiation of high-risk individuals from average-risk individuals also affects surveillance.

Recent breast cancer screening modalities for average-risk women include mammography, clinical breast examination, and patient self-screening. The efficacy of screening mammography in the early detection of breast cancer and reduction of mortality is well supported by data from randomized controlled trials and observational studies. However, the relative value of clinical and self-breast examination, appropriate age of initiation and discontinuation of screening, and screening intervals has remained controversial. Currently there is insufficient evidence to support doing clinical examinations and teaching self-breast examinations. Taking into account the benefits, harms, limitations of screening, and end points for detection, **Table 4** summarizes the current guidelines of the American Cancer Society and the USPSTF for screening in average-risk women.[25,26]

Identifying women at high risk for breast cancer

In 2013, The USPSTF recommended that primary care providers screen women who have family members with breast, ovarian, tubal, or peritoneal cancer with one of several screening tools designed to identify a family history consistent with the presence of potentially harmful mutations in breast cancer susceptibility genes (BRCA1 or BRCA2). Women with positive screening results should receive genetic counseling and, if indicated after counseling, BRCA testing. Breast cancer risk tools include the Breast Cancer Risk Assessment (Gail), BRCAPRO, and International Breast Cancer Intervention Study models.

Screening Adjuncts

MRI

In 2007, the American Cancer Society convened an expert panel that reviewed evidence and presented updated recommendations for the use of MRI as an adjunct to screening mammography in high-risk populations. Screening MRI is recommended for women with a 20% to 25% or greater lifetime risk of breast cancer. Evidence was insufficient to make recommendations for some risk subgroups.[27] **Box 2** summarizes the recommendations of the panel.

Ultrasound

When performed carefully, ultrasonography may detect occult breast cancer in dense breasts.[28,29] However, the high rate of false-positive findings limits the usefulness of ultrasound for screening purposes. ACOG does not recommend routine use of alternative tests to screening mammography in asymptomatic women with dense breasts and no additional risk factors.[30] Likewise, the USPSTF cites insufficient evidence to support routine use for screening of women with dense breasts identified on an otherwise negative screening mammogram.[26]

Table 4
Breast cancer screening recommendations for women at average risk

Source of Recommendation	Mammography	Clinical Breast Examination	Self-Breast Examination
American Cancer Society (updated 2015)	Age 40–44: women should have the choice to start annual breast cancer screening with mammograms if they wish to do so. The risks of screening and the potential benefits should be considered. Age 45 to 55: annually. Age 55 and older: mammograms every 2 y, or have the choice to continue yearly screening.	Insufficient evidence.	Not recommended, but self-awareness suggested.
USPSTF 2016	Before the age of 50: the decision to start regular, biennial screening mammography should be an individual one and take patient context into account, including the patient's values regarding specific benefits and harms. Age 50–74: biennially. Age 75 or older: current evidence is insufficient to assess the benefits and harms of screening.	Insufficient evidence to assess the additional benefits and harms of in women 40 y or older.	Teaching self-breast examination not recommended.

Data from U.S. Preventive Services Task Force. Screening for breast cancer: U.S. preventive services task force recommendation statement. Ann Intern Med 2009;151:716–26. Available at: http://www. uspreventiveservicestaskforce.org/Page/Document/RecommendationStatementFinal/breast-cancer-screening. Accessed January 15, 2016; and Oeffinger K, Fontham ETH, Etzioni R, et al. Breast cancer screening for women at average risk 2015 guideline update from the American Cancer Society. JAMA 2015;314(15):1599–614.

Three-dimensional mammography

According to the USPSTF, current evidence is insufficient to assess the benefits and harms of tomosynthesis (three-dimensional mammography) as a screening modality for breast cancer.[26] ACOG also recommends further study to confirm whether three-dimensional mammography may replace digital mammography alone as first-line screening.[31]

CHEMOPREVENTION

Chemoprevention implies pharmacotherapy to prevent disease. Many examples of chemoprevention exist. Medical management of osteopenia is considered here as an example.

According to the National Osteoporosis Foundation more than 10 million people in the United States have osteoporosis.[32] This disorder disproportionately affects women partly because of female longevity because it is a disorder primarily seen in the elderly. With the predicted increase in life span the sequalae of fracture and medical care costs will continue to exceed 17 billion dollars per year.[33]

Box 2
American Cancer Society recommendations for breast MRI screening

Annual MRI Screening (Based on Evidence)

- BRCA mutation
- First-degree relative of BRCA carrier, but untested
- Lifetime risk approximately 20% to 25% or greater as defined by BRCAPRO or other models that are largely dependent on family history

Annual MRI Screening (Based on Expert Consensus Opinion)

- Radiation to chest between age 10 and 30 years
- Li-Fraumeni syndrome, Cowden disease, and Bannayan-Riley-Ruvalcaba syndrome and first-degree relatives

Insufficient Evidence to Recommend for or Against MRI Screening

- Lifetime risk 15% to 20% as defined by risk assessment tools that are based mainly on family history
- Increased risk based on personal history
  - Breast cancer
  - Ductal carcinoma in situ
  - Lobular carcinoma in situ or atypical lobular hyperplasia
  - Atypical ductal hyperplasia
- Heterogeneously or extremely dense breast on mammography

Recommend Against MRI Screening (Based on Expert Consensus Opinion)

- Women at less than 15% lifetime risk

From Saslow D, Boetes C, Burke W, et al. American Cancer Society guidelines for breast screening with MRI as an adjunct to mammography. CA Cancer J Clin 2007;57:76; with permission.

Age is a major determinant of osteoporosis. Although osteoporosis is generally a disease of the elderly, healthy habits starting as early as adolescence including adequate dietary calcium optimize peak bone mass, which is achieved in the 30s (**Table 5**).[34]

Primary prevention focuses on maximizing peak bone mass and minimizing loss in subsequent years. There are many influences on optimal bone health including hereditary, medical disorders, hormonal, and environmental factors outlined fully in the

---

Table 5
Institute of Medicine dietary recommendations for calcium and vitamin D intake in female adolescence and adulthood

Age	Recommended Dietary Allowance Calcium (mg/d)	Recommended Dietary Allowance Vitamin D (IU/d)
9–18 y old	1300	600
19–50 y old	1000	600
51–70 y old	1200	600
71 and older	1200	800

Data from Institute of Medicine. Dietary reference intakes for calcium and vitamin D. Washington, DC: The National Academies Press; 2011.

article on endocrine disorders elsewhere in this issue. Modifiable lifestyle factors include appropriate exercise, avoidance of cigarette smoking, limiting alcohol consumption, and fall prevention.[35]

In addition to optimizing peak bone mass, and modifying factors that contribute to bone loss, early intervention after low bone density is diagnosed also plays an important role in prevention. Dual-energy X-ray absorptiometry of the hip and spine is the most commonly used method to measure bone mineral density and the only one validated for the diagnosis. USPSTF recommends screening for osteoporosis in women aged 65 years and older and in younger women whose fracture risk is equal to or greater than that of a 65-year-old white woman with average risk.[36] Women can be screened for osteoporosis at an earlier age than 65 if they have increased risk of fracture including medical history of fragility fracture, low body weight, disorders or medications that cause bone loss, smoker, excessive alcohol consumption, rheumatoid arthritis, and parental history of hip fracture. Baseline screening at the initiation of menopause is not recommended.

Low bone density is identified by DEXA as a T-score between -1.0 and -2.5 at the lumbar spine or femoral neck measurements. In combination with the DEXA, the Fracture Risk Assessment Tool can help identify postmenopausal women with low bone mass who should be treated prophylactically. The FRAX tool, developed in 2008 by the World Health Organization, uses clinical risk factors to estimate the 10-year risk of hip fracture.[37] Individual variables including age, gender, body mass index, prior history of fracture, parental hip fracture history, current smoking, alcohol use, glucocorticoid use, the presence of a disorder strongly associated with osteoporosis, rheumatoid arthritis, combined with femoral neck bone mineral density are used in the calculation. The 10-year probability of hip fracture greater than or equal to 3% or the 10-year probability of a major osteoporosis-related fracture greater than or equal to 20% on the FRAX score is a guideline to initiate therapy.[37]

Once low bone mass is noted, chemoprevention of osteoporosis includes several classes of medications. These include estrogen, selective estrogen receptor modulators, and bisphosphonates.[30] Continued surveillance of bone density with DEXA is recommended but should be at least 2-year intervals.

SUMMARY

This overview of well-woman care defines the major types of prevention and highlights major organizations that provide guidelines for care. It also gives brief examples of clinical interventions supporting prevention with a focus on the leading causes of morbidity and mortality in women. Behavioral interventions in the context of unintentional accidents, suicides, and homicides are reviewed. Vaccination for high-risk subtypes of HPV is an example of immunization that impacts cervical cancer. Breast imaging as a form of cancer screening is highlighted. Finally, optimized bone health in prevention of osteoporosis is also considered. These examples of prevention may impact quality of life and duration of health.

REFERENCES

1. Stormo A, Saralya M, Hing E, et al. Women's clinical preventive services in the United States who is doing what? JAMA Intern Med 2014;174(9):1512–4.
2. Available at: http://www.cdc.gov/women/lcod/2013/WomenAll_2013.pdf. Accessed October 10, 2015.
3. Conry JA, Brown H. Well-Woman Task Force: components of the well-woman visit. Obstet Gynecol 2015;126(4):697–701.

4. Available at: http://www.cdc.gov/nchs/fastats. Accessed October 10, 2015.
5. Williams SB, Whitlock EP, Edgerton EA, et al. Counseling about proper use of motor vehicle occupant restraints and avoidance of alcohol use while driving: a systematic evidence review for the US Preventive Services Task Force. Ann Intern Med 2007;147:194–206.
6. Hjorthoj CR, Madsen T, Agerbo E, et al. Risk of suicide according to level of psychiatric treatment: a nationwide nested case-control study. Soc Psychiatry Psychiatr Epidemiol 2014;49:1357–65.
7. Pignone MP, Gaynes BH, Rushton JL, et al. Screening for depression in adults: a summary of the evidence for the U.S. Preventive Services Task Force. Ann Intern Med 2002;136:765–76.
8. Kerr LK, Kerr LD. Screening tools for depression in primary care: the effects of culture, gender, and somatic symptoms on the detection of depression. West J Med 2001;175(5):349–52.
9. Bolton J, Gunnell D, Gustavo T. Suicide risk assessment and intervention in people with mental illness. BMJ 2015;351:h4978.
10. Centers for Disease Control and Prevention, National Center for Injury Prevention and Control. Strategic direction for the prevention of suicidal behavior: Promoting individual, family and community connectedness to prevent suicidal behavior. 2008. Available at: http://www.cdc.gov/nchs/deaths.htm. Accessed October 10, 2015.
11. Bureau of Justice Statistics. Homicide trends in the U.S. 2014. Available at: https://www.fbi.gov/about-us/cjis/ucr/crime-in-the-u.s/2014/crime-in-the-u.s.-2014/tables/expanded-homicide-data/expanded_homicide_data_table_2_murder_victims_by_age_sex_and_race_2014.xls; https://www.fbi.gov/about-us/cjis/ucr/crime-in-the-u.s/2014/crime-in-the-u.s.-2014/tables/expanded-homicide-data/expanded_homicide_data_table_10_murder_circumstances_by_relationship_2014.xls. Accessed January 12, 2016.
12. Campbell JC, Webster D, Koziol-McLain J, et al. Risk Factors for femicide in abusive relationships: results from a multisite case control study. Am J Public Health 2003;93:1089–97.
13. Gonzalez-Guarda RM, Luke B. Contemporary homicide risks among women of reproductive age. Womens Health Issues 2009;19:119–25.
14. U.S. Preventive Services Task Force. 2016. Available at: http://www.uspreventiveservicestaskforce.org. Accessed October 15, 2015.
15. Lipsky S, Caetano R, Roy-Byrne P. Racial and ethnic disparities in police-reported intimate partner violence and risk of hospitalization among women. Womens Health Issues 2009;19:109–18.
16. American College of Obstetricians and Gynecologists. Integrating immunizations into practice. Committee Opinion No. 558. Obstet Gynecol 2013;121:897–903.
17. Kim DK, Bridges CB, Harriman KH. Advisory Committee on Immunization Practices recommended immunization schedule for adults aged 19 years or older: United States, 2015. Ann Intern Med 2015;162(3):214–23.
18. U.S. Cancer Statistics Working Group. United States cancer statistics: 1999–2012 incidence and mortality Web-based report. Atlanta (GA): Department of Health and Human Services, Centers for Disease Control and Prevention, and National Cancer Institute; 2015.
19. Carmichael JA, Jeffrey JF, Steele HD, et al. The cytologic history of 245 patients developing invasive cervical carcinoma. Am J Obstet Gynecol 1984;148(5):685–90.

20. Saslow D, Solomon D, Lawson HW, et al. American Cancer Society, American Society for Colposcopy and Cervical Pathology and American Society for Clinical Pathology Screening guidelines for the prevention and early detection of cervical cancer. CA Cancer J Clin 2012;62(3):147–72.

21. Leval A, Herweijer E, Arnheim-Dahlstrom L, et al. Incidence of genital warts in Sweden before and after quadravalent human papillomavirus vaccine availability. J Infect Dis 2012;206:860–6.

22. Available at: http://www.cancer.gov/about-cancer/what-is-cancer/statistics. Accessed December 15, 2015.

23. American Cancer Society. Cancer facts and figures 2015. Atlanta (GA): American Cancer Society; 2015. Available at: http://www.cancer.org/acs/groups/content/@editorial/documents/document/acspc-044552.pdf. Accessed August 10, 2015.

24. Howlader N, Noone AM, Krapcho M, et al, editors. SEER cancer statistics review, 1975-2012. Bethesda (MD): National Cancer Institute. Available at: http://seer.cancer.gov/csr/1975_2012/. based on November 2014 SEER data submission, posted to the SEER web site, April 2015. Accessed August 15, 2015.

25. U.S. Preventive Services Task Force. Screening for breast cancer: U.S. preventive services task force recommendation statement. Ann Intern Med 2009; 151:716–26. Available at: http://www.uspreventiveservicestaskforce.org/Page/Document/RecommendationStatementFinal/breast-cancer-screening. Accessed January 15, 2016.

26. Oeffinger K, Fontham ETH, Etzioni R, et al. Breast cancer screening for women at average risk guideline update from the American Cancer Society. JAMA 2015; 314(15):1599–614.

27. Saslow D, Boetes C, Burke W, et al. American Cancer Society guidelines for breast screening with MRI as an adjunct to mammography. CA Cancer J Clin 2007;57:75–89.

28. Kolb TM, Lichy J, Newhouse JH. Occult cancer in women with dense breasts: detection with screening US–diagnostic yield and tumor characteristics. Radiology 1998;207(1):191–9.

29. Buchberger W, Niehoff A, Obrist P, et al. Clinically and mammographically occult breast lesions: detection and classification with high-resolution sonography. Semin Ultrasound CT MR 2000;21(4):325–36.

30. American College of Obstetricians and Gynecologists. Digital breast tomosynthesis. Technology assessment in obstetrics and gynecology No. 9. American College of Obstetricians and Gynecologists. Obstet Gynecol 2013;121: 1415–7.

31. American College of Obstetricians and Gynecologists. Management of women with dense breasts diagnosed by mammography. Committee Opinion No. 625. American College of Obstetricians and Gynecologists. Obstet Gynecol 2015; 125:750–1.

32. National Osteoporosis Foundation. Clinician's guide to prevention and treatment of osteoporosis. Washington, DC: National Osteoporosis Foundation; 2010.

33. Burge R, Dawson-Hughes B, Solomon DH, et al. Incidence and economic burden of osteoporosis-related fractures in the United States, 2005–2025. J Bone Miner Res 2007;22(3):465–75.

34. Institute of Medicine. Dietary reference intakes for calcium and vitamin D. Washington, DC: The National Academies Press; 2011.

35. Management of osteoporosis in postmenopausal women: 2010 position statement of the North American Menopause Society. Menopause 2010;17(1):25–54.

36. U.S. Preventive Services Task Force. Screening for osteoporosis: U.S. Preventive Services Task Force recommendation statement. Ann Intern Med 2011;154(5): 356–64.
37. Kanis JA, McCloskey E, Johansson H, et al. FRAX® with and without bone mineral density. Calcif Tissue Int 2012;90(1):1–13.

Primary Care of Adult Women

Common Dermatologic Conditions

Arlene M. Ruiz de Luzuriaga, MD, MPH[a],*, Julie Mhlaba, BS[b],
Carly Roman, MD[a]

KEYWORDS

- Skin disease • Skin cancer • Pigmentation disorders • Alopecia • Acne • Rosacea

KEY POINTS

- Melasma is a disorder of skin pigmentation. Vitiligo is an autoimmune condition leading to skin depigmentation.
- Rosacea is a chronic, inflammatory condition of the eyes and face and can be managed with trigger-avoidance and pharmacologic therapies. Acne presents with inflammatory papules, nodules, cysts and comedones.
- Alopecia is a common condition with multiple etiologies that may be primarily cutaneous, or involve systemic disease. This can be elucidated using a careful history and physical examination.
- Nonmelanoma skin cancers (NMSCs) occur in sun-exposed areas on fair-skinned. Melanoma is a malignant melanocytic tumor that may occur in sun-exposed and sun-protected areas.
- Eczema or dermatitis is an inflammatory skin condition. Lichen sclerosus is an inflammatory disease that presents with pruritus, and can result in scarring.

MELASMA
Epidemiology

Melasma is a disorder of skin pigmentation that affects nearly 5 million people in the United States with 90% of cases occurring in women.[1] It predominately affects premenopausal women with medium to darker skin tones.[2] In 1 study of Latino women in Texas, 8.8% of women reported a current self-diagnosis of melasma and an additional 4% reported a previous self-diagnosis of melasma.[3] Although the underlying pathogenesis of melasma has not yet been elucidated, it has been associated with sun exposure, family

---

Conflicts of Interest: None.
[a] Section of Dermatology, University of Chicago, 5841 S. Maryland Avenue, Chicago, IL 60637, USA; [b] Pritzker School of Medicine, University of Chicago, Chicago, IL, USA
* Corresponding author.
E-mail address: aruizde@medicine.bsd.uchicago.edu

history, pregnancy, and oral contraceptive pill use.[4] In addition, there may be an association between melasma and thyroid abnormalities, particularly in women who develop the condition during pregnancy or with oral contraceptive pill use.[5]

Presentation

- Melasma is usually asymptomatic.
- Patients often seek medical attention owing to cosmetic concerns.
- Melasma typically presents as symmetric, hyperpigmented macules and patches on the face and usually has well-demarcated borders (**Fig. 1**).
- A centrofacial distribution involving the forehead, cheeks, nose upper lip, and chin is most common. However, melasma may also present in a malar pattern (cheeks and nose) or a mandibular pattern.
- The areas of pigmentation appear over several weeks to months, and almost always in the setting of sun exposure.

Diagnosis

- Diagnosis of melasma is usually based on clinical examination and history.
- Other diagnoses that may present similarly should be explored via a careful history and physical examination:
  ○ Postinflammatory hyperpigmentation: The patient will have history of preceding dermatitis or alternative dermatologic condition that was present in the affected areas.
  ○ Drug-induced pigmentation: The patient will have history of recent drug exposure with a known causative agent (eg, antipsychotics, anticonvulsants, amiodarone, minocycline).
  ○ Solar lentigines ("sun spots"): Common lesions usually involve both face and other sun-exposed areas and occur usually in 50 to 60-year-olds.
  ○ Ephelides ("freckles"): These lesions usually appear as smaller brown discrete macules. They often occur early in life or with sun exposure and fade over time.[5]
- Laboratory tests or procedures are often unnecessary. Occasionally, a skin biopsy may be helpful for diagnosis.

Treatment

- All patients with melasma should practice rigorous sun protective measures including daily application and reapplication of SPF 50+ sunscreen with physical block, hat wearing, and sun avoidance measures.

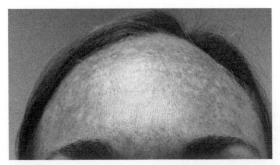

Fig. 1. Melasma: well-defined, coalescent, hyperpigmented macules and patches diffusely distributed on the forehead.

- If the development of melasma is associated with recent oral contraceptive pill use, consideration of discontinuation of this medication should be reviewed with the prescriber, although the resolution is not guaranteed.
- Several treatment modalities are available that should all be combined with rigorous sun protection as above (**Table 1**).

Prognosis

The clinical course of patients with melasma is variable. Areas of hyperpigmentation may fade spontaneously over months to years or may persist. For patients who developed melasma during pregnancy, pigmentation often fades postpartum. The most important aspect of prevention is rigorous sun protection as melasma may return with subsequent sun exposure.

ROSACEA
Epidemiology

Rosacea is a common, inflammatory condition that affects approximately 16 million Americans.[9] The condition peaks in incidence between the ages of 30 and 50 and equally affects women and men. Risk factors for the development of rosacea include fair to medium skin complexions, family history and ultraviolet (UV) light exposure. Alcohol intake, heat exposure, and consumption of spicy foods have been described as exacerbating factors.[10]

Presentation

- Onset of symptoms is usually gradual and may follow the onset of acne.
- Patients often present with facial dryness and facial skin that is easily irritated, as well as redness, stinging, or a burning sensation.
- In addition, patients may note a "gritty" sensation in the eyes, simulating a foreign body sensation.

Table 1 Management of melasma	
Method	**Comments**
Sun protection	• SPF 30+ sunscreen with physical block • Sun avoidance and protective wear • Used alone or in combination with topical therapy
Makeup/concealment	• Dermablend • Covermark/CM Beauty • Cover FX
Topical	• 4% hydroquinone • 20% azelaic acid • 5% ascorbic acid • Combination creams (eg, hydroquinone, tretinoin, low-potency topical corticosteroid)
Laser	• Fractional resurfacing • Intense pulsed light therapy • Copper bromide lasers
Chemical peels	• Alpha hydroxy acid peels • Salicylic acid peels

Data from Refs.[6–8]

Diagnosis

- The diagnosis of rosacea is based on criteria divided into primary and secondary features (**Table 2**).
- Initially, there is symmetric erythema of the cheeks, followed by telangectasias (**Fig. 2**).
- Some patients subsequently develop small papules and pustules, which can progress to larger papules and nodules.
- Over time, chronic rosacea may cause thickening of the nose (rhinophyma), forehead, eyelids, and chin.
- Rarely, the chest, neck, back, and scalp are involved.
- Rosacea can be distinguished from acne vulgaris by the absence of comedones, onset in middle age, and a central facial distribution.
- Rosacea can be distinguished from seborrheic dermatitis by its involvement of the concave surfaces of the face compared with the convex surfaces (nasolabial folds) of seborrheic dermatitis.
- Diagnosis is made clinically, and biopsy is usually not necessary.
- Clinicians may consider bacterial culture of pustules to rule out concurrent *Staphylococcus aureus* infection in patients at increased risk for infection or are refractory to standard treatments.

There are 4 clinical subtypes of rosacea[11]:

- Erythematotelangiectatic rosacea (subtype I)
  - Characterized by nontransient episodes of flushing and central facial erythema.
  - Telangiectasia is common.
- Papulopustular rosacea (subtype II)
  - Similar to erythematotelangiectatic rosacea, but addition of papules and pustules in central face distribution.
- Phymatous rosacea (subtype III)
  - Characterized by thickened skin with irregular surface.
  - Most commonly affects the nose, but can affect any sebaceous region.
  - Rare in women.
- Ocular rosacea (subtype IV)
  - Characterized by the presence of watery or bloodshot eyes, foreign body sensation, burning or stinging, dryness, itching, light sensitivity, blurred vision, telangiectasia of the conjunctiva and lid margin or lid, and periocular erythema.

Table 2 Primary and secondary features of rosacea	
	Features
Primary (≥1 required for diagnosis)	Transient erythema, nontransient erythema, telangiectasia, papules and pustules
Secondary (not required for diagnosis)	Burning or stinging, plaque, dryness, edema, ocular manifestations, peripheral location, phymatous changes

Adapted from Two AM, Wu W, Gallo RL, et al. Rosacea: part I. introduction, categorization, histology, pathogenesis, and risk factors. J Am Acad Dermatol 2015;72(5):749–58.

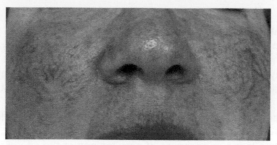

Fig. 2. Rosacea: malar cheeks with background erythema with overlying telangectasias.

Treatment

- Patients should be educated regarding the chronic and relapsing nature of the condition.
- Avoidance of common triggers, including alcohol use, heat exposure, and spicy food consumption, may be helpful.
- In addition, discontinuation of medications that exacerbate flushing (eg, niacin, topical steroids) may be helpful when possible.
- Patients should use a gentle skin cleanser, daily moisturizer, and sun protection, which have been shown to improve skin hydration and decrease sensitivity.
- Pharmacologic therapies include the following.
  - Topical preparations of metronidazole, sodium sulfacetamide, and azaleic acid can be particularly useful in patients with a papulopustular component to their disease.
  - Topical brimonidine gel, an alpha-adrenergic agonist, has been approved to treat facial redness owing to rosacea.
  - Systemic tetracyclines have been shown to be effective owing to their antiin-flammatory properties.
- Telangiectasias associated with rosacea may be treated with lasers that target blood vessels such as the pulsed dye laser. Rhinophymatous changes may be improved by surgery or laser therapy in certain circumstances.

Prognosis

Rosacea is a chronic condition, but often responds to treatment both for acute flares and for chronic maintenance. Telangectasias may persist despite therapy.

VITILIGO
Epidemiology

Vitiligo is presumed to be an autoimmune disorder of melanocytes leading to depigmentation. The prevalence of the disease is 1% in the United States.[12] Symptoms can begin at any age with roughly one-half of patients developing symptoms before the age of 20. It is believed to occur equally in men and women, but female patients have an earlier age of onset and are more likely to seek treatment. Although the exact method of genetic inheritance is unclear, there is a strong familial link, with greater than 30% of patients reporting an immediate family member with vitiligo. In addition, associations have been noted with systemic autoimmune and endocrine abnormalities. Although the condition affects all Fitzpatrick skin types, it is particularly challenging in patients with darker skin, because the areas of depigmentation are more evident. Importantly, the condition can lead to severe psychological disturbance and social isolation in all skin types.[13]

Presentation

- Depigmentation usually occurs gradually.
- Triggers, including pregnancy, sunburn, and emotional stress, may be associated with onset.
- Patients may report that lesions itch, but they are usually asymptomatic.
- Lesions appear as white macules or patches within normally pigmented skin (**Fig. 3**).
- The face, hands, elbows, knees, and the anogenital region are frequent areas of involvement.
- Koebnerization is the appearance of new lesions at the site of injury or irritation and may be reported.

Diagnosis

- Vitiligo can usually be diagnosed clinically after a careful history and physical examination.
- A Wood's lamp examination may be helpful in enhancing areas of depigmentation and defining the extent of involvement.
- Association with endocrine and autoimmune abnormalities has been reported. As such, thyroid-stimulating hormone levels, antinuclear antibody titer, and a complete blood count may be considered in adults.[12]
- Biopsy is rarely required for diagnosis of vitiligo. When done, it may be helpful to have adjacent normally pigmented skin for comparison.

Treatment

- Treatment can be challenging.
- Conservative treatment options include the use of cosmetic concealers and the use of sunscreen, which prevents further pigmentation of uninvolved areas and protects depigmented areas from UV light exposure.
- Several topical therapies that have been helpful with repigmentation include topical glucocorticoids, calcineurin inhibitors, and vitamin D_3 analogs.[13]

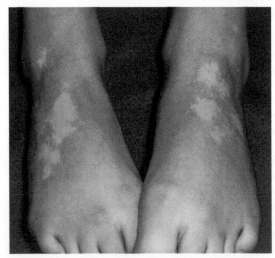

Fig. 3. Vitiligo. Depigmented patches on dorsum of feet extending to ankles bilaterally. (*Courtesy of* S. Stein, MD, Chicago, IL.)

- Phototherapy may be used in patients who fail topical monotherapy. Both UVA light therapy with psoralen or narrowband UVB light therapy have been shown to be effective. Excimer laser therapy may be used in treatment of limited lesions.
- Surgical treatment may be used in patients who fail nonsurgical therapy. Grafting of skin from normal donor sites and transplanting to affected sites has been performed with good results. In addition, autologous melanocyte suspension transplant, which involves suspending normal cells from donor sites and injecting them into deepithelialized recipient sites, has shown promising results.[14]
- Finally, for patients with extensive vitiligo, bleaching of normally pigmented skin may be considered using topical monobenzone or hydroquinone. This is a permanent and irreversible treatment method, and should be discussed thoroughly with the patient before initiation.[15]
- Younger patients with recent onset of disease, darker skin types, and lesions on face, neck, and trunk have a better response to therapy.

Prognosis

Vitiligo is a chronic disease with a variable course. Spontaneous repigmentation may occur for some patients, whereas others may experience progressive depigmentation. Management of vitiligo should be patient centered, focusing on the patient's desired outcome and frequently evaluating psychosocial well-being.

ACNE
Epidemiology

Acne is a chronic inflammatory condition affecting the pilosebaceous unit. It is the most common skin disorder and affects roughly 85% of people between the ages of 12 and 24. Although it is most frequently associated with adolescents, acne may appear at age 25 years or older and persist into adulthood. This is particularly applicable to women; the prevalence of female acne is estimated to be between approximately 40% in women between the ages of 25 and 40.[16] Proposed triggers include stress, hormones, cosmetics, and tobacco, although these associations are inconsistent. Additionally, acne in women may be a result of hormonal abnormalities, including polycystic ovarian syndrome and congenital adrenal hyperplasia.[17]

Presentation

- Acne is often self-diagnosed by patients before presentation to a physician.
- Acne can be classified as noninflammatory and inflammatory.
  - Noninflammatory lesions include both open and closed comedones ("blackheads" or "white-heads," respectively)
  - Inflammatory lesions include papules, pustules, and nodules (**Fig. 4**).
- Acne may result in depressed or hypertrophic scarring.
- Lesions may flare premenstrually.[18]
- Affected areas usually include the face, specifically the chin and mandibular region. If a hyperandrogenic state is the cause of acne, signs of irregular menses, excess facial hair, hyperhidrosis, and acanthosis nigricans may be present.

Diagnosis

- Careful medication reconciliation should be performed to evaluate for drug-induced acne (eg, phenytoin, lithium, isoniazid) or steroid-induced acne.
- Acne may be confused with folliculitis or rosacea, but can be distinguished by the presence of comedones.

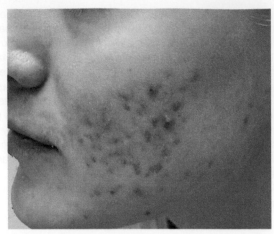

Fig. 4. Acne vulgaris. Inflammatory papules and pustules on the cheek of a young woman. Postinflammatory erythema (red macules) are noted at the sites of prior lesions.

- If there is concern for endocrine disorder the following may be ordered: free testosterone, follicle-stimulating hormone, luteinizing hormone, and dehydroepiandrosterone sulfate.

Treatment

- Selection of therapy differs depending on the type and severity of acne.
- For mild or moderate, noninflammatory or comedonal acne, therapy begins with topical retinoids (tretinoin, adapalene, and tazarotene).
- For patients with inflammatory acne that involves mostly papules and pustules, a combination of benzoyl peroxide in the morning and topical retinoid in the evening is recommended.
- Systemic tetracyclines may be added if clinical improvement is not noted after 2 to 3 months of topical therapy.
- For severe, nodular acne, a combination of topical therapy and systemic antibiotic is usually necessary for resolution.
- Alternative therapies include hormonal treatment.
  - Although data are mixed, spironolactone is an antiandrogenic, antihypertensive agent that has been used in the management of female acne.
  - In addition, combined oral contraceptives have been shown to decrease androgen receptor activation and decrease levels of circulating testosterone.[18]
  - A detailed medical and family history should be performed before beginning hormonal therapy.
- The oral retinoid isotretinoin can be used for severe acne. This is a highly effective medication that produces lasting improvement in symptoms. However, side effects are common and include dry skin, chapped lips, and increased liver enzymes among others. Importantly, isotretinoin is teratogenic and requires patients use strict birth control and comply with frequent follow-up appointments.

Prognosis

With treatment, the prognosis is good. Adult-onset acne may be more persistent than typical adolescent acne. Systemic antibiotics should be discontinued after several months of use if possible, but topical therapies may be continued for months to years.

The goal of treatment is to prevent the formation of new lesions as scars can develop from even small comedones.

ALOPECIA
Epidemiology

Alopecia is a common condition that may cause significant distress and embarrassment. Alopecia can be described as either nonscarring, which is devoid of inflammation and atrophy, or scarring, which displays evidence of tissue destruction. This discussion focuses on nonscarring alopecia.

Alopecia can affect different stages of the hair follicle cycle (**Table 3**). Hair loss may be diffuse or localized (**Table 4**). In women, the 2 most common causes of diffuse hair loss are female pattern hair loss (FPHL) and telogen effluvium (TE). FPHL describes the loss of hair on the central and bitemporal region of the scalp (**Fig. 5**). Also known as androgenetic alopecia, FPHL affects roughly one-half of women in their 50s.[19] The role of heredity in the development of FPHL has not been established. TE is an acute, generalized hair loss that typically presents several months after a physical or psychological stressor. Common triggers include childbirth, thyroid abnormalities, nutritional deficiencies, rapid weight loss, major surgery, medications, or depression or anxiety. In a large portion of cases, no clear cause can be determined.[19,20]

Some common localized causes of hair loss include alopecia areata (**Fig. 6**), an autoimmune disorder that causes patches of nonscarring alopecia, tinea capitis, and trichotillomania.[21] Finally, damage from hair care practices and hairstyles may result in hair loss.

Presentation

- Patients presenting with diffuse hair loss should undergo a thorough history and scalp examination.
  - Determine whether hair loss is occurring at the roots or along the shaft of the hair. Hair breakage along the shaft should prompt an investigation into the patient's hair care practices; common culprits include chemical relaxers, permanent waves, or hair straighteners.[22]
  - With complaints of hair shedding, the patient's health and well-being over the preceding 6 to 12 months should be elucidated. Any recent hospitalizations, new medications, or life stressors should be elicited because these factors have been associated with TE. In addition, the patient's diet should be considered to rule out a nutritional deficiency.

Table 3
Features of the hair follicle cycle

Stage	Behavior	Duration	Distribution of Total Hairs (%)	Microscopic Features
Anagen	Growth phase	2–6 y	80–90	Club-shaped hair bulb
Telogen	Resting phase	~3 mo	10–15	Attached root sheath, pigmented and distorted bulb
Catagen	Apoptotic phase	2–3 wk	<1	Club shaped bulb with "Tail" of soft, clear tissue trailing from bulb

Adapted from Sperling, LC, Cowper SE, Knopp EA. An atlas of hair pathology with clinical correlations. 2nd edition. Boca Raton (FL): CPC Press; 2012.

Table 4
Common causes of alopecia

Etiology	Clinical Morphology
Scarring alopecia	Absent follicular orifices
Female pattern hair loss	• Hair loss affects central and bitemporal region • Hair becomes finer and eventually atrophies
Telogen effluvium	• Diffuse hair loss • Newly growing hairs are finer than previous hairs
Alopecia areata	• Single or multiple, sharply demarcated patches of hair loss on any hair-bearing area (rarely, diffuse hair loss) • Patches are surrounding by fractured hairs • Associated with nail pitting
Tinea capitis	• Patchy hair loss with broken shafts leaving "black dots" • May demonstrate pustules within areas of hair loss • May lead to infected plaque (kerion), which can scar
Trichotillomania	• Ill-defined patchy areas of hair loss • Hair feels comparable to coarse stubble

○ In patients where FPHL is suspected, additional signs of androgen excess should be assessed including acne, hirsutism, irregular menses, and virilization.

Diagnosis

- Clinical
  ○ A detailed history and careful examination of the scalp will usually result in a preliminary diagnosis.
  ○ A hair-pull test may be performed, which involves grasping a group of hairs and applying gentle traction from the base to the tip of hair. Removal of more than 3 telogen hairs consistently from different areas of the scalp is consistent with excessive shedding from TE.
  ○ Lymphadenopathy may be present with tinea capitis.

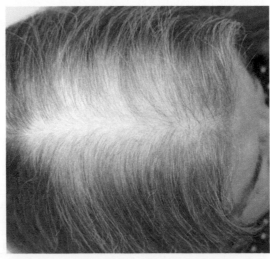

Fig. 5. Female pattern hair loss/androgenetic alopecia: widening of the midline part with decreased hair volume at the crown.

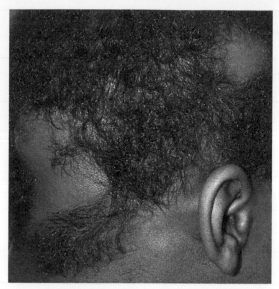

Fig. 6. Alopecia areata: round, well-circumscribed areas of alopecia. (*Courtesy of* S. Stein, MD, Chicago, IL.)

- Ancillary tests
  - Tinea capitis: potassium hydroxide preparation and culture may be helpful for confirmation.
  - Androgen excess: testosterone, dehydroepiandrosterone sulfate, and prolactin may be ordered to evaluate hormonal abnormalities.
  - Additional testing: thyroid function tests, iron studies, a complete blood count, and antinuclear antibodies.
  - Scalp biopsy: not typically necessary for nonscarring alopecia; however, a biopsy may be helpful to demonstrate the presence, character, and location of inflammation.

Treatment

Common treatments for alopecia are presented in **Table 5**.

Prognosis

The prognosis of hair loss depends on the cause and responsiveness to available treatments. The degree of hair loss in FPHL is most severe between ages 30 and 50, with subsequent slowing of hair loss. With regard to therapy, FPHL can be treated but not cured. Importantly, hair regrowth often requires continuous use of therapy. TE is a self-limiting condition that usually resolves within 2 to 6 months, although it may be prolonged if the trigger is not resolved. In some patients, chronic TE (ie, TE lasting >6 months) can develop. Alopecia areata has a variable and unpredictable course. The majority of patients have a spontaneous recovery, but may go on to have relapses. Approximately 5% of cases will progress to complete hair loss of the scalp (alopecia totalis) or complete hair loss of the body (alopecia universalis). With treatment, tinea capitis resolves within 1 to 3 months. Inflammatory tinea capitis that develops into a kerion may result in permanent scarring. Trichotillomania has a variable disease course. In children, the condition is usually self-limited and resolves without lasting effects. However, in adults, the condition is often difficult to treat.

Table 5
Common treatments for alopecia

Etiology	Treatment
Scarring alopecia	Consultation with hair specialist or dermatologist
Female pattern hair loss	• Topical minoxidil (2% or 5%) • Spironolactone (50–200 mg)
Telogen effluvium	• Identification and treatment of any inciting factors • Reassurance
Alopecia areata	• Intralesional corticosteroids (triamcinolone acetonide 3-7 mg/mL every 4 wk to affected areas) • Topical corticosteroids • Diphenylcyclopropenone • Cyclosporine • Photochemotherapy
Tinea capitis	• Oral griseofulvin • Oral terbinafine • Oral itraconazole
Trichotillomania	• Emotional support • Behavioral counseling

Data from Refs.[19,20,23,24]

BASAL CELL CARCINOMA AND SQUAMOUS CELL CARCINOMA
Epidemiology

Basal cell carcinoma and squamous cell carcinoma (SCC) are the 2 most common NMSC with the lifetime incidence in the United States reported 28% to 33% and 7% to 11%, respectively. In 2012, it was estimated that more than 3 million people in the US population were treated for NMSC. NMSC commonly presents in the sixth decade and beyond, and there is a slight predominance in men.[25] Risk factors include intermittent and intense sun exposure, radiation therapy, a fair complexion, immuno-suppression, and a positive family history.

Presentation

- NMSC is most common in areas that are frequently exposed to UV light. Patients may present with a nonhealing ulcer, rapidly growing nonresolving lesion, or sometimes pain and neuropathy.
- Basal cell carcinoma.[26]
  ○ Basal cell carcinoma favors the face, most often the forehead, ears, periocular areas, and cheeks.
  ○ Basal cell carcinoma presents commonly as waxy, semitranslucent papules or nodules that can be ulcerated, crusted, or bleeding (**Fig. 7**)
  ○ Basal cell carcinoma often has a rolled border and appears shiny or "pearly"
  ○ Basal cell carcinoma is often reported bleeding with minor trauma.
- SCC.[27]
  ○ SCC favors chronically sun-exposed sites such as the dorsal hands, forearms, and face.
  ○ SCC neoplasms most often present as erythematous, scaly and crusted lesions (**Fig. 8**).

Diagnosis

Diagnosis is typically made by skin biopsy and histologic analysis.

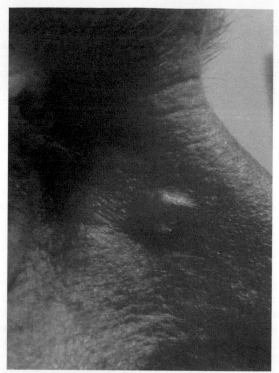

Fig. 7. Nodular basal cell carcinoma. Pink, pearly nodule on nasal sidewall with telangecta-sias and overlying scaling.

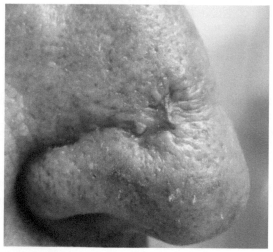

Fig. 8. Invasive squamous cell carcinoma of the nose: erythematous hyperkeratotic nodule with central ulceration.

Treatment

- Treatment is based on the size, site, and histologic pattern of the lesion.[26,27]
- Treatment of SCC most often includes Mohs micrographic surgery for appropriate cases or complete excision.
- Other therapies include electrodessication and curettage, cryosurgery with liquid nitrogen, or application of a topical immunomodulator therapy where indicated for a course of several weeks.

Prognosis

The prognosis for NMSC is excellent with proper management (cure rate based on treatment type is >90%). Metastasis is very rare in basal cell carcinomas, occurring in 0.0028% to 0.55% of cases.[28] In SCCs, metastasis has been reported in 2% to 5% of cases.[27] Importantly, there is an increased risk of developing a subsequent NMSC after initial diagnosis and annual total body skin examinations are recommended.[29]

MELANOMA
Epidemiology

Melanoma is a malignant tumor that arises from melanocytes and is most commonly of cutaneous origin, but can also arise from the oral, conjunctival, and vagina mucosa. The lifetime risk of melanoma is about 1 in 40 for whites, 1 in 500 for Hispanics, and 1 in 1000 for blacks. It is estimated that in 2015, about 31,200 women will be diagnosed with melanoma and 3300 women will die of melanoma.[30] Risk factors for melanoma include age (mean age of 62), UV light exposure (history of blistering sun burns), atypical moles, family history of melanoma, and fair skin tone and hair color (red or blonde hair, blue or green eyes, freckling). Indoor tanning is believed to be a significant contributor to the increased rate of melanoma in young women.[31]

Presentation

- Classically, the ABCDEs of melanoma are used to describe symptoms[32]:
  - Asymmetry in shape;
  - Border irregularity;
  - Color variegation (eg, red, white and blue);
  - Diameter (>6 mm); and
  - Evolution.
- Melanoma typically presents on the legs of women and the trunk of men between 40 and 60 years.
- Melanoma can arise in a preexisting nevus or de novo.
- Clinically, it presents as an enlarging, asymmetric macule, papule, or nodule with irregular borders, asymmetry, and color variation (**Fig. 9**).
- Lesions may become ulcerated or bleed.

Diagnosis

- Diagnosis is usually made by biopsy and histopathologic analysis.
- Dermoscopy may be helpful to identify concerning lesions.[33]
- Suspicious pigmented lesions should be biopsied via excision with margin of normal skin or deep shave to ensure that the deep margin can be assessed.

Treatment

- When melanoma is detected early, cure may be achieved through surgical excision.

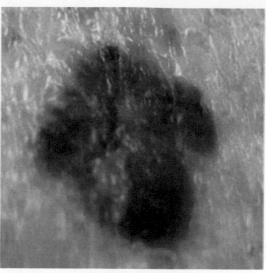

Fig. 9. Melanoma: asymmetric, unevenly pigmented brown–black nodule with irregular borders. (*Courtesy of* J. Basko-Plluska, MD, Chicago, IL.)

- Tumors are characterized by depth of invasion, which serves as the basis for the size of normal skin margin excised.
- In addition, sentinel lymph node mapping and biopsy may be considered in melanomas greater than 1 mm in thickness in patients with clinically negative node status.
- If clinically palpable nodes are detected, therapeutic nodal dissection is recommended.[34]
- For patients with a high risk of recurrence, adjuvant systemic therapy may be considered. Systemic therapies are also used for patients with disseminated disease and include chemotherapies, immunotherapies and kinase inhibitors.[35] Radiation therapy may be used for bone or brain metastases or for large tumors in which surgical excision would be challenging.

Prognosis

Detected early, melanoma is largely curable by surgical excision. Prognosis depends on tumor thickness. The 10-year survival is greater than 95% for patients with thin tumors (stage IA) and approximately 50% for tumors greater than 4 mm in thickness. The 5-year survival rates for melanoma are largely dependent on stage at presentation, ranging from 97% for stage IA to 15% to 20% for stage IV.[30] For patients with primary melanoma, follow-up depends on tumor stage, thickness, and lymph node status, but generally includes physical examination every 3 to 6 months with imaging and blood work performed for patients with more advanced tumors.

DERMATITIS: CONTACT AND ATOPIC
Epidemiology

Eczema or dermatitis is a general term used to describe a common, chronic inflammatory skin process. The most common types of eczema are contact dermatitis and atopic dermatitis (AD). Contact dermatitis – both irritant and allergic – can affect individuals of all ages and is often related to occupational exposures in professions such as housekeeping, hairdressing, medical/dental work, food service, and construction. Additional exposures include makeup products, jewelry, and detergents. An epidemiologic analysis of hand eczema found a lifetime prevalence of 17.6% in women compared with 11% in men, which they attributed to different domestic/occupational exposures and an increased prevalence of AD in women.[36]

Irritant contact dermatitis results from a localized direct toxic effect on the skin owing to contact with irritant chemicals. Allergic contact dermatitis (ACD) results from a delayed-type hypersensitivity reaction to a chemical to which there has been previous sensitization. The diagnosis of contact dermatitis may be relevant in patients with chronic pruritus or irritation of the vulva. In the vulvar area irritant contact dermatitis is more common than ACD.[37] Causes of irritant contact dermatitis in the vulvar area include excessive washing, bodily fluids, hygiene products, soaps/detergents, and topical medications.[37] Fragrances, medicaments, and preservatives are the most common categories of topical agents that can cause ACD in the vulvar area.[38]

AD is typically presents in infancy, but can persist into adulthood. In 1 study, 50% of patients with AD in childhood had persistence of symptoms at age 29.[39] Common triggers for exacerbations of atopic dermatitis include aeroallergens, microbial agents, foods, cold climates, and wool clothing.[40]

Presentation

- Contact dermatitis
  - Contact dermatitis may be acute or chronic.
  - Exposure to irritant contact will precede dermatitis by hours to days, while exposure to allergic contact will precede by 1 to 4 days.
  - Erythematous patches or plaques, vesicles may arise in more severe cases.
  - Distribution of lesion may depend on nature of exposure (eg, linear streaks in poison ivy exposure).
  - Contact dermatitis may burn, sting, or itch.
- AD
  - AD presents with dry, itchy skin.
  - Acute lesions are erythematous patches, papules, and plaques. Linear erosions may be present from scratching.
  - Chronic lesions are lichenified – thickened skin with accentuation of skin markings.
  - In adults, distribution is mostly on flexural surfaces as well as face and neck.

Diagnosis

- The diagnosis of eczema is usually clinical based on careful history and evaluation of the lesion.
- For ACD, patch testing may be helpful in identifying a causative agent to avoid.
- Alternative diagnoses to consider include seborrheic dermatitis, psoriasis, fixed drug eruption, or soft tissue infection.
- Although rare in adults, occasionally lesions may be come colonized with S aureus or herpes simplex virus, requiring appropriate cultures.

Treatment

- For contact dermatitis, identification and avoidance of causative agents is essential to clinical improvement. Additionally, protective clothing (eg, gloves) or barrier creams may be used.
- For AD, patient education on avoidance of rubbing or scratching is key.

- For acute dermatitis, a short course of topical corticosteroid creams may be used along with systemic antihistamines for symptomatic relief.
- For severe or chronic dermatitis, topical calcineurin inhibitors may be prescribed by a specialist.
- Occasionally, a short course of systemic steroids is required to control disease.

Prognosis

AD is a chronic disease with one-half of patients with childhood AD experiencing symptoms into adulthood.[39] Contact dermatitis typically subsides within 3 to 4 weeks of removal of irritant or allergic stimuli. Importantly, chronic dermatitis may develop in individuals with repeated occupational exposure and occasionally requires a change in occupation.

LICHEN SCLEROSUS
Epidemiology

Lichen sclerosus (LS) is a chronic inflammatory condition seen in the anogenital area. The exact incidence of LS is unknown; however, women are more commonly affected than men. In women, the mean age of onset is between 45 and 55 years, but 9% to 23% of females experience prepubertal symptom onset. An association between LS and autoimmune diseases has been described, including autoimmune thyroiditis, vitiligo, alopecia areata, and pernicious anemia.[41] LS can lead to severe pruritus, scarring, and cosmetic disfigurement. Dyspareunia and malignant transformation are long-term sequelae of LS, and thus early treatment and monitoring are important.

Presentation

- Nongenital lesions typically present on trunk and extremities as white, guttate ("drop-like") papules or plaques.
- Anogenital lesions typically present in the "figure-of-8" distribution affecting both the vulva and the perineum.
- Initially begins as erythema progressing to hypopigmented, sclerotic plaques, often with "cigarette-paper" epidermis.
- Plaques may erode and scar leading to dysuria and dyspareunia.
- Severe pruritus is common.

Diagnosis

- The differential for genital LS includes lichen planus and lichen simplex chronicus; a biopsy may be required to distinguish these conditions.
- Histopathologic changes on biopsy include epidermal atrophy, hyalinization of the papillary dermis, and a bandlike lymphocytic infiltrate in the deeper dermis.
- When genital LS appears eroded, biopsy is required to rule out SCC.
- Nongenital LS may be confused with morphea, a localized scleroderma.

Treatment

- Treatment includes the avoidance of irritants, including urinary contact, and topical emollients.
- Potent topical steroids (eg, clobetasol propionate 0.05% cream) applied for 3 to 6 months on alternating days help to reduce skin breakdown.
- Topical macrolides (tacrolimus or pimecrolimus) may be applied twice daily for 3 to 6 months.[27]

Prognosis

LS is a chronic condition with a relapsing and remitting course. Long-standing vulvar disease in the female may result in vulvar scarring, fusion of the labia minora, clitoral entrapment, and narrowing of the introitus. Rarely, LS may be complicated by SCC. Treatment may reduce pruritus and inflammation and improve appearance.[42]

REFERENCES

1. Grimes PE. Melasma: etiologic and therapeutic considerations. Arch Dermatol 1995;131(12):1453–7.
2. Sheth VM, Pandya AG. Melasma: a comprehensive update: part I. J Am Acad Dermatol 2011;65(4):689–97.
3. Werlinger KD, Guevara IL, Gonzalez CM, et al. Prevalence of self-diagnosed melasma among pre-menopausal Latino women in Dallas and Forth Worth, Tex. Arch Dermatol 2007;143(3):424–5.
4. Handel AC, Lima PB, Tonolli VM, et al. Risk factors for facial melasma in women: a case–control study. Br J Dermatol 2014;171(3):588–94.
5. Lutfi RJ, Fridmanis M, Misiunas AL, et al. Association of melasma with thyroid autoimmunity and other thyroidal abnormalities and their relationship to the origin of the melasma. J Clin Endocrinol Metab 1985;61(1):28–31.
6. Rodrigues M, Pandya AG. Melasma: clinical diagnosis and management options. Australas J Dermatol 2015;56(3):151–63.
7. Jutley GS, Rajaratnam R, Halpern J, et al. Systematic review of randomized controlled trials on interventions for melasma: an abridged Cochrane review. J Am Acad Dermatol 2014;70(2):369–73.
8. Sheth VM, Pandya AG. Melasma: a comprehensive update: part II. J Am Acad Dermatol 2011;65(4):699–714.
9. Two AM, Wu W, Gallo RL, et al. Rosacea: part I. Introduction, categorization, histology, pathogenesis, and risk factors. J Am Acad Dermatol 2015;72(5):749–58.
10. Tan J, Berg M. Rosacea: Current state of epidemiology. J Am Acad Dermatol 2013;69(6 Suppl 1):S27–35.
11. Wilkin J, Dahl M, Detmar M, et al. Standard classification of rosacea: Report of the National Rosacea Society Expert Committee on the Classification and Staging of Rosacea. J Am Acad Dermatol 2002;46(4):584–7.
12. Alikhan A, Felsten LM, Daly M, et al. Vitiligo: a comprehensive overview part I. Introduction, epidemiology, quality of life, diagnosis, differential diagnosis, associations, histopathology, etiology, and work-up. J Am Acad Dermatol 2011;65(3):473–91.
13. Felsten LM, Alikhan A, Petronic-Rosic V. Vitiligo: a comprehensive overview part II: treatment options and approach to treatment. J Am Acad Dermatol 2011;65(3):493–514.
14. Whitton ME, Pinart M, Batchelor J, et al. Interventions for vitiligo. Cochrane Database Syst Rev 2015;(2):CD003263.
15. Grau C, Silverberg NB. Vitiligo patients seeking depigmentation therapy: a case report and guidelines for psychological screening. Cutis 2013;91(5):248–52.
16. Preneau S, Dreno B. Female acne – a different subtype of teenager acne? J Eur Acad Dermatol Venereol 2012;26(3):277–82.
17. Zouboulis CC. Acne as a chronic systemic disease. Clin Dermatol 2014;32(3):389–96.

18. Lam C, Zaenglein AL. Contraceptive use in acne. Clin Dermatol 2014;32(4): 502–15.
19. Harfmann KL, Bechtel MA. Hair loss in women. Clin Obstet Gynecol 2015;58(1): 185–99.
20. Torres F, Tosti A. Female pattern alopecia and telogen effluvium: figuring out diffuse alopecia. Semin Cutan Med Surg 2015;34(2):67–71.
21. Alkhalifah A, Alsantali A, Wang E, et al. Alopecia areata update: part I. Clinical picture, histopathology, and pathogenesis. J Am Acad Dermatol 2010;62(2): 177–88.
22. Sperling LC, Cowper SE, Knopp EA. An atlas of hair pathology with clinical correlations. 2nd edition. Boca Raton (FL): CPC Press; 2012.
23. Alkhalifah A, Alsantali A, Wang E, et al. Alopecia areata update: part II. Treatment. J Am Acad Dermatol 2010;62(2):191–202 [quiz: 203–4].
24. Hordinsky M, Donati A. Alopecia areata: an evidence-based treatment update. Am J Clin Dermatol 2014;15(3):231–46.
25. Rogers HW, Weinstock MA, Feldman SR, et al. Incidence estimate of nonmelanoma skin cancer (keratinocyte carcinomas) in the US PoV. JAMA Dermatol 2015;151(10):1081–6.
26. Maruka AG, Book SE. Basal cell carcinoma: pathogenesis, epidemiology, clinical features, diagnosis, histopathology and management. Yale J Biol Med 2015; 88(2):167–79.
27. Kallini JR, Hamed N, Khachemoune A. Squamous cell carcinoma of the skin: epidemiology, classification, management and novel trends. Int J Dermatol 2015;54(2):130–40.
28. James W, Elston D. Andrews' diseases of the skin: clinical dermatology. 11th edition. London: Saunders/Elsevier; 2011.
29. Krueger H, Williams D. Burden of malignancy after a primary skin cancer: recurrence, multiple skin cancers and second primary cancers. Can J Public Health 2010;101(4):I23–7.
30. American Cancer Society. Cancer facts and figures 2015. Atlanta: American Cancer Society; 2015.
31. Mayer JE, Swetter SM, Fu T, et al. Screening, early detection, education, and trends for melanoma: current status (2007-2013) and future directions: part I. Epidemiology, high-risk groups, clinical strategies, and diagnostic technology. J Am Acad Dermatol 2014;71(4):599.e1–12.
32. Tsao H, Olazagasti JM, Cordoro KM, et al. Early detection of melanoma: reviewing the ABCDEs. American Academy of Dermatology Ad Hoc Task Force for the ABCDEs of Melanoma. J Am Acad Dermatol 2015;72:717–23.
33. Vestergaard ME, Macaskill P, Holt PE, et al. Dermoscopy compared with naked eye examination for the diagnosis of primary melanoma: a meta-analysis of studies performed in a clinical setting. Br J Dermatol 2008;159(3):669–76.
34. Kimbrough CW, McMasters KM, Davis EG. Principles of surgical treatment of malignant melanoma. Surg Clin North Am 2014;94:973–88.
35. Niezgoda A, Niezgoda P, Czajkowski R. Novel approaches to treatment of advanced melanoma: a review on targeted therapy and immunotherapy. Biomed Res Int 2015;2015:851387.
36. Thyssen JP, Johansen JD, Linneberg A, et al. The epidemiology of hand eczema in the general population–prevalence and main findings. Contact Derm 2010; 62(2):75–87.
37. Schlosser BJ. Contact dermatitis of the vulva. Dermatol Clin 2010;28(4):697–706.

38. O'Gorman SM, Torgerson RR. Allergic contact dermatitis of the vulva. Dermatitis 2013;24(2):64–72.
39. Mortz CG, Andersen KE, Dellgren C, et al. Atopic dermatitis from adolescence to adulthood in the TOACS cohort: prevalence, persistence and comorbidities. Allergy 2015;70(7):836–45.
40. National Collaborating Centre for Women's and Children's Health (UK), editor. Atopic eczema in children: management of atopic eczema in children from birth up to the age of 12 years. London: RCOG Press; 2007. National Institute for Health and Clinical Excellence: Guidance.
41. Fistarol SK, Itin PH. Diagnosis and treatment of lichen sclerosus: an update. Am J Clin Dermatol 2013;14(1):27–47.
42. Chi C-C, Kirtschig G, Baldo M, et al. Systematic review and meta-analysis of randomized controlled trials on topical interventions for genital lichen sclerosus. J Am Acad Dermatol 2012;67(2):305–12.

Clinical Management of Obesity in Women

Addressing a Lifecycle of Risk

Nadia N. Ahmad, MD, MPH[a,b,*], Winfield Scott Butsch, MD, MSc[c], Sabina Aidarous, MBBS[a]

KEYWORDS

- Weight loss • Overweight • Lifestyle • Antiobesity pharmacotherapy
- Bariatric surgery • Energy regulation • Obesity treatment

KEY POINTS

- Adiposity is a highly regulated physiologic parameter with a complex biology that can be disrupted by microlevel and macrolevel factors (eg, genetics, developmental factors, lifestyle, psychosocial factors, environment).
- Obesity is a chronic and heterogenous disease disproportionately affecting women; primary care providers caring for women have an opportunity to prevent and treat obesity at multiple stages in women's lives when they are most at risk of weight gain.
- Addressing obesity in the clinical setting requires understanding and assessing the multifactorial nature of the condition and applying rational and practical therapeutic strategies designed to restore normal energy regulation.
- Targeted and individualized lifestyle therapy is the foundational step in treatment, but given high variability in treatment response, pharmacotherapy, surgery, and/or multimodal combination therapy is often required.
- An unbiased stepwise approach allows provider and patient engagement in addressing obesity, with the option to refer to obesity medicine specialists or multidisciplinary weight management centers at any step in the treatment process.

The obesity epidemic is currently one of the most pressing public health issues. Given that two-thirds of the population in the United States is at least overweight and one-third has obesity,[1] it is of paramount importance for health care providers to become well versed in the latest understanding of this condition and its current assessment and management strategies. This article addresses the obesity education

[a] Obesity Medicine Institute, Armada Towers, P2, Floor 19, Jumeirah Lake Towers, Dubai, United Arab Emirates; [b] Armada Medical Center, Internal Medicine, Armada Towers, P2, Floor 19, Jumeirah Lake Towers, Dubai, United Arab Emirates; [c] MGH Weight Center, Massachusetts General Hospital, 50 Staniford Street, Boston, MA 02114, USA
* Corresponding author. Obesity Medicine Institute, Armada Towers, P2, Floor 19, Jumeirah Lake Towers, Dubai, United Arab Emirates.
E-mail address: drahmad@obesitymedicineinstitute.com

Obstet Gynecol Clin N Am 43 (2016) 201–230
http://dx.doi.org/10.1016/j.ogc.2016.01.007
0889-8545/16/$ – see front matter © 2016 Elsevier Inc. All rights reserved.

obgyn.theclinics.com

gap in medical practice, which has been cited by providers as one of the key barriers to proper obesity management.[2] It discusses the physiologic basis of obesity, the multiple potential drivers of excess adiposity, key components of assessment, and rational treatment strategies that are feasible in the context of a busy clinical practice. This article focuses specifically on these issues as they relate to women's health. The female population is disproportionately affected by obesity and its consequences[3] and obstetrician-gynecologists are in a pivotal position to affect obesity diagnosis and management in women.

THE GENDER GAP

There is a global gender disparity in obesity.[3] The prevalence of obesity is higher in women than in men in all regions of the world, placing women at greater risk of morbidity and mortality caused by diabetes, cardiovascular disease, cancer, and a host of other obesity-related conditions.[4] Although the disparity is most notable in developing regions where women carry double to triple the risk of obesity, the developed world is also affected by the gender gap (**Fig. 1**).

Wang and Beydoun[5] found that there are more adult women than men with obesity in the United States across all age groups, income levels, and ethnicities (with the exception of Asian Americans). The relationships among gender, age, ethnicity, socioeconomic status, and obesity prevalence are complex and dynamic. In general, the gender gap seems to worsen with increasing age, minority status, and greater severity of obesity.[5] Notably, a body mass index (BMI) greater than 25 kg/m^2 is more common among men, but twice as many women than men have a BMI greater than 40 kg/m^2.[6]

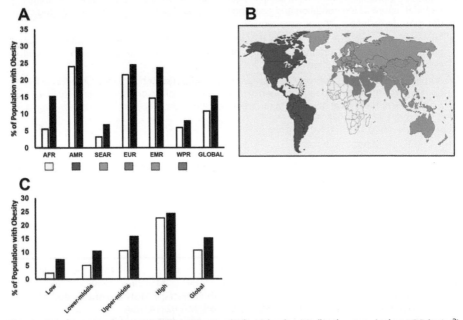

Fig. 1. Percentage of women (■) and men (□) with obesity (body mass index >30 kg/m^2) according to (*A, B*) World Health Organization region and (*C*) World Bank income groups. AFR, Africa; AMR, Americas; EMR, eastern Mediterranean; EUR, Europe; SEAR, southeast Asia; WPR, western Pacific. (*Data from* Global Health Observatory data repository. World Health Organization Web site. Available at: http://apps.who.int/gho/data/view.main. 2480A?lang=en. Accessed December 15, 2015.)

CONSEQUENCES

Obesity causes, worsens prognosis, or reduces treatment efficacy in more than 65 medical conditions.[7] The gender disparity in obesity extends to its complications. In a survey-based study, Muennig and colleagues[8] found that overweight women and men lose 1.8 million and 270,000 quality-adjusted life years, respectively, compared with their normal-weight counterparts. The numbers are 3.4 million and 1.9 million, respectively, for obese women and men. Overweight and obese women have a disproportionate burden of disease compared with men and much of the difference seems to be in health-related quality of life and late-life mortality.

The specific comorbidities associated with obesity are shown in **Fig. 2** and span the categories of metabolic, structural, inflammatory, degenerative, neoplastic, and psychological disease.[9] Of particular concern in women are metabolic syndrome and type 2 diabetes mellitus, cardiovascular disease, polycystic ovarian syndrome and infertility, musculoskeletal issues (arthritis and foot problems), urinary incontinence, obesity-related complications in pregnancy, breastfeeding issues, breast and ovarian cancer, depression, and eating disorders.[10–12]

WHAT IS OBESITY?

Obesity is a chronic condition of excess adiposity that is both biopsychosocially complex in its origins and clinically heterogeneous in its presentation. The causal contributors to this condition are shown in **Fig. 3**. The causes of obesity range from genetic and developmental factors that determine the intricate physiology of energy balance to broader environmental, social, and political factors that can influence and alter that physiology. The increased prevalence of obesity among women must be understood

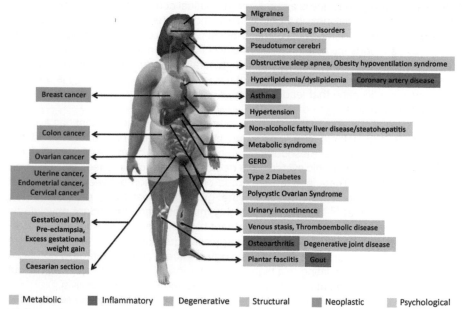

Fig. 2. Common obesity-related comorbidities in women. [a] Increased risk of cervical adenocarcinoma, and increased mortality possibly related to lower rates of screening in women with obesity. DM, diabetes mellitus; GERD, gastroesophageal reflux disease.

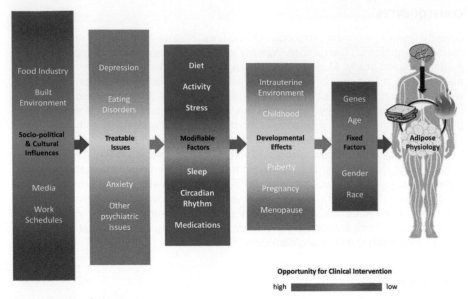

Opportunity for Clinical Intervention

high ▬▬▬▬▬▬▬▬▬ low

Fig. 3. Causes of obesity.

in terms of both biological and social drivers of the condition so that clinically relevant treatment approaches can be introduced.

BIOLOGICAL BASIS OF EXCESS ADIPOSITY

The idea that energy balance is a purely mathematical construct dependent on the net difference between calories in (food intake) and calories out (physical activity) is outdated. The preponderance of scientific investigation on energy intake, expenditure, and storage supports the notion that adiposity is a highly regulated physiologic parameter.[13] Hence, to construe obesity as a behaviorally determined condition of simple energy imbalance (ie, voluntary excess intake and/or inadequate activity) is an erroneous oversimplification that leads to narrow assessments and ineffective treatment strategies for patients.

Energy regulation refers to the complex neurohormonal physiology that has evolved to determine and defend an adiposity set point. Neurohormonal pathways at the level of the hypothalamus, mesocorticolimbic system, and cognitive brain define the homeostatic system, hedonic system, and decisions/behaviors, respectively, involved in energy regulation. There is extensive cross-communication between these central processes and peripheral signals from the gastrointestinal tract, pancreas, liver, muscle, bone, and fat.[13] The result is a highly integrated and redundant physiologic network that regulates appetitive drive, nutrient handling, metabolic rate, and fat storage within an optimal range for survival. Energy dysregulation may therefore be a more apt term to broadly refer to the pathophysiology of excess energy storage, a condition in which the body is regulating to a high level of adiposity that is no longer optimal but rather places the person at risk of myriad diseases and decreases survival.

Within the broader framework of energy regulatory biology, changes in sex-specific hormones can predispose women to obesity. Estrogen and progesterone have clear effects on energy regulation.[14] Estrogen decreases food intake, increases physical activity and energy expenditure, and favors a femoral versus central body fat distribution. Estrogen is also associated with decreased lipogenesis and increased catecholamine-induced lipolysis in adipose tissue. Moreover, estrogen leads to heightened hepatic and muscle insulin sensitivity, decreased tissue lipid accumulation, and enhanced oxidative capacity in skeletal muscle.[14] In contrast, progesterone counters most of these effects. Thus, the changing balance of these hormones over the menstrual cycle and over the course of the female life cycle should be taken into account when evaluating obesity risk in women.[15]

A basic understanding of the normal physiology of energy regulation leads clinicians to consider those factors that determine, modulate, or disrupt that physiology in their patients. Most biological processes are influenced by certain immutable factors, namely genetics, age, gender, and race. There are also modifiable factors that play significant roles in modulating energy regulatory physiology to increase adiposity. Of these, developmental, lifestyle, behavioral, psychological, and environmental modulators are each discussed separately in this article and shown in **Fig. 3**.

DEVELOPMENTAL CONSIDERATIONS

There are developmental considerations that may or not be amenable to clinical intervention depending on the developmental stage at which the patient is treated. Pregnancy is the prime example of the long-lasting effects that developmental exposures and processes can have on both mothers and offspring. It has been well established through epidemiologic and basic science studies that intrauterine and early life exposures can modify the genome to metabolically program energy regulatory pathways in favor of excess energy storage.[16] Hence, fetal exposures to maternal factors including diet,[17–19] activity,[20] stress,[21] toxins,[22] and increased adiposity[23] have been linked with 1 or more of the following: distinct alterations in metabolic pathways in oocytes, embryos, and offspring[24]; rapid fetal growth[25]; high birthweight[25]; rapid infant growth[17]; childhood obesity[18,21]; and obesity and chronic disease later in life.[19] Similarly, early life exposures (0–12 months), including infant nutrition and feeding,[26] maternal-infant attachment,[27,28] infant sleep,[29] and maternal stress,[30] have been associated with childhood and adult obesity and chronic disease.[31,32] Because the plasticity of human physiology and reversibility of detrimental effects are greatest early in life, it is of paramount importance to target the fetal and infancy periods in order to halt the transgenerational spread of obesity and chronic disease. Obstetricians can play a pivotal role by identifying and beginning to address the maternal side of the equation.

Pregnancy is also a recognized risk factor for obesity among women.[33] More than half of US women exceed the Institute of Medicine's BMI-specific guidelines for weight gain during pregnancy, with women from ethnic minorities experiencing the greatest gain.[34] Excess gestational weight gain is associated with postpartum maternal weight retention and the development of obesity and its complications in women of reproductive age.[35] Moreover, weight retention augments interpregnancy BMI such that women are at increased risk of obesity, gestational diabetes, and its complications with every subsequent pregnancy.[33]

Other developmental periods of particular relevance to overweight and obesity in women are menarche and menopause. These stages are also clinically associated with obesity onset or significant weight gain in a subset of women.[36] Again, changes in estrogen and progesterone levels may play a role in the mechanism of weight gain in concert with other lifestyle, behavioral, psychological, or environmental factors. So far, there are no conclusive studies showing a specific underlying pathophysiology in women with menarchal onset of obesity, excess gestational weight gain, postpartum weight retention, or menopause-associated weight gain. Thus, similar therapeutic strategies apply across all these phenotypes.

In short, developmental changes can increase obesity risk. The female life cycle is in some ways a lifecycle of risk (**Fig. 4**). Therefore, it is important for clinicians caring for women during peripubertal, perinatal, and perimenopausal stages to be proactive and pay heightened attention to the modifiable factors that can influence weight gain during these susceptible periods.

LIFESTYLE DRIVERS

Lifestyle factors such as unhealthy diet,[37] lack of activity,[38] increased stress,[39,40] inadequate sleep,[41] and circadian rhythm disturbances[42] have well-documented associations with obesity, and need to be screened for in clinical practice. The contribution of these factors to the development of obesity should be reframed in light of recent advancements in the understanding of energy regulatory physiology. For example, an unhealthy diet does not simply lead to obesity because of its caloric contribution; individual nutrients have varying effects on neurohormonal pathways at the level of the gastrointestinal tract, central nervous system, and other organs.[43] Chronic nutrient-induced disturbances of key signaling pathways and subsequent alteration of the adiposity set point have been shown in animal models.[44] Further research is needed to translate these findings to humans. **Table 1** details the energy regulatory effects of diet and the other specific modifiable components of lifestyle that guide lifestyle assessment and treatment.

BEHAVIORAL DRIVERS

With regard to behavioral contributors to obesity, emerging evidence suggests that individuals with obesity, compared with normal-weight controls, may have alterations in the decision-making functions of the prefrontal cortex that guide behavior.[45,46] It is unclear whether these changes are a cause or result of obesity; some reversal has

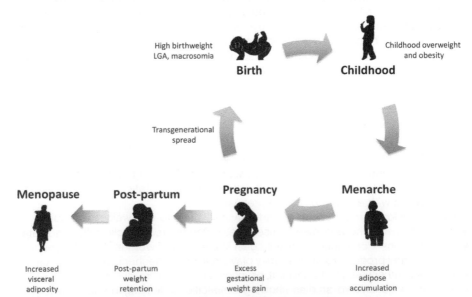

High birthweight
LGA, macrosomia

Birth

Childhood overweight
and obesity

Childhood

Transgenerational
spread

Menopause   **Post-partum**   **Pregnancy**   **Menarche**

Increased
visceral
adiposity

Post-partum
weight
retention

Excess
gestational
weight gain

Increased
adipose
accumulation

Fig. 4. The female lifecycle and obesity risk. LGA, large for gestational age.

been documented with weight loss.[45,46] Behavioral assessments and treatment strategies are relevant to obesity in as much as the targeted behavioral issues affect the implementation of lifestyle therapy, pharmacotherapy, or surgical therapy. For example, motivational interviewing and goal-oriented behavioral therapy may enable patients to implement a healthy diet, improve their sleep, or become compliant with a medication.[47] Key obesity treatments in this case are related to diet, sleep, or medication, and behavioral therapy is a strategy used to apply the treatment.

PSYCHOLOGICAL DRIVERS

Psychological issues such as depression, anxiety, binge eating, emotional eating, night-eating syndrome, and other psychiatric illnesses co-occur frequently with obesity, particularly in women.[48,49] There is also evidence of a relationship between obesity and adverse childhood events or trauma.[50] The complex relationships between a broad range of mental health issues and obesity are difficult to untangle. There is mechanistic overlap between obesity and some psychological disorders, with the dopaminergic and serotonergic systems that affect mood also playing critical roles in homeostatic and hedonic pathways of energy balance, which in turn drive food intake patterns, propensity for activity, energy expenditure, and fat storage.[51] Psychological issues also affect other lifestyle components, such as sleep, stress, and circadian rhythm, either through a shared physiologic mechanism or via effects on individual behaviors that in turn affect lifestyle. Adding to the complexity is the weight gain–promoting effect of many commonly used psychotropic medications, which can initiate a downward spiral of worsening obesity and psychological distress.[52] Therefore, in most cases, the cause-effect question remains unresolved in patients who have obesity complicated by psychological conditions. The critical clinical consideration is that each condition (obesity and psychological illness) usually worsens the other, so addressing both is essential. Most often underlying mental health issues need to be addressed before implementation of lifestyle therapy, pharmacotherapy, or surgery.

ENVIRONMENTAL DRIVERS

It is well-recognized that myriad environmental factors are contributing to the obesity epidemic. Many health care systems and practices that focus on addressing obesity are beginning to move toward more community engagement to target the environmental and social drivers of obesity faced by their patient populations.[53] However, for individual clinicians, sociopolitical, economic, and cultural trends in areas such as the food industry or built environment are beyond the scope of clinical care. Nevertheless, these larger scale societal issues are relevant to the lives of individual patients. During history taking, clinicians treating obesity should briefly assess the patient's local environment, access to healthy foods, recreational options, and work hours so that therapeutic interventions may be realistically tailored to the individual's life.

DIAGNOSIS

The formal diagnosis of a weight issue is the first step in obesity prevention and treatment. Srivastava and colleagues[54] found that, over 1 year at an academic hospital, internal medicine residents failed to record obesity as a diagnosis in every patient with a BMI greater than 30. In the outpatient setting obesity is diagnosed more often, but there is still considerable room for improvement.[55]

Table 1
Lifestyle factors contributing to energy dysregulation

Factor	Contribution to Energy Dysregulation	Assessment	Treatment
Diet	Ingested nutrients and their breakdown products interact directly with metabolic processes in the brain and peripheral organs to influence energy intake, expenditure, and storage An obesogenic diet is not one that is simply high in calories, but is one in which the nutrients (based on their type, form, and quantity) are increasing the adiposity set point	Obtain information about food quality, meal structure and timing, and quantity (24-h recalls are practical in the clinical setting) Pay attention to consumption of processed foods, fried foods, sugar-sweetened beverages, alcohol Consider asking about hunger, fullness, taste preferences, cravings, and other non–hunger-related eating	Physician-led nutritional counseling Focus on healthy diet: Attention to hunger/satiety cues Incorporating whole foods, fresh fruits and vegetables, nuts, lean protein, complex carbohydrates, polyunsaturated/monounsaturated fats Avoid processed foods Avoid sugar-sweetened beverages Promote structured meals and snacks Referral to dietitian at any time: at onset, if no improvement, or in complex cases
Activity	Activity is crucial not simply for burning calories but for releasing muscle growth factors and building healthy muscle By building healthy muscle, activity improves insulin sensitivity and increases fat oxidation Exercise also releases myokines that may play a role in improved central leptin signaling, thereby reducing appetitive drive and increasing energy expenditure	Obtain information on type, duration, and frequency of activity Ask about work-related activity vs recreational activity, and preference for different types of activity Pay attention to barriers (eg, time, finances, built environment, physical limitations such as pain) and facilitative factors	Physician-led counseling to achieve a mix of aerobic and resistance exercise, plus balance and flexibility exercises especially for postmenopausal women Recommendations need to fit into daily routine, be physically practical and medically safe Can be done in conjunction with wearable devices (eg, pedometers) Apply behavioral strategies as needed Referral to exercise physiologist in complex cases
Stress	Stress is associated with increased cortisol levels, which cause hyperinsulinemia and insulin resistance, which in turn increase leptin resistance Leptin resistance in the brain's homeostatic circuitry leads to increased appetitive drive and decreased energy expenditure Leptin resistance in the brain's hedonic, or reward-based, circuitry increases hedonic drive and consumption of palatable foods, which further worsen hyperinsulinemia	Stress assessment tools are currently lacking in clinical practice In the absence of tools, information on the degree of stress can be obtained through patient self-report Try to identify work stress vs other social stressors Patients can be asked to rate the amount of daily stress to give some idea of whether high stress is a significant issue	Stress management strategies may include referral for cognitive behavior therapy, yoga, meditation, and/or breathing exercises

Sleep	Inadequate sleep (fragmentation, deprivation, OSA) leads to: Increased fatigue and altered thermoregulation causing a decrease in energy expenditure. Changes in leptin and ghrelin levels leading to a decrease in energy expenditure and increase in appetitive drive. Hyperinsulinemia resulting in altered sugar metabolism and more storage of fats. High cortisol levels producing a catabolic state and inhibition of muscle building	Obtain information on duration and quality of sleep and screen for OSA. Identify bedtime, sleep latency (difficulty falling asleep), nocturnal awakenings, wake time, snoring, fatigue on awakening, morning headaches, daytime sleepiness and so forth. Can use tools such as Beck Sleep Inventory, Epworth Sleepiness Scale	Counsel on sleep hygiene. Low threshold to refer to sleep medicine if issue unresolved by counseling
Circadian rhythm	Inappropriate light exposure and feeding patterns disrupt the central biological clock (housed in the suprachiasmatic nucleus of the hypothalamus) and thereby alter the timing of cellular metabolic process throughout the body, leading to increased adiposity. Night shift workers and flight personnel are thus prone to weight gain	Assess for shift work, frequent travel across time zones, exposure to light late at night, and irregular feeding patterns	Physician-led counseling to improve nighttime light exposure and meal timings. Can consider melatonin, particularly for jet lag and shift work

Abbreviation: OSA, obstructive sleep apnea.

Nonpregnant Women

In nonpregnant women, diagnosis involves determining both the percentage of body fat and its distribution because both the amount of fat and its location are independent determinants of disease risk.

The World Health Organization defines obesity in women as greater than 35% body fat.[56] However, the most accurate methods to measure percent body fat (dual-energy X-ray absorptiometry, air-displacement plethysmography) are costly and currently restricted to the research setting. Bioelectrical impedance is used in some clinical practices but decreases in accuracy with increasing obesity. BMI remains the most practical method of estimating body fat in the clinical setting, and its routine use as a vital sign for every patient has been advocated to improve the diagnosis and treatment of obesity in clinical practice.[57]

BMI calculation, categories, associated health risks, and limitations are detailed in **Table 2**. Although BMI correlates with percentage body fat, its diagnostic sensitivity is lower in individuals who are in the normal and overweight categories (BMI 18–24.9, and BMI 25–29.9, respectively).[57]

It is therefore highly recommended that a second measure of adiposity be used routinely in clinical practice to assess body fat distribution, particularly in individuals who are in the normal to intermediate BMI categories. Waist circumference (WC) is a simple and practical measure for routine diagnosis in the office. WC reflects visceral adiposity and is independently associated with increased cardiovascular risk up to a BMI of 35 kg/m^2 (see **Table 2**). The WC should be obtained at the level of the iliac crest or at 1 fingerbreadth above the umbilicus; gender-specific cutoffs vary by ethnicity, but in general a WC greater than 88 cm (35 inches) in women is considered high.[57]

Pregnant Women

The diagnostic measures discussed earlier may be applied to women in early pregnancy in the absence of a prepregnancy baseline. In addition to diagnosing overweight and obesity at the onset of pregnancy, the amount and rate of weight gain during

Table 2
Classifying obesity to determine disease risk and weight gain in pregnancy

Weight Status		BMI (kg/m^2)	Disease Risk*		Recommended Weight Gain in Pregnancy (kg)
			WC Normal	WC >88 cm	
Underweight		<18.5	—	—	12.5–18.0
Normal		18.5–24.9	—	Increased	11.5–16.0
Overweight		25–29.9	Increased	High	7.0–11.5
Obesity	Class I	30–34.9	High	Very high	5.0–9.0
	Class II	35–39.9	Very high	Very high	5.0–9.0
	Class III	>40	Extremely high	Extremely high	5.0–9.0

* Risk for development of type 2 diabetes, hypertension and coronary artery disease.
BMI = weight (kg)/height (m^2) or weight (lb) × 703/height (inches). Waist circumference: at the level of the iliac crest, greater than 88 cm (35 inches) = high in women.
Abbreviation: WC, waist circumference.
Adapted from Rasmussen KM, Yaktine AL, Institute of Medicine (Committee to Reexamine IOM Pregnancy Weight Guidelines, Food and Nutrition Board and Board on Children, Youth, and Families). Weight gain during pregnancy: reexamining the guidelines. Washington, DC: National Academy Press; 2009; *Adapted from* National Institutes of Health NHLBI and North American Association for the Study of Obesity. The Practical Guide: Identification, Evaluation and Treatment of Overweight and Obesity in Adults. Washington, DC; 2000.

pregnancy need to be measured and tracked. The Institute of Medicine guidelines have established BMI-specific cutoffs for gestational weight gain, as detailed in **Table 2**.[58] There is also evidence to suggest that rapid weight gain in early pregnancy predicts excess gestational weight gain and related complications.[59–61]

ASSESSMENT

The purpose of the history and physical examination is to identify underlying conditions contributing to weight gain and to assess for potential complications of excess body fat. The history should begin with obtaining a weight history, in particular the age of onset of obesity, any identifiable circumstances (eg, menarche, menopause, pregnancy, smoking cessation, medications) associated with weight changes, and response to prior weight loss attempts. Details of key lifestyle factors described in **Table 1** should be assessed. Social and cultural routines as well as psychological and situational stressors may influence lifestyle factors and should be explored both for their possible contribution to weight gain and as potential barriers to lifestyle modification. Family history should include history of overweight states and obesity in first-degree and second-degree relatives. The review of systems should screen for the most common obesity-related comorbidities (see **Fig. 2**).

The physical examination of a patient with obesity may be challenging for multiple reasons, ranging from the amount and distribution of adiposity to the physical environment of the examination room. Therefore, it is essential to overcome potential environmental barriers (eg, by providing gowns that can fit larger patients and using large blood pressure cuffs when appropriate).[62] Routine physical examination includes the search for both causes and possible complications of obesity. Ruling out organic causes of obesity, such as Cushing syndrome, may be difficult because signs and symptoms of hypercortisolemia (eg, striae and central adiposity) may overlap with some hyperinsulinemic obesity phenotypes. A careful breast examination as well as examination of the skin and lower extremities (in particular, potential unreachable areas like the feet) are suggested because these areas may be less frequently addressed.[63]

Laboratory testing should complement the physical examination in elucidating the diagnosis of an underlying medical cause and the detection of the metabolic consequences of obesity. Hypothyroidism is rarely a direct cause of obesity, but thyroid function should still be checked. Screening for metabolic syndrome is also essential and, therefore, fasting glucose level and lipid profile should be routinely measured. Serum insulin levels provide a more direct measurement of hyperinsulinemia, but assays are not well standardized.

TREATMENT STRATEGY

The goals of obesity treatment are to reduce adiposity, decrease cardiovascular risk and mortality, and improve comorbidities and quality of life using safe, evidence-based approaches. Treatment strategies are in 1 of 3 therapeutic modalities, namely lifestyle, pharmacotherapy, and surgery, and in most cases multimodal combination therapy is required. **Fig. 5** outlines a working algorithm for antiobesity treatment based on patient assessment.

STEP 1: REMOVAL OF WEIGHT GAIN–PROMOTING MEDICATIONS

There are a host of commonly prescribed medications that may interfere with the normal functioning of the energy regulatory system and promote weight gain.[64] Occasionally, chronologic evidence on history can help identify whether a medication

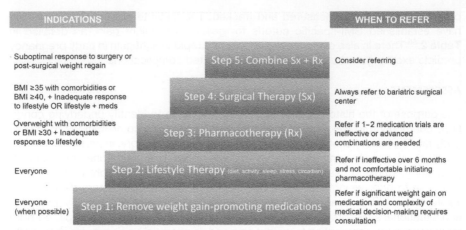

Fig. 5. Working algorithm for obesity treatment. (*Adapted from* Corey KE, Kaplan LM. Obesity and liver disease: the epidemic of the twenty-first century. Clin Liver Dis 2014;18(1):1–18.)

is the cause of significant gain. However, even in the absence of obvious weight gain on a medication, weight gain–promoting medications may have insidious and cumulative effects, and/or may hinder the weight loss effects of other therapies. The first step in obesity treatment is therefore to discontinue weight gain–promoting medications or switch to an alternative that is weight neutral or weight loss promoting, or at least associated with less weight gain.[63] Weight gain–promoting medications and potential alternatives are detailed in **Table 3**.

STEP 2: LIFESTYLE THERAPIES

As mentioned earlier and shown in **Fig. 3**, there are several interrelated aspects of individual lifestyle that can adversely affect energy regulation, including diet, activity, sleep, stress, and circadian rhythm. Patients may present with a need for improvement in all, none, or only some of these issues. Improving all identified factors as a whole is not only overwhelming for patients and providers but also impractical within the time and resource constraints of a clinical visit. Hence, a sequential approach based on a targeted assessment of modifiable lifestyle factors and spread over several clinical visits is advocated. Therapeutic strategies for each lifestyle component are summarized in **Table 1** and detailed later.

DIET

Historically, diets for weight reduction have been described or categorized according to macronutrient composition (low-carbohydrate, low-fat, or high-protein diets), specific nutrient content (low glycemic index or low glycemic load diets), or specific combinations of foods (Mediterranean, plant-based, South Beach, or DASH [dietary approaches to stop hypertension] diets). Although some of these diets may be superior to others for certain health effects, such as improvements in lipid levels, glucose homeostasis, blood pressure, inflammation, or cardiovascular risk,[65,66] there is no single diet that has proved most effective for weight loss.[67] Multiple comparative trials and meta-analyses have shown a similar and modest average weight loss across all diets.[68,69] The conclusion has been that caloric reduction is more critical for weight loss than diet composition.

Table 3
Medications associated with weight gain

Weight Gain Promoting	Weight Neutral or Weight Loss Promoting
Atypical Antipsychotics	
Clozapine (Clozaril)	Ziprasidone
Olanzapine (Zyprexa)	
Quetiapine (Seroquel)	
Risperidone (Risperdal)	
Aripiprazole (Abilify)	
Haloperidol (Haldol)	
Perphenazine (Trilafon)	
Chlorpromazine (Thorazine)	
Anticonvulsants/Mood Stabilizers	
Lithium	Topiramate
Valproic acid (Valproate)	Zonisamide
Carbamazepine (Tegretol)	Lamotrigine
Vigabatrin (Sabril)	
Gabapentin (Neurontin)	
Phenytoin (Dilantin)	
Divalproex sodium (Depakote)	
Oxcarbazepine (Trileptal)	
Antidepressants	
Selective serotonin reuptake inhibitors	Bupropion
Paroxetine (Paxil)	
Citalopram (Celexa)	
Fluoxetine (Prozac)	
Sertraline (Zoloft)	
Tricyclic antidepressants	
Amitriptyline (Elavil)	
Nortriptyline (Pamelor)	
Imipramine (Tofranil)	
Monoamine oxidase inhibitors	
Phenelzine (Nardil)	
Other antidepressant	
Mirtazapine (Remeron)	
Trazadone (Desyrel)	
Antidiabetic Agents	
Insulin	Metformin
Sulfonylureas	Pramlintide
Glyburide (DiaBeta)	GLP-1 analogues
Glipizide (Glucotrol)	DPP4 inhibitors
Glimepiride (Amaryl)	SGLT-2 inhibitors
Thiazolidinediones	Acarbose
Pioglitazone (Actos)	
Rosiglitazone (Avandia)	
Antihypertensive Medications	
β-Blockers	Other antihypertensives
Propranolol (Inderal)	Carvedilol
Metoprolol (Lopressor, Toprol)	
Atenolol (Tenormin)	
α-Blockers	
Clonidine (Catapres)	
Prazosin (Minipress)	
Terazosin (Hytrin)	

(continued on next page)

Table 3 (continued)	
Weight Gain Promoting	**Weight Neutral or Weight Loss Promoting**
Corticosteroids	
Prednisone	Cytotoxic agents
Hydrocortisone	
Dexamethasone	
Antihistamines	
Diphenhydramine (Benadryl)	Loratadine
Hormonal Contraceptives	
Depo-medroxyprogesterone acetate (Depo-Provera)	Nonhormonal contraception
Oral contraceptives	
Hormonal intrauterine device	
Hormone vaginal ring	
Sleep Aids	
Zolpidem	Melatonin
	Sleep hygiene counseling

Alternative medications are weight neutral or cause less weight gain.

Drugs are listed in order from greatest to least weight gain. Bold drugs have the greatest degree of weight gain.

Abbreviations: DPP4, dipeptidyl-peptidase 4; GLP-1, glucagon-like peptide-1; SGLT-2, sodium glucose cotransporter-2.

Caloric reduction does yield weight loss, although primarily in the short-term. A moderate caloric reduction typically provides 500 to 1000 fewer calories to achieve a weight loss of 0.5 to 1.0 kg/wk and an average 5% to 10% weight loss over 6 months. A very low calorie diet, usually prescribed for a period of 8 to 12 weeks under physician supervision, provides less than 800 calories/d through commercially available products (shakes, soups, bars) and results in up to 25% total weight loss. In both cases, weight regain over 1 to 5 years is the rule rather than the exception.[70]

Physiologic studies in humans have shown that caloric reduction alone leads to metabolic adaptation with neurohumoral responses that promote hunger, reduced energy expenditure, and ultimate restoration of the adiposity set point.[71,72] In this regard, caloric reduction in obesity is analogous to fluid restriction in heart failure. It works in the short-term but, once normal intake is resumed, the excess returns. As with heart failure or other chronic diseases, addressing the underlying physiologic dysfunction in obesity is critical for long-term results. Studies combining caloric reduction with pharmacotherapy to counter metabolic adaptation are ongoing and future results may provide a strategy to use reduced calorie diets for long-term weight loss.[73] At present, the authors advocate restricting the use of caloric reduction strategies to scenarios in which short-term weight loss is medically indicated (**Box 1**). Otherwise, caloric reduction as a general antiobesity therapy sets the stage for so-called yo-yo dieting, failure, frustration, and self-blame.

Because specific nutrients, including sugars, fatty acids, and amino acids, have neurohumoral effects, diet therapy for long-term weight loss may be designed to improve nutrient composition in an attempt to achieve a neurohumoral reduction in the set point.[74] Theoretically, this would limit metabolic adaptation, reduce appetite, and increase compliance. Previous trials that showed similar average responses to different diets also showed that there is wide variability in weight loss response to

---

Box 1
Medical situations in which calorie reduction for short-term weight loss is appropriate

Caloric restriction leads to short-term weight loss. Gradually weight regain after restrictive dieting occurs because of metabolic adaptations.

Weight loss through caloric restriction (low or very low calorie diets) may be indicated in the following circumstances:
1. Before a therapeutic procedure or operation, in order to medically qualify for procedure or improve prognosis after treatment.
   Examples:
      Orthopedic surgery
      Transplant surgery
      In vitro fertilization
2. Before a diagnostic or therapeutic procedure in which weight and/or size is prohibitive because of equipment limitations.
   Examples:
      Computed tomography scan or MRI
      Radiation therapy
      Interventional cardiology procedure
      Interventional radiology procedure

---

any given diet.[75] A recent study by Zeevi and colleagues[76] found that the glucose response to the same nutrient intake varies considerably from person to person, further supporting the need for individualized nutritional therapies. Obesity is a heterogeneous condition and it is likely that different individuals respond better to specific diets. In light of the scarcity of data to guide providers in prescribing individualized diet therapy for specific obesity phenotypes, the authors recommend aiming for a metabolically healthy balanced diet (see **Table 1**), for which there seems to be a general consensus. More specific healthy diets (eg, Mediterranean, DASH, plant-based) can be considered in the context of the patient's comorbidities and risk factors.

EXERCISE

Exercise plays an important role in obesity management in women. The benefits of exercise can be defined in terms of weight loss, weight maintenance, and comorbidity improvement.

The weight loss response to exercise varies broadly among individuals and the average weight loss is modest at best.[77,78] As with calorie-restricted diets, attempts at increasing the expenditure side of the energy balance equation through short-term vigorous activity regimens can be countered by metabolic adaptations that reduce resting metabolic rate and preserve adiposity.[79,80] The goal of exercise therapy for obesity is, therefore, not increased short-term expenditure, but sustained improvement in muscle mass and its metabolic function over time.[81]

Relative to its variable effect on weight loss, exercise seems to be a stronger predictor of weight maintenance.[82] Exercise helps to preserve lean body mass and may increase resting energy expenditure in the weight-reduced state.[83] The weight-independent effects of exercise on obesity-related conditions such as diabetes, cardiovascular risk, cancer, osteoporosis, arthritis, depression, and dementia, as well its beneficial effects on quality of life, are further reasons that exercise therapy should be a critical component of any obesity management strategy.[84]

Data on the type, dose, and frequency of activity needed for weight loss, weight maintenance, and disease risk reduction continue to emerge. Although resistance training has positive effects on body composition, aerobic exercise seems to be more beneficial for weight loss. Both types of exercise improve diabetes and cardio-vascular risk and should be a part of any exercise routine.[85,86] For postmenopausal women, flexibility and balance exercises are recommended in addition to resistance and aerobic activities.[87]

Recommendations for prevention of weight gain are at least 150 minutes per week or 30 to 60 minutes 5 days per week of moderately intense physical activity, or 20 to 60 minutes per week of vigorous activity. However, researchers estimate more than 200 minutes per week of moderately intense physical activity are needed for weight loss and more than 250 minutes are needed for weight maintenance.[88]

Achieving the amount of exercise recommended by the guidelines mentioned earlier is difficult. Behavioral strategies that include goal setting, exercise prescriptions and follow-up, self-monitoring, and social support are often key to implementation. Most importantly, recommendations should be physically realistic, medically safe, and able to fit into the patient's daily routine.

SLEEP

Individuals with obesity have more disordered and inadequate sleep than their normal-weight counterparts.[89] However, targeting sleep as a part of lifestyle therapy for weight loss has yet to be formally studied. In our clinical experience, there are patients whose energy regulatory systems seem to be more sensitive to the effects of sleep disruption than others. Improving sleep in these patients leads to weight loss, whereas in others the weight loss effect may not be noticeable but the remaining health benefits of sleep therapy are still substantial and should be pursued. For patients with sleep fragmentation or sleep deprivation, sleep hygiene counseling in combination with psychological-behavioral approaches is recommended.[90] Because many sleeping aids can contribute to weight gain, these should be avoided whenever possible.[91] Melatonin has been shown to have only modest effects on sleep, but can be considered as treatment because it is not associated with weight gain.[92] If the goal of 7 to 8 hours of uninterrupted sleep per night is not achieved with conservative measures, referral to sleep medicine should be considered. For patients who screen positive for sleep apnea, appropriate diagnosis and treatment in conjunction with a sleep medicine specialist is indicated.

STRESS

Stress reduction as a discrete therapy for weight loss has not been studied and there is a dearth of data guiding clinical intervention in this area. In light of the correlation between work stress and obesity and the adverse physiologic response to stress that contributes to the onset or worsening of obesity and chronic disease, the authors recommend addressing stress if patient assessment reveals high stress levels. Stress reduction strategies may include mindfulness, meditation, yoga, other structured exercise, and cognitive behavior therapy.[93] The chosen strategy should involve shared decision making and fit into the patient's routine.

STEP 3: PHARMACOTHERAPY

When the benefits of reducing adiposity outweigh the potential risks of medication, and the patient has had an inadequate response to conservative lifestyle therapy, antiobesity pharmacotherapy should be initiated. A similar rationale is used in the treatment of other chronic conditions, such as type 2 diabetes, hypertension, and hyperlipidemia.

According to clinical guidelines, pharmacotherapy for obesity is recommended for a BMI greater than 30 kg/m² or BMI greater than 27 kg/m² with obesity-related comorbidities.[91] In general, lifestyle change should have been attempted and yielded inadequate results before starting an antiobesity medication. There may be cases in which the severity of the condition warrants initiation of pharmacotherapy in conjunction with, rather than after, lifestyle changes. Providers should rely on a thorough patient assessment and their best clinical judgment in such cases. Efforts should still be made to optimize the patient's lifestyle, and a follow-up and monitoring plan should be in place.

Table 4 details current US Food and Drug Administration–approved antiobesity medications, as well as some medications that are used off-label by obesity medicine specialists.[91] Choice of medication depends on a combination of factors, including type of obesity (eg, medication-induced weight gain or evidence of a strong hedonic drive), patient characteristics (eg, age and comorbidities), side effect profile, cost, and patient preference. It is also suggested that clinicians should aim for a double benefit whenever possible, such as the use of topiramate in the presence of migraines, or metformin in the setting of polycystic ovarian syndrome (PCOS).[91]

One of the pitfalls of using antiobesity medications is the tendency to prematurely terminate pharmacotherapy based on the patient's response to the first prescribed medication. There is substantial variability in response to treatment, as shown in antiobesity medication trials.[94–96] The average response to any medication is often modest, and there are many patients who do not respond. However, for each medication, a significant number of patients experience at least 5% weight loss, with some achieving 10% weight loss and a few having a robust response (>20% weight loss). Because each medication has a different mechanism of action, it is unlikely that a response to one predicts response to another. A medication that has not been effective in the first 1 to 3 months should therefore be switched to a reasonable alternative. Patient education regarding the variability in response needs to be provided to better manage expectations and ensure compliance.

To minimize side effects while maximizing efficacy, slow-titration regimens and combination treatments are recommended (see **Table 4**). Follow-up is usually 1 month for any new medication or change in dosage, and every 3 months thereafter. Weight regain does ensue on cessation of medication because the drug-induced biological changes responsible for the weight loss revert to baseline with discontinuation of therapy. Hence, long-term therapy is recommended.[91]

STEP 4: SURGERY

Weight loss surgery for obesity is recommended for individuals with a BMI greater than or equal to 40, or BMI greater than or equal to 35 and at least 2 obesity-related comorbidities, such as type 2 diabetes, PCOS, hypertension, sleep apnea and other respiratory disorders, nonalcoholic fatty liver disease, osteoarthritis, lipid abnormalities, gastrointestinal disorders, heart disease, or infertility.[97,98] Surgery should be considered if prior weight loss efforts have been unsuccessful. Although surgery is the most invasive treatment option for obesity and has a broad distribution of response, it remains the most effective therapy, achieving significant and durable weight loss in most patients.[97]

Profound physiologic effects on energy regulation through surgical manipulation of the gastrointestinal tract are thought to underlie the weight loss and metabolic effects of procedures such as sleeve gastrectomy and Roux-en-Y gastric bypass.[99]

Bariatric surgery has been found to have positive effects on PCOS and infertility.[100] There is also a suggestion of a maternal epigenetic effect because offspring born to

Table 4
Pharmacotherapy for obesity

Drug Name (Brand Name): Mechanism of Action in Weight Loss	Dosage Range	Adverse Effects/Cautions[a]	Contraindications[a]	Comments
FDA-approved Medications for Treatment of Obesity				
Benzphetamine (Didrex): Induces synaptic vesicular amine transporter to increase NE in synapse; α-1A, 1B adrenergic receptor agonist	25–50 mg TID	Similar to phentermine	Similar to phentermine	• FDA approved for short-term use (~12 wk) • DEA schedule III drug[b] • Pregnancy category X
Diethylpropion (Tenuate): Inhibits Na+-dependent NE transporter and serotonin transporter and serotonin (less)	75 mg/d (75 mg QD XR caps)	Similar to phentermine	Similar to phentermine	• FDA approved for short-term use (~12 wk) • Immediate release not studied • DEA schedule IV drug[b] • Pregnancy category X
Liraglutide (Saxenda): Acylated human GLP-1 receptor agonist; weight loss mechanism unknown	0.6–3.0 mg/d	Nausea, vomiting hypoglycemia, cholecystitis, pancreatitis	History of medullary thyroid carcinoma, MEN type II	• Animal (not human) studies: increased risk of thyroid C-cell tumors • Injectable medication • Expensive • Pregnancy category X
Lorcaserin (Belviq): Selective serotonin 2c receptor agonist; activates POMC neurons via 5HT2c receptor	10 mg BID	Nasopharyngitis, HA, dizziness, fatigue	Preexisting depression. Caution in CHF, on SSRI	• Monitor for depression, serotonin syndrome, priapism • Expensive • Pregnancy category X
Naltrexone-Bupropion XR (Contrave): Combination of weak DA and NE reuptake inhibitor and opioid receptor agonist	8/90–32/360 mg/d	Constipation, HA, nausea, vomiting, dizziness, insomnia Avoid coadministration with MAOIs, high-fat meals because of increased risk of seizures	Seizures, uncontrolled HTN, bulimia, chronic opioid use, liver failure, glaucoma	• Expensive • Pregnancy category X

Medication	Dose	Side Effects	Contraindications	Comments
Orlistat (Xenical, Alli): Lipase inhibitor	120 mg/d–120 mg TID	Flatulence, diarrhea, bloating/cramping, liver failure	Chronic malabsorption; liver failure, cholestasis	• Take with fat-containing meal • Monitor fat-soluble vitamins • Expensive • Alli is an OTC form of orlistat, less expensive
Phendimetrazine (Bontril, others): Inhibits Na+-dependent NE transporter; α-1A,1B adrenergic receptor agonist	17.5–70 mg TID	Similar to phentermine	Similar to phentermine	• FDA approved for short-term use (~12 wk) • DEA schedule III drug[b] • Pregnancy category X
Phentermine (Adipex-P, Ionamin, others): Sympathomimetic amine, increased NE activity in HT; reduces appetite, possible increase EE	15–30 mg/d 18.75–37.5 mg/d	Dry mouth, constipation, insomnia, headache, ↑BP/HR Caution: ↑ risk of serotonin syndrome with SSRIs	CAD, CVA, cardiac arrhythmia, hyperthyroidism, uncontrolled HTN, seizures	• FDA approved for short-term use (~12 wk) • DEA schedule IV drug[b] • Inexpensive • Most widely prescribed anti-obesity medication • Pregnancy category X
Phentermine-Topiramate XR (Qsymia): Combined effects of phentermine and topiramate	3.75/23–15/92 mg/d	Paresthesias, dry mouth, constipation, dysgeusia, others similar to phentermine and topiramate	Similar to phentermine and topiramate	• Increased risk of congenital fetal oropalatal clefts • Expensive • Robust weight loss • Pregnancy category X
Medications That May Cause Weight Loss				
Bupropion (Wellbutrin): Weak DA and NE reuptake inhibitor; Activates POMC and modulates reward pathways	150–450 mg/d	Insomnia, anxiety, HA, diarrhea, dry mouth	Seizures, bulimia, cardiac arrhythmia	• Monitor HR, BP • Avoid in bipolar disorders
Canagliflozin (Invokana): Inhibition of SGLT-2 in renal tubules, which blocks glucose reabsorption in the proximal tubule	100–300 mg/d	Increased creatinine, hypotension, dehydration, hyperkalemia, UTIs, candidiasis	Renal failure (GFR<30 mL/min)	• Weight loss is modest • Has insulin-sparing effects • Expensive

(continued on next page)

Table 4
(continued)

Drug Name (Brand Name): Mechanism of Action in Weight Loss	Dosage Range	Adverse Effects/Cautions[a]	Contraindications[a]	Comments
Exenatide (Byetta, Bydureon): Synthetic analogue of GLP-1; weight loss mechanism not known	5–10 μg BID Bydureon (2 mg q7d)	Nausea, hypoglycemia pancreatitis; possibly pancreatic ductal neoplasia	Medullary thyroid carcinoma, MEN type II	• Injectable medication • Take before meals (2 meals) • Bydureon is an exenatide XR • Expensive
Metformin (Glucophage, Glumetza): Reduces hepatic glucose production; enhances insulin sensitivity	500–2000 mg/d	Nausea, diarrhea, vitamin B_{12} deficiency Increased risk of lactic acidosis in combination with topiramate	Renal insufficiency, CHF, or other hypovolemic state	• Useful in antipsychotic-induced weight gain • Useful in PCOS
Pramlintide (Symlin): Synthetic amylin analogue; weight loss mechanism not known	60–120 μg TID	Hypoglycemia, nausea, vomiting, HA	Gastroparesis	• Useful in diabetics on insulin • Take before meals
Topiramate (Topamax): Enhances GABA receptor activity; inhibits carbonic anhydrase	25–150 mg/d	Paresthesias, dysgeusia, somnolence, memory impairment, acute angle glaucoma Increased risk of lactic acidosis in combination with metformin	Kidney stones, glaucoma	• Useful in antipsychotic-induced weight gain • Useful in binge eating • Increased risk of congenital fetal oropalatal clefts • Pregnancy category D
Zonisamide (Zonegran): Enhances serotonin and DA activity	100–400 mg/d	Dysgeusia, HA, impaired memory, gastrointestinal and musculoskeletal problems	Sulfa allergy, kidney stones, glaucoma	• Interactions with naproxen and *Ginkgo biloba* • Monitor renal function (serum Cr)

Abbreviations: 5HT, serotonin; BID, 2 times a day; BP, blood pressure; CAD, coronary artery disease; CHF, congestive heart failure; Cr, creatinine; CVA, cerebrovascular accident; DA, dopamine; DEA, Drug Enforcement Administration; EE, energy expenditure; FDA, US Food and Drug Administration; GABA, gamma-aminobutyric acid; GFR, glomerular filtration rate; HA, headache; HR, heart rate; HTN, hypertension; MAOI, monoamine oxidase inhibitor; MEN, multiple endocrine neoplasias; NE, norepinephrine; OTC, over-the-counter; PCOS, polycystic ovarian syndrome; POMC, pro-opiomelanocortin; QD, every day; SSRI, serotonin reuptake inhibitor; TID, 3 times a day; UTI, urinary tract infections; XR, extended release.

[a] This is an incomplete list of all the adverse effects and contraindications of the medications.

[b] DEA schedule III drugs are associated with a proposed higher risk of abuse compared with schedule IV drugs.

Adapted from Apovian CM, Aronne LJ, Bessesen DH, et al. Pharmacological management of obesity: an Endocrine Society clinical practice guideline. J Clin Endocrinol Metab 2015;100:342–62.

Table 5
Surgery for obesity

Procedure	Description	Mechanism	Response	Indications	Considerations
RYGB	Laparoscopic (rarely open) Stomach is divided into a small pouch (15–30 mL) and large remnant 80–150 cm of proximal small intestine are bypassed by the creation of a Roux limb that connects to the pouch	Alterations in neurohumoral signaling, including dramatic changes in the basal and postprandial release of key gut peptides involved in energy regulation Effects include diminished appetitive drive, changes in food preference, increase in energy expenditure shown in rodent models, and weight loss–independent improvements in glucose homeostasis	Mean: 60%–80% EBWL Broad variation	BMI $\geq$30 kg/m^2 with type 2 diabetes[103] BMI $\geq$35 kg/m^2 with comorbidities Or BMI $\geq$40 kg/m^2 Prior failed weight loss attempts	Monitoring and long-term repletion of micronutrients required May affect absorption of oral contraceptives May be more effective than VSG for type 2 diabetes remission Improved fertility and reduced metabolic disease in offspring reported
VSG	Laparoscopic (rarely open) Surgical removal of 75% of the stomach along the greater curvature resulting in a sleeve or tubelike stomach	Alterations in neurohumoral signaling similar to RYGB despite no intestinal component to the procedure. Dramatic changes in gut peptides thought to be related to rapid transit of food through tubelike stomach	Mean: 50%–60% EBWL Broad variation	BMI $\geq$30 kg/m^2 with type 2 diabetes[103] BMI $\geq$35 kg/m^2 with comorbidities Or BMI $\geq$40 kg/m^2 Prior failed weight loss attempts	Can worsen GERD; contraindicated in severe reflux disease
AGB	Laparoscopic Inflatable silicon device implanted around the top of the stomach to create a small pouch. Inflation of the band occurs through injecting fluid through a small port placed under the skin	Restrictive procedure causing early satiety. Does not seem to result in neurohumoral alterations that would affect energy regulation as in RYGB or VSG	50% of patients have 40%–60% EBWL The other 50% have minimal response	BMI $\geq$30 kg/m^2 with comorbidities Or BMI $\geq$40 kg/m^2 Prior failed weight loss attempts	Least invasive but also least effective and falling out of favor Contraindicated in immunosuppressed states Band slippage and erosion, GERD and esophageal dysmotility are possible side effects

Abbreviations: AGB, adjustable gastric band; EBWL, excess body weight loss; GERD, gastroesophageal reflux disease; RYGB, Roux-en-Y gastric bypass; VSG, vertical sleeve gastrectomy.

Table 6
Approved weight loss devices

	Mechanism	Indication	Results	Side Effects	Contraindications
Gastric pacemaker Maestro by Enteromedics	Intermittently blocks afferent vagal signals from the gastrointestinal tract to the brain. The afferent vagus is involved in regulating hunger and satiety but the precise mechanism of weight loss with the device is unknown	BMI 35–39.9 kg/m^2 with at least 1 comorbidity, or BMI ≥40 kg/m^2 Prior failed supervised weight loss attempt in the past 5 y	Clinical trial results showed 8.5% greater excess weight loss at 12 mo with gastric electrical stimulation compared with control	Pain at neuroregulator site, nausea, vomiting, abdominal pain, heartburn, problems swallowing, belching, and chest pain	Cirrhosis, portal hypertension, esophageal varices, or clinically significant hiatal hernia Patients needing MRI or those with another permanently implanted electrically powered medical device or prosthesis
Gastric balloons Orbera by Apollo Endosurgery Reshape dual balloon by Allergan	Placed endoscopically and filled with saline. Promotes satiety and weight loss by occupying space in the stomach	BMI 30–40 kg/m^2 Failed prior lifestyle therapy. (approved for use for 6 mo in conjunction with a supervised diet and exercise program)	Orbera: 10.5% weight loss vs 4.7% with diet and exercise alone ReShape: 25% excess weight loss compared with 11.3% with diet and exercise alone	Nausea, vomiting, abdominal pain, gastric ulcers, indigestion, and balloon migration with obstruction	Pregnancy Previous gastrointestinal or bariatric surgery, inflammatory intestinal or bowel disease, large hiatal hernia, symptoms consistent with delayed gastric emptying, or active *Helicobacter pylori* infection Avoided in patients on anticoagulants, aspirin, or antiinflammatory agents

Data from Obesity treatment devices. US Food and Drug Administration Web site. Available at: http://www.fda.gov/MedicalDevices/ProductsandMedicalProcedures/ObesityDevices/ucm20036251.htm. Accessed December 15, 2015.

women after gastrointestinal weight loss surgery have significantly less obesity and metabolic disease in childhood and adulthood.[101]

Although surgery does not interfere with the normal physiology and weight gain of pregnancy, it is recommended that pregnancy be avoided in the initial weight loss phase up to 18 months after the procedure.[98] Women of childbearing age, including those with prior infertility, should be advised to use contraception during the first 18 months. During any pregnancy following bariatric surgery, particularly Roux-en-Y gastric bypass, micronutrient deficiencies and supplementation should be monitored closely.[98]

The most commonly performed evidence-based procedures and considerations for practitioners are detailed in **Table 5**. After an initial discussion with their primary providers, patients should be referred to surgical practices or centers of excellence that provide multidisciplinary evaluations and support as recommended by current practice guidelines.

WEIGHT LOSS DEVICES

Over the past decade, obesity therapeutics has expanded considerably in the device development arena, with a focus on the gastrointestinal tract. After the failure of early devices, several have been approved for clinical trials in the United States and 3 were approved for use in 2015 (**Table 6**).[102]

Practitioners treating obesity should anticipate the addition of more weight loss devices to the therapeutic options that will be available for patients in the future. For appropriate medical management, clinicians will need to be well versed in the efficacy and side effect profile of each device to be able to appropriately channel patients to the best therapy, monitor their prognosis, and exploit the full potential of device therapy using multimodal combinatorial approaches. In general, referral to a multidisciplinary weight loss center performing endoscopic procedures should be considered.

REFERRAL

When to refer a patient to an obesity medicine specialist or a multidisciplinary weight loss clinic (consisting of 1 or more of the following providers: dietician, psychologist, exercise trainer, obesity medicine specialist, bariatric surgeon) is not clear, but should be considered when treatment decisions become complex, as outlined in **Box 2**.

Box 2
When to refer a patient to an obesity medicine specialist or a multidisciplinary weight loss clinic

Consider referral to multidisciplinary weight management centers[a] or obesity medicine specialists for the following:
1. Patients with medically complex obesity who are resistant to lifestyle modification after 6 to 12 months and/or have not had an adequate response to 1 or 2 medication trials
2. Patients requiring more intensive weight loss treatments (eg, very low calorie diets, combination pharmacotherapy, weight loss surgery, or weight loss devices)
3. Weight loss before surgery (eg, general, orthopedic, or transplant surgeries)
4. Weight loss before pregnancy or in vitro fertilization
5. Patients with medication-induced weight gain
6. Patients with a BMI greater than 50 kg/m²

  [a] Multidisciplinary (eg, exercise trainer, dietitian, psychologist, physician, surgeon).

SUMMARY

The neurohumoral regulation of energy balance may be disrupted by a host of developmental and biopsychosocial factors, leading to states of excess adiposity referred to collectively as obesity. Rather than a lifestyle choice or characterological flaw, obesity is a chronic medical condition in which biological complexity results in clinical heterogeneity and great variability in treatment response. The management of this condition requires a basic understanding of energy regulatory physiology, factors that affect that physiology, and how to assess and address those factors in individual patients in clinical practice.

Biological, developmental, and psychosocial factors specific to women may be placing them at greater risk of obesity and obesity-related comorbidities. Obstetrician-gynecologists have the opportunity to prevent and treat obesity at multiple critical stages in women's lifecycles. This article reviews a stepwise approach to long-term obesity management involving removal of weight gain–promoting medications and targeted lifestyle therapy, followed by pharmacotherapy, surgical therapy, and/or referral to an obesity medicine specialist when clinically indicated. By applying the current working algorithm, clinicians can engage their patients in an unbiased and supportive weight management process, and keep the patients engaged by being both realistic about the variability in results with any 1 treatment and reassuring that more treatment options exist if initial steps are ineffective. As obesity medicine continues to evolve, newer and better evidence-based therapies and treatment strategies will emerge that will require adoption and implementation by a medical community that is already actively engaged in primary obesity care.

ACKNOWLEDGMENTS

The authors thank Sriram Machineni, MD for his contribution to **Fig. 2**.

REFERENCES

1. Ogden CL, Carroll MD, Kit BK, et al. Prevalence of childhood and adult obesity in the United States, 2011-2012. JAMA 2014;311:806–14.
2. Mauro M, Taylor V, Wharton S, et al. Barriers to obesity treatment. Eur J Intern Med 2008;19:173–80.
3. Kanter R, Caballero B. Global gender disparities in obesity: A review. Adv Nutr 2012;3:491–8.
4. Global Health Observatory data repository. World Health Organization Web site. Available at: http://apps.who.int/gho/data/view.main.2480A?lang=en. Accessed December 15, 2015.
5. Wang Y, Beydoun MA. The obesity epidemic in the United States–gender, age, socioeconomic, racial/ethnic, and geographic characteristics: A systematic review and meta-regression analysis. Epidemiol Rev 2007;29:6–28.
6. Flegal KM, Carroll MD, Kit BK, et al. Prevalence of obesity and trends in the distribution of body mass index among US adults, 1999-2010. JAMA 2012;307: 491–7.
7. Guh DP, Zhang W, Bansback N, et al. The incidence of co-morbidities related to obesity and overweight: a systematic review and meta-analysis. BMC Public Health 2009;9:88.
8. Muennig P, Lubetkin E, Jia H, et al. Gender and the burden of disease attributable to obesity. Am J Public Health 2006;96:1662–8.

9. Corey KE, Kaplan LM. Obesity and liver disease: the epidemic of the twenty-first century. In: Younossi ZM, editor. The impact of obesity and nutrition on chronic liver diseases. Philadelphia: Elsevier; 2014. p. 1–18.

10. Kulie T, Slattengren A, Redmer J, et al. Obesity and women's health: an evidence-based review. J Am Board Fam Med 2011;24:75–85.

11. Jones-Johnson G, Johnson WR, Frishman N. Race and gender differences in obesity and disease. Sociol Mind 2014;4:233–41.

12. Hudson JI, Hiripi E, Pope HG Jr, et al. The prevalence and correlates of eating disorders in the National Comorbidity Survey Replication. Biol Psychiatry 2007; 61:348–58.

13. Richard D. Cognitive and autonomic determinants of energy homeostasis in obesity. Nat Rev Endocrinol 2015;11:489–501.

14. Mauvais-Jarvis F, Clegg DJ, Hevener AL. The role of estrogens in control of energy balance and glucose homeostasis. Endocr Rev 2013;34:309–38.

15. Davidsen L, Vistisen B, Astrup A. Impact of the menstrual cycle on determinants of energy balance: a putative role in weight loss attempts. Int J Obes 2007;31: 1777–85.

16. Cottrell EC, Ozanne SE. Early life metabolic programming of obesity and metabolic disease. Physiol Behav 2008;94:17–28.

17. Parlee SD, MacDougald OA. Maternal nutrition and risk of obesity in offspring: The Trojan horse of developmental plasticity. Biochim Biophys Acta 2014; 1842:495–506.

18. Okubo H, Crozier SR, Harvey NC, et al. Maternal dietary glycemic index and glycemic load in early pregnancy are associated with offspring adiposity in childhood: the Southampton Women's Survey. Am J Clin Nutr 2014;100:676–83.

19. Maslova E, Rytter D, Bech BH, et al. Maternal protein intake during pregnancy and offspring overweight 20 y later. Am J Clin Nutr 2014;100:1139–48.

20. Hayes L, Bell R, Robson S, et al, Upbeat Consortium. Association between physical activity in obese pregnant women and offspring health. Pregnancy Hypertens 2014;4:234.

21. Entringer S. Impact of stress and stress physiology during pregnancy on child metabolic function and obesity risk. Curr Opin Clin Nutr Metab Care 2013;16: 320–7.

22. Valvi D, Casas M, Mendez MA, et al. Prenatal bisphenol a urine concentrations and early rapid growth and overweight risk in the offspring. Epidemiology 2013; 24:791–9.

23. Heerwagen MJ, Miller MR, Barbour LA, et al. Maternal obesity and fetal metabolic programming: a fertile epigenetic soil. Am J Physiol Regul Integr Comp Physiol 2010;299:R711–22.

24. Wu LL, Russell DL, Wong SL, et al. Mitochondrial dysfunction in oocytes of obese mothers: transmission to offspring and reversal by pharmacological endoplasmic reticulum stress inhibitors. Development 2015;142:681–91.

25. Siega-Riz AM, Viswanathan M, Moos MK, et al. A systematic review of outcomes of maternal weight gain according to the Institute of Medicine recommendations: birthweight, fetal growth and postpartum weight retention. Am J Obstet Gynecol 2009;201:339.e1–14.

26. Young BE, Johnson SL, Krebs NF. Biological determinants linking infant weight gain and child obesity: Current knowledge and future directions. Adv Nutr 2012; 3:675–86.

27. Anderson SE, Gooze RA, Lemeshow S, et al. Quality of early maternal–child relationship and risk of adolescent obesity. Pediatrics 2012;129:132–40.

28. Mazzeschi C, Pazzagli C, Laghezza L, et al. The role of both parents' attachment pattern in understanding childhood obesity. Front Psychol 2014;5:791.
29. Taveras EM, Rifas-Shiman SL, Oken E, et al. Short sleep duration in infancy and risk of childhood overweight. Arch Pediatr Adolesc Med 2008;162:305–11.
30. Tate EB, Woo W, Liao Y, et al. Do stressed mothers have heavier children? A meta-analysis on the relationship between maternal stress and child body mass index. Obes Rev 2015;16:351–61.
31. Andersen LG, Holst C, Michaelson KF, et al. Weight and weight gain during early infancy predict childhood obesity: a case-cohort study. Int J Obes 2012;36:1306–11.
32. Wien M, Biro FM. Childhood obesity and adult morbidities. Am J Clin Nutr 2010;91:1499S–505S.
33. Leddy MA, Power ML, Schulkin J. The impact of maternal obesity on maternal and fetal health. Rev Obstet Gynecol 2008;1:170–8.
34. Deputy NP, Sharma AJ, Kim SY. Gestational weight gain- United States, 2012 and 2013. MMWR Morb Mortal Wkly Rep 2015;64:1215–20.
35. Widen EM, Whyatt RM, Hoepner LA, et al. Excessive gestational weight gain is associated with long-term body fat and weight retention at 7 y postpartum in African American and Dominican mothers with underweight, normal, and overweight prepregnancy BMI. Am J Clin Nutr 2015;102:1460–7.
36. Davis SR, Castelo-Branco C, Chedraui P, et al. Understanding weight gain at menopause. Climacteric 2012;15:419–29.
37. Swinburn BA, Caterson I, Seidell JC, et al. Diet, nutrition and the prevention of excess weight gain and obesity. Public Health Nutr 2004;7:123–46.
38. Wilks DC, Besson H, Lindroos AK, et al. Objectively measured physical activity and obesity prevention in children, adolescents and adults: a systematic review of prospective studies. Obes Rev 2011;12:e119–29.
39. Dallman MF. Stress-induced obesity and the emotional nervous system. Trends Endocrinol Metab 2010;21:159–65.
40. Bose M, Olivan B, Laferrere B. Stress and obesity: the role of the hypothalamic-pituitary-adrenal axis in metabolic disease. Curr Opin Endocrinol Diabetes Obes 2009;16:340–6.
41. Beccuti G, Pannain S. Sleep and obesity. Curr Opin Clin Nutr Metab Care 2011;14:402–12.
42. Froy O. Metabolism and circadian rhythms: implications for obesity. Endocr Rev 2010;31:1–24.
43. Obici S, Rossetti L. Minireview: nutrient sensing and the regulation of insulin action and energy balance. Endocrinology 2003;144:5172–8.
44. Woods SC, D'Alessio DA, Tso P, et al. Consumption of a high-fat diet alters the homeostatic regulation of energy balance. Physiol Behav 2004;83:573–8.
45. Smith E, Hay P, Campbell L, et al. A review of the association between obesity and cognitive function across the lifespan: implications for novel approaches to prevention and treatment. Obes Rev 2011;9:740–55.
46. Brooks SJ, Cedernaes J, Schioth HB. Increased prefrontal and parahippocampal activation with reduced dorsolateral prefrontal and insular cortex activation to food images in obesity: a meta-analysis of fMRI studies. PLoS One 2013;8:e60393.
47. Butryn ML, Webb V, Wadden TA. Behavioral treatment of obesity. Psychiatr Clin North Am 2011;34:841–59.

48. Simon GE, Von Korff M, Saunders K, et al. Association between obesity and psychiatric disorders in the US adult population. Arch Gen Psychiatry 2006; 63:824–30.

49. Stunkard AJ, Allison KC. Two forms of disordered eating in obesity: binge eating and night eating. Int J Obes 2003;27:1–12.

50. Danese A, Tan M. Childhood maltreatment and obesity: systematic review and meta-analysis. Mol Psychiatry 2014;19:544–54.

51. Nousen EK, Franco JG, Sullivan EL. Unraveling the mechanisms responsible for the comorbidity between metabolic syndrome and mental health disorders. Neuroendocrinology 2013;98:254–66.

52. White W, Elmore L, Luthin DR, et al. Psychotropic-induced weight gain: a review of management strategies. Consultant 2013;53:153–60.

53. Cheadle A, Schwartz PM, Rauzon S, et al. The Kaiser Permanente community health initiative: overview and evaluation design. Am J Public Health 2010; 100:2111–3.

54. Srivastava G, Guanaga DP, Kaplan LM. Underrecognition and underreporting of obesity by medical residents. 761-P. Poster Presented at the Obesity Society 30th Annual Scientific Meeting. San Antonio (TX), September 20–24, 2012.

55. Bardia A, Holtan SG, Slezak JM, et al. Diagnosis of obesity by primary care physicians and impact on obesity management. Mayo Clin Proc 2007;82: 927–32.

56. World Health Organization (WHO). Physical status: the use and interpretation of anthropometry: report of a WHO Expert Committee: WHO Technical Report Series 854. Geneva (Switzerland): 1995. Available at: http://whqlibdoc.who.int/trs/WHO_TRS_854.pdf Accessed January 18, 2016.

57. Cornier MA, Depres JP, Davis N, et al. Assessing adiposity: a scientific statement from the American Heart Association. Circulation 2011;124:1996–2019.

58. Rasmussen KM, Yaktine AL, Institute of Medicine (Committee to Reexamine IOM Pregnancy Weight Guidelines, Food and Nutrition Board and Board on Children, Youth, and Families). Weight gain during pregnancy: reexamining the guidelines. Washington, DC: National Academy Press; 2009.

59. Carreno CA, Clifton RG, Hauth JC, et al. Excessive early gestational weight gain and risk of gestational diabetes mellitus in nulliparous women. Obstet Gynecol 2012;119:1227–33.

60. Overcash RT, Hull AD, Moore TR, et al. Early second trimester weight gain in obese women predicts excessive gestational weight gain in pregnancy. Matern Child Health J 2015;19:2412–8.

61. Knabl J, Riedel C, Gmach J, et al. Prediction of excessive gestational weight gain from week-specific cutoff values: A cohort study. J Perinatol 2014;34: 351–6.

62. Silk AW, McTigue KM. Reexamining the physical examination for obese patients. JAMA 2011;305:193–4.

63. Butsch WS. Evaluation of overweight and obesity. In: Gorrol AH, Mulley AG, editors. Primary care medicine. 7th edition. New York: Lippincott Williams & Wilkins; 2014. p. 57–64.

64. Leslie WS, Hankey CR, Lean MEJ. Weight gain as an adverse effect of some commonly prescribed drugs: a systematic review. QJM 2007;100:395–404.

65. Moore TJ, Conlin PR, Ard J, et al. DASH (dietary approaches to stop hypertension) diet is effective treatment for stage 1 isolated systolic hypertension. Hypertension 2001;38:155–8.

66. Brand-Miller J, Hayne S, Petocz P, et al. Low-glycemic index diets in the management of diabetes: a meta-analysis of randomized controlled trials. Diabetes Care 2003;26:2261–7.
67. Dansinger ML, Tatsioni A, Wong JB, et al. Meta-analysis: the effect of dietary counseling for weight loss. Ann Intern Med 2007;147:41–50.
68. Franz MJ, VanWormer JJ, Crain AL, et al. Weight-loss outcomes: a systematic review and meta-analysis of weight-loss clinical trials with a minimum 1-year follow-up. J Am Diet Assoc 2007;107:1755–67.
69. Johnston BC, Kanters S, Bandayrel K, et al. Comparison of weight loss among named diet programs in overweight and obese adults: a meta-analysis. JAMA 2014;312:923–33.
70. Wadden T. Treatment of obesity by moderate and severe caloric restriction. Results of clinical research trials. Ann Intern Med 1993;119:688–93.
71. Leibel RL, Rosenbaum M, Hirsch J. Changes in energy expenditure resulting from altered body weight. N Engl J Med 1995;332:621–8.
72. Sumithran P, Prendergast LA, Delbridge E, et al. Long-term persistence of hormonal adaptations to weight loss. N Engl J Med 2011;365:1597–604.
73. Leptin in human energy and neuroendocrine homeostasis. Clinical Trials.gov Web site. Available at: https://clinicaltrials.gov/ct2/show/NCT00265980?term=leibel&rank=3. Accessed January 18, 2016.
74. Levin BE. Metabolic sensing neurons and the control of energy homeostasis. Physiol Behav 2006;89:486–9.
75. Dansinger ML, Gleason JA, Griffith JL, et al. Comparison of the Atkins, Ornish, Weight Watchers, and Zone diets for weight loss and heart disease risk reduction. JAMA 2005;293:43–53.
76. Zeevi D, Korem T, Zmora N, et al. Personalized nutrition by prediction of glycemic responses. Cell 2015;163:1079–94.
77. King NA, Hopkins M, Caudwell P, et al. Individual variability following 12 weeks of supervised exercise: identification and characterization of compensation for exercise-induced weight loss. Int J Obes 2008;32:177–84.
78. Bouchard C, Rankinen T. Individual differences in response to regular physical activity. Med Sci Sports Exerc 2001;33(6 Suppl):S446–51.
79. Johanssen DL, Knuth ND, Huizenga R, et al. Metabolic slowing with massive weight loss despite preservation of fat-free mass. J Clin Endocrinol Metab 2012;97:2489–96.
80. Speakman JR, Selman C. Physical activity and resting metabolic rate. Proc Nutr Soc 2003;62:621–34.
81. Pederson BK, Febbraio MA. Muscles, exercise and obesity: skeletal muscle as a secretory organ. Nat Rev Endocrinol 2012;8:457–65.
82. Anderson JW, Konz EC, Frederich RC, et al. Long-term weight-loss maintenance: a meta-analysis of US studies. Am J Clin Nutr 2001;74:579–84.
83. Stiegler P, Cunliffe A. The role of diet and exercise for the maintenance of fat-free mass and resting metabolic rate during weight loss. Sports Med 2006;36:239–62.
84. Warburton DE, Nicol CW, Bredin SS. Health benefits of physical activity: the evidence. CMAJ 2006;174:801–9.
85. Thorogood A, Mottillo S, Shimony A, et al. Isolated aerobic exercise and weight loss: a systematic review and meta-analysis of randomized controlled trials. Am J Med 2011;124:747–55.

86. Williams MA, Haskell WL, Ades PA, et al. Resistance exercise in individuals with and without cardiovascular disease: 2007 update. Circulation 2007;116:572–84.
87. Asikainen TM, Kukkonen-Harjula K, Miilunpalo S. Exercise for health for early postmenopausal women: a systematic review of randomized controlled trials. Sports Med 2004;34:753–78.
88. Donnelly JE, Blair SN, Jakicic JM, et al. American College of Sports Medicine Position Stand. Appropriate physical activity intervention strategies for weight loss and prevention of weight regain for adults. Med Sci Sports Exerc 2009; 41:459–71.
89. Vorona RD, Winn MP, Babineau TW, et al. Overweight and obese patients in a primary care population report less sleep than patients with a normal body mass index. Arch Intern Med 2005;165:25–30.
90. Morgenthaler T, Kramer M, Alessi C, et al. Practice parameters for the psychological and behavioral treatment of insomnia: an update. An American Academy of Sleep Medicine Report. Sleep 2006;29:1415–9.
91. Apovian CM, Aronne LJ, Bessesen DH, et al. Pharmacological management of obesity: an Endocrine Society Clinical Practice Guideline. J Clin Endocrinol Metab 2015;100:342–62.
92. Ferracioli-Oda E, Qawasmi A, Bloch MH. Meta-analysis: melatonin for the treatment of primary sleep disorders. PLoS One 2013;8:e63773.
93. Barlow DH, Lehrer PM, Woolfolk RL, et al. Principles and practice of stress management. New York: Guilford Press; 2007.
94. Astrup A, Rössner S, Van Gaal L, et al. Effects of liraglutide in the treatment of obesity: a randomized, double-blind, placebo-controlled study. Lancet 2009; 374:1606–16.
95. Gadde KM, Allison DB, Ryan DH, et al. Effects of low-dose, controlled-release, phentermine plus topiramate combination on weight and associated comorbidities in overweight and obese adults (CONQUER): a randomized, placebo-controlled, phase 3 trial. Lancet 2011;377:1341–52.
96. Smith SR, Prosser WA, Donahue DJ, et al. Lorcaserin (ADP356), a selective 5-HT$_{2C}$ agonist, reduces body weight in obese men and women. Obesity 2009;17:494–503.
97. Buchwald H, Avidor Y, Braunwald E, et al. Bariatric surgery: a systematic review and meta-analysis. JAMA 2004;292:1724–37.
98. Mechanick JI, Youdim A, Jones DB, et al. Clinical practice guidelines for the perioperative nutritional, metabolic, and nonsurgical support of the bariatric surgery patient–2013 update: cosponsored by American Association of Clinical Endocrinologists, the Obesity Society, and American Society for Metabolic & Bariatric Surgery. Endocr Pract 2013;19:337–72.
99. Stefater MA, Wilson-Pérez HE, Chambers AP, et al. All bariatric surgeries are not created equal: insights from mechanistic comparisons. Endocr Rev 2012;33: 595–622.
100. Maggard MA, Yermilov I, Li Z, et al. Pregnancy and fertility following bariatric surgery: a systematic review. JAMA 2008;300:2286–96.
101. Guenard F, Deshaies Y, Cianflone K, et al. Differential methylation in glucoregulatory genes of offspring born before vs. after maternal gastrointestinal bypass surgery. Proc Natl Acad Sci U S A 2013;110:11439–44.
102. Obesity treatment devices. US Food and Drug Administration Web site. Available at: http://www.fda.gov/MedicalDevices/ProductsandMedicalProcedures/ ObesityDevices/ucm20036251.htm. Accessed December 15, 2015.

103. Mechanick JI, Youdim A, Jones DB, et al. Clinical Practice Guidelines for the Perioperative Nutritional, Metabolic, and Nonsurgical Support of the Bariatric Surgery Patient—2013 Update: Cosponsored by American Association of Clinical Endocrinologists, The Obesity Society, and American Society for Metabolic & Bariatric Surgery. Obesity (Silver Spring, Md.) 2013;21(1):S1–27. PMC. Web. 22 Mar. 2016.

Evaluation and Management of Behavioral Health Disorders in Women

An Overview of Major Depression, Bipolar Disorder, Anxiety Disorders, and Sleep in the Primary Care Setting

Elizabeth Fitelson, MD*, Cheryl McGibbon, MD

KEYWORDS

- Depression • Women • Behavioral health • Reproductive • Mental health
- Bipolar disorder • Anxiety disorders • Sleep disorders

KEY POINTS

- Women are twice as likely to develop anxiety, depressive, and insomnia disorders as men, and presentation or exacerbation often correlate with times of hormonal change.
- Evaluation of women with behavioral health concerns should include a medical and psychiatric history as well as screening for substance use, domestic violence, and suicide risk.
- Clinicians treating behavioral health problems in women in primary care or obstetric/gynecologic (OB/GYN) settings should be familiar with the range of both nonpharmacologic and pharmacologic treatment options and gear treatment according to patients' goals, comorbidities, and medication profiles.
- Perinatal women may be particularly vulnerable to mood, anxiety, and insomnia disorders. Decisions about pharmacologic management should be made by carefully weighing the risks faced by a patient and her family related to the psychiatric illness with the known risks of available treatments.

INTRODUCTION

Mental health disorders, such as depression and anxiety, are nearly twice as common in women compared with men.[1,2] The etiology of this gender gap in risk for anxiety and depressive disorders is likely multifactorial, including biologic

Disclosure Statement: The authors have nothing to disclose.
The Women's Program, Columbia University Department of Psychiatry, 710 West 168th Street, 12th Floor, New York, NY 10032, USA
* Corresponding author.
E-mail address: eem36@cumc.columbia.edu

vulnerability, socioeconomic status, conflict in women's roles as providers and caregivers, and risk for trauma and gender-based violence. Increasingly, research is pointing to an important role for female sex hormones in the regulation of affect, anxiety, cognition, and sleep,[3,4] with clinically relevant consequences for women through the reproductive life cycle. Risk for episodes of affective disorders is higher in women at times of hormonal transition, such as at menarche,[5] childbirth,[6] and perimenopause.[7]

Providers of OB/GYN care are often the most commonly seen medical providers for adult women, providing both primary and reproductive care.[8] Even in places where psychiatric care is readily available, obstetric and gynecologic are frequently the front line for recognition, education, and initial management of many mental health problems. In settings where psychiatric treatment is a more scarce resource, obstetricians/gynecologists often are responsible for ongoing treatment of these disorders as well. This review focuses on the impact of the female reproductive life cycle on the presentation and management of some of the most common behavioral health problems in women: major depression, bipolar disorder (BD), anxiety disorders and primary sleep disorders.

ASSESSMENT AND DIFFERENTIAL DIAGNOSIS

Assessment of women presenting with psychiatric symptoms should include a history of prior episodes and treatment, medical and reproductive history, social supports and stressors, comorbidities, and a risk assessment:

- Psychiatric differential diagnosis: affective or sleep dysregulation may occur in adjustment disorders (after a significant life stressor), bereavement, posttraumatic stress disorder (PTSD), personality disorders, dysthymia, and premenstrual dysphoric disorder.[9]
- Substance use: screening for substance use disorders is essential, because they are highly comorbid with psychiatric illness, increase risk for suicide, and predict poorer response to treatment if the substance issues are not addressed. Women with mood and anxiety disorders are more likely to use substances, including during pregnancy and lactation.[10]
- General medical conditions: many behavioral health problems can be early manifestations of, or comorbid with, several medical conditions, including Cushing syndrome, thyroid disorders, hyperparathyroidism, malignancies, cardiac disease, diabetes, stroke, kidney disease, anemia, Wilson disease, and AIDS.[11] Based on presentation, work-up should include laboratory or other diagnostic evaluation to rule out these disorders.
- Prescription medications: many medications can cause psychiatric symptoms and insomnia, including steroids, anticholinergics, antihistamines, benzodiazepines, and anticonvulsants, among others.[9]
- Interpersonal violence (IPV) and trauma: women with depression, anxiety, or PTSD are 3 to 7 times more likely to have been victims of IPV in the past year or in their lifetimes.[12] Recent IPV is strongly correlated with new onset of psychiatric disorders.[13]
- Suicide risk assessment: suicide is a leading cause of death in women ages 15 to 44[14] as well as a leading cause of maternal mortality.[15] Patients should be asked about suicidal thoughts and other risk factors for suicide. Comorbid anxiety, agitation, sleep problems, poor concentration, hopelessness, social isolation, and excessive or increasing use of alcohol or drugs are modifiable warning signs that merit increased concern.[16]

MAJOR DEPRESSIVE DISORDER

The lifetime prevalence of depression in women is more than 20%,[17] and depression is the most common psychiatric disorder encountered by obstetricians/gynecologists.[18] A diagnosis of major depression requires low mood or loss of interest as well as at least 4 other neurovegetative symptoms to be present for 2 weeks or more, causing significant loss of function. Anxiety may be prominent, and severe depression can cause psychotic symptoms, such as hallucinations, delusions of guilt or worthlessness, and paranoia. Many women with depression in OB/GYN settings present with a primarily somatic complaint, leading to a high rate of missed diagnosis. Only 20% to 40% of depression cases were identified by obstetricians/gynecologists in clinical practice in several studies.[19]

Depression screening measures are often recommended in primary care or OB/GYN settings. Unless screening is matched with enhanced access to appropriate treatment, however, screening alone does not improve outcomes for patients. Commonly used screening measures include:[20]

- Patient Health Questionnaires, 9-question (PHQ-9) and 2-question (PHQ-2) versions: most used in primary care, but they have been validated in perinatal patients in some studies.
- Edinburgh Postnatal Depression Scale: often recommended for obstetric patients, because it does not emphasize somatic symptoms that are often normal in the perinatal period.

Nonpharmacologic Treatments

Psychotherapy

Recommended as a first-line treatment of mild to moderate major depression and usually in combination with medications for moderate to severe depression.[21] Cognitive behavioral therapy (CBT): an evidence-based structured treatment of depression, teaches patients to challenge distorted thoughts and modify unhelpful behaviors. Interpersonal psychotherapy: a time-limited psychotherapy, focuses on disruptions in important relationships that occur in depression. Other psychotherapies of potential benefit in depression include problem-solving therapy, behavioral activation therapy, and psychodynamic psychotherapy.[9]

Other nonpharmacologic treatments

- Electroconvulsive therapy: recommended for severe depression when there has been an inadequate response to medications and psychotherapy or when a patient displays psychotic features, catatonia, or severe suicidality.
- Bright light therapy: effective for both seasonal and nonseasonal depression with appropriate light and timing.[22]
- Transcranial magnetic stimulation is a newer technique of brain stimulation with efficacy in depression.
- Exercise
- Dietary changes
- Relaxation techniques[23]

Pharmacotherapy

First-line medications for depression include

- Selective serotonin reuptake inhibitors (SSRIs): fluoxetine, sertraline, citalopram, escitalopram, paroxetine

- Serotonin-norepinephrine reuptake inhibitors (SNRIs)
- Bupropion
- Mirtazapine

These medications have similar efficacy, with a 60% to 70% response rate. Side effects differ between agents and classes and help guide treatment choice. For example, bupropion may worsen comorbid anxiety or agitation, whereas weight gain is a significant side effect of mirtazapine, potentially limiting its utility in women with concerns about weight.[24] Most patients start to feel relief of symptoms within 2 to 4 weeks, although the full benefit of medication may take as long as 10 weeks. Most experts recommend tracking symptoms with a standardized assessment (the PHQ-9 can be used for this purpose), and it is important to dose adequately if symptoms persist.[9]

Major Depression and the Female Reproductive Life Cycle

Menstrual cycle

Approximately two-thirds of menstruating women with depression experience premenstrual worsening of symptoms.[25] Between 2% and 5% of women meet criteria for premenstrual dysphoric disorder (PMDD), a severe form of premenstrual syndrome that has significant adverse effects on functioning. Treatment of severe premenstrual syndrome or PMDD includes

- SSRIs: continuous or luteal phase dosing
- Hormonal contraceptives: drospirenone/ethinyl estradiol combination pill is the best studied. Risks of oral hormones should be considered.
- Exercise
- CBT
- Vitamin supplements: calcium, magnesium
- Herbal medicine: vitex agnus-castus[26]

Perinatal

Between 10% and 15% of women experience depression during or after pregnancy. Women with a history of major depression, in particular those with more than 1 prior episode, remain at risk for relapse during pregnancy. In a study by Cohen[27] among women who had previously been stable on an antidepressant, those who stopped the medication for pregnancy had a 68% relapse rate during pregnancy compared with 26% of those who remained on antidepressants. Depression (and other mental illness) in the perinatal period carries significant risks for the mother, the fetus, the future child, and the family. Studying the effects of antidepressant treatment in pregnancy is complicated by the reliance on observational data, which are subject to important confounders, such as rates of depression and anxiety, adherence to prenatal care, use of substances, nutrition, and psychosocial stressors. A full discussion of the risks and benefits of prescribing psychotropic medication in pregnancy and lactation is beyond the scope of this review, but important resources for clinicians evaluating and treating pregnant women with psychiatric symptoms includes American College of Obstetricians and Gynecologists guidelines[28,29] as well as several online information sources and databases (**Box 1**).

Menopause and perimenopause

The hormonal fluctuations of perimenopause seem to trigger an increased risk for depression, even among women with no prior history of major depression. Women with a history of premenstrual mood worsening or postpartum depression may be at particular risk. In postmenopausal women, the risk for first-episode depression

> **Box 1**
> **Online resources for information about perinatal mental health disorders and medications in pregnancy and lactation**
>
> - MedEdPPD: www.mededppd.org
>   National Institute of Mental Health–funded, Web-based education for perinatal depression
> - Postpartum Support International: www.postpartum.net
> - Massachusetts General Hospital Center for Women's Mental Health www.womensmentalhealth.org
> - Reprotox: www.reprotox.org
> - Teratogen Information System (TERIS) http://depts.washington.edu/terisweb/teris/index.html
> - LactMed: http://toxnet.nlm.nih.gov/newtoxnet/lactmed.htm
> - Developmental and Reproductive Toxicology Database (DART) http://toxnet.nlm.nih.gov/newtoxnet/dart.htm
> - Motherisk: www.motherisk.org
> - MotherToBaby www.mothertobaby.org

decreases.[30] First-line treatments are generally considered SSRIs or SNRIs, although SNRIs may have more effect on vasomotor symptoms. Hormone therapy has not consistently been found to alleviate depression, but it may be beneficial as an augmenting agent for perimenopausal women.[31]

BIPOLAR DISORDER

BD is a chronic, episodic mood disorder consisting of periods of major depression, periods of euthymia, and periods of mania (in BD I disorder) or hypomania (in BD II). It is associated with high rates of psychosocial morbidity, psychiatric and medical comorbidity, and mortality.[32] Patients with bipolar illness are more likely to present with depressive symptoms than mania or hypomania. In primary care settings, up to 9% of patients presenting with depression or other psychiatric complaints meet criteria for BD.[33]

Women in particular have predominantly depressive symptoms and are more vulnerable to mixed states, with both manic and depressive symptoms present at the same time.[34] Because antidepressants can precipitate mania and mood cycling in patients with bipolar susceptibility, it is important to screen women presenting with depression for a personal and family histories of manic or hypomanic symptoms prior to initiating treatment with antidepressants. Screening tools, such as the Mood Disorder Questionnaire, can be helpful in identifying women at risk of bipolar mood cycling.[35]

Common medical comorbidities in women include obesity, migraine headaches, hypertension, hyperlipidemia, asthma, thyroid disease, and type 2 diabetes mellitus. There are also high rates of psychiatric comorbidity, in particular substance use disorders and anxiety disorders.[36]

Nonpharmacologic Treatments

Psychosocial treatments are increasingly recognized as important for achieving and maintaining remission in BD, usually as adjuncts to pharmacologic or other somatic treatments.

Psychotherapy

- Psychoeducation about the importance of monitoring mood, regular sleep-wake cycles, medication adherence, and management of stress.[37]
- Interpersonal and social rhythm therapy
- CBT
- Family-focused therapy

Other nonpharmacologic treatments

- Electroconvulsive therapy: effective in both depressive and manic phases of BD, can be used safely with adequate precautions in pregnancy[38]
- Bright light therapy: effective for bipolar depression but risk of switching to a manic or mixed state[39]

Pharmacotherapy for bipolar disorder

The mainstay of pharmacologic treatment of BD is mood stabilization with lithium, anticonvulsant medications, and/or second-generation antipsychotic agents.[37] These mood-stabilizing medications carry risks for adverse effects, medication interactions, and side effects, and patients require ongoing monitoring.[22] **Table 1** lists the major classes of mood stabilizers and some of the most common monitoring and safety issues in women.

Bipolar Disorder and the Female Reproductive Life Cycle

Menstrual cycle

Although many women note increased symptoms at different phases of the menstrual cycle, there is no one consistent pattern of mood shifts with the menstrual cycle in BD. There are higher rates of menstrual cycle irregularity in women with BD compared with women with unipolar depression.[40] Some medications also interfere with fertility and menstruation: valproate is associated with an increased risk of polycystic ovarian syndrome, and antipsychotic agents may cause elevated prolactin levels.[34]

Women with BD are at higher risk for unintended pregnancy.[41] Given this risk, it is particularly important for clinicians to discuss appropriate contraception as well as the potential risks of a patient's medications in pregnancy. Many mood-stabilizing medications have significant interactions with hormonal contraceptive agents, which can result in either contraceptive failure or breakthrough psychiatric symptoms (see **Table 1**).

Perinatal

Women with BD remain at risk for relapse during pregnancy. In 1 study, 50% of previously stable women who stopped lithium treatment of pregnancy relapsed to a mood episode during the course of pregnancy, similar to nonpregnant women who stopped lithium; risk was highest in women with more prior mood episodes and with rapid discontinuation of medication.[42] Maintaining mood stabilizers during pregnancy seems to protect against relapse.[43] Mood-stabilizing medication, however, alone or in combination with other medications, confers some risk of adverse fetal and pregnancy outcomes (see **Table 1**). Given the potential for severe morbidity with mood relapse in bipolar illness as well as the adverse effects of psychiatric illness on outcomes for the pregnancy, the child, and the mother, it is particularly important to carefully weigh the risks of medications in pregnancy with the risks of undertreatment on an individual basis.[28]

The postpartum period is a time of particular risk for bipolar women. Even in women who are able to maintain euthymic mood through pregnancy, the risk of relapse is

Table 1
Safety and monitoring of major mood stabilizers

Medication	Interaction with Hormonal Contraception	Maintenance Monitoring	Pregnancy	Other Considerations
Lithium	None known	• Serum level q 3-6 mo • Thyroid function q 6 mo • Renal function q 6 mo	• Cardiac defects (0.05%–0.1%) • Polyhydramnios • Fetal nephrogenic diabetes insipidus • Preterm birth • Transient hypothyroidism • Decreased muscle tone in neonate • Decreased serum levels 2nd and 3rd trimesters	• Narrow therapeutic index • Potential interactions with diuretics, ACE-inhibitors, NSAIDs
Valproate	HC decreases VPA levels 30%	Serum level, CBC, LFTs q 6 mo	• NTD (3%–5%) • Craniofacial anomalies • IUGR • Neonatal hypoglycemia • Neurodevelopmental effects (decreased IQ)	• Increased risk of polycystic ovarian syndrome • Not first line for women at risk of unintended pregnancy
Lamotrigine	• HC decreases LMG levels 50% (not when coadministered with VPA) • Slight decrease of progesterone, of uncertain clinical significance	—	Decreased serum levels 2nd and 3rd trimesters	• In sensitive women, some recommend decrease of 25%–50% LMG dose during placebo HC • Risk of serious rash (Stevens-Johnson syndrome) 0.3%
Carbemazepine/ oxcarbazepine	Decrease in HC efficacy	CBC, LFT, electrolytes q 3 mo	• NTD 1% • Craniofacial anomalies • Vitamin K deficiency in neonate	Use alternate form of contraception Multiple drug interactions
Second-generation antipsychotic agents: risperidone, olanzapine, quetiapine, aripirazole	—	• Fasting blood glucose • BMI • Lipid profile	• Neonatal EPS (FDA warning) • Maternal BMI, possible increased risk for GDM • Possible LBW, PTB	• Risk of weight gain and metabolic dysregulation • Elevation of prolactin (especially risperidone)

Abbreviations: ACE, angiotensin-converting enzyme; BMI, body mass index; CBC, complete blood cell count; EPS, extrapyramidal sign; FDA, Food and Drug Administration; GDM, gestational diabetes mellitus; HC, hormonal contraception; IUGR, inrauterine growth restriction; LBW, low birth weight; LFT, liver function test; LMG, lamotrigine; NSAID, nonsteroidal anti-inflammatory drug; NTD, neural tube defect; PTB, preterm birth; VPA, valproate.
   Data from Refs.[22,81–85]

significantly elevated in the first 3 months postpartum.[42] This elevation in risk may result from a combination of the dramatic hormonal shifts at parturition, sleep deprivation (which is particularly destabilizing for individuals with BD), and the psychological effects of motherhood on the patient and family system.[44] Women presenting with a first episode of major depression in the immediate postpartum period are more likely than women presenting with depression at other times to eventually meet criteria for a bipolar diagnosis.[45] Mood-stabilizing medications have variable levels in breast milk (see the link for LactMed in **Box 1**). Significant consideration should be given to the importance of sleep in maintaining mood stability in postpartum women with bipolar illness; in some cases, women may choose not to breastfeed or to supplement with formula both to reduce the infant's exposure to medications as well as to optimize sleep.[34] Social and family support are particularly important for women with BD in the postpartum period.

Women with a prior diagnosis of BD have a significantly elevated risk of experiencing postpartum psychosis (PP): although the rate of PP is 1 to 2 per 1000 live births in the general population, for women with BD the risk is as high as 20%.[44] PP is a severe manifestation of postpartum affective illness and is considered a psychiatric emergency because it is associated with significantly elevated rates of suicide and infanticide.[46] PP is typically described as having a waxing and waning course, often with delirium-like confusion in addition to symptoms of paranoia, ideas of reference, hallucinations, and other psychotic symptoms. Any woman manifesting new-onset psychotic symptoms in the postpartum period should be evaluated immediately in a monitored setting and organic causes of postpartum delirium ruled out.[44]

Menopause and perimenopause

Few data are available about the course of BD in perimenopause and menopause. Women with BD are likely to be at higher risk for mood instability through the hormonal fluctuations of perimenopause, particularly if they have demonstrated mood sensitivity at other times of hormonal change. One study found higher rates of depressive symptoms in women with BD in late perimenopause and early menopause compared with reproductive age women, although no clear correlation with hormone status was found.[47]

ANXIETY DISORDERS

The broad category of anxiety disorders encompasses several diagnoses, including generalized anxiety disorder (GAD), panic disorder, social phobia, specific phobia, obsessive-compulsive disorder (OCD), PTSD, and body dysmorphic disorder. One of 4 Americans fulfills diagnostic criteria for at least 1 anxiety disorder in their lifetime.[1] Women are at increased risk for anxiety disorders and twice as likely to have GAD as men.[48] GAD and panic disorder are two of the most commonly seen anxiety disorders in primary care settings.

Generalized Anxiety Disorder

GAD is defined as the excessive and uncontrollable worry and anxiety about everyday life situations, accompanied by physical complaints, such as fatigue, muscle tension, irritable mood, and restlessness. Lifetime prevalence of GAD ranges from 6% to 9%, and it has a chronic, waxing and waning course. GAD is highly comorbid with other psychiatric and medical conditions; up to 90% of patients with GAD also have another lifetime psychiatric condition, in particular depression.[1] Because anxiety has many associated physical symptoms, many patients have high rates of doctor visits, emergency room visits, hospitalizations, and diagnostic tests.[49]

Panic Disorder

The core feature of panic disorder is recurrent, unexpected attacks of fear or discomfort with subsequent worry about when the next attack will occur. Like GAD, panic disorder is a chronic condition with a waxing and waning course. Prevalence rates in the general population are estimated to be up to 22%.[1,50] Common medical or physical conditions that mimic panic include cardiovascular (arrhythmia, tachycardia, and myocardial infarction), respiratory (bronchitis, asthma, chronic obstructive pulmonary disease, and pulmonary embolism), endocrine (hyperthyroidism, hypoglycemia, and pheochromocytoma), and drug related (benzodiazepine withdrawal, alcohol withdrawal, and excessive caffeine).[51]

Evaluation and Management

Assessment of complaints of anxiety should include physical and laboratory testing as well as questions about current use of prescription and over-the-counter medications, caffeine, alcohol, and illicit drugs. Commonly used, validated screening tools include the Hamilton Anxiety Rating Scale[52] and the Beck Anxiety Inventory.[53]

Nonpharmacologic Treatment

- CBT: equally or more effective than medication treatment of many anxiety disorders[54]
- Mindfulness-based stress reduction
- Exercise
- Yoga
- Biofeedback
- Meditation

Pharmacotherapy for Anxiety Disorders

Davidson and colleagues[55] have proposed a useful algorithm flowchart for treatment of GAD. It is recommended that medication be continued for GAD or panic at least 1 year because early discontinuation is associated with higher relapse rates.

- SSRIs and SNRIs[55]: first-line treatment. Side effects include increased activation at initiation.
- Benzodiazepines: first-line treatment when anxiety is of short duration, for acute relief of panic or somatic symptoms and anxiety-related sleep disruption or to mitigate side effects of agitation with antidepressant initiation.[56] Risks include dependency, tolerance, and long-term effects on cognition and memory.
- Tricyclic antidepressants: effective for both panic disorder and GAD; side effects limit use.
- Buspirone: some effect for GAD, no demonstrated benefit for panic disorder.
- Other medications: quetiapine, pregabalin, and hydroxazine have shown some benefit for anxiety, but safety and effectiveness data are limited relative to first-line therapies.[54]

Anxiety Disorders and the Female Reproductive Life Cycle

Menstrual cycle

Anxiety disorders can be exacerbated during the late luteal phase, and premenstrual worsening of symptoms has been shown in various retrospective and prospective studies in women with GAD, panic disorder, OCD, or social anxiety.[57]

Perinatal

Rates of anxiety are high in pregnant women.[58] Anxiety symptoms during pregnancy may be associated with perinatal complications, premature rupture of membranes, preeclampsia, caesarian section, and fetal complications.[59] The presence of an antenatal anxiety disorder is predictive of postpartum depression.[58] New mothers may be acutely vulnerable to anxiety disorders; panic disorder and OCD can be exacerbated or emergent during the postpartum period.[60] The development of PTSD in women with traumatic deliveries occurs in 2% to 6% of women.[61] Currently, the safety of benzodiazepines during pregnancy remains controversial in light of conflicting results regarding their teratogenicity. A recent review of the topic concludes that benzodiazepines do not seem overall to significantly increase rates of malformations, but the studies are limited and benzodiazepines should be used with caution, for the briefest time period possible.[62]

Menopause and perimenopause

Many symptoms of menopause are similar to those of anxiety (ie, rapid onset of physical symptoms, fatigue, and sleep disturbance) and can make distinguishing between the two difficult.[63] SSRIs are effective in improving vasomotor symptoms of menopause and remain first-line treatment of women with anxiety disorders in perimenopause.

SLEEP DISORDERS

Disturbed sleep affects all areas of life and can impair work performance, pose safety risks, and be detrimental for interpersonal relationships, mood, anxiety, and overall quality of life. The complaint of poor sleep may be the result of a broad range of primary sleep disorders or medical or psychiatric conditions. Sleep concerns fall into 3 broad categories: (1) insomnia; (2) abnormal movement, behaviors, or sensations during sleep or during nocturnal awakenings; and (3) excessive daytime sleepiness. This section focuses on the most common sleep disorder: insomnia.

The prevalence of insomnia disorder among the adult population is estimated to be 6%, with 12% reporting insomnia symptoms with daytime impairment and an additional 15% reporting dissatisfaction with their sleep.[64] Women are estimated to be twice as likely as men to develop insomnia, with a predominance of symptoms presenting during the menstrual cycle, pregnancy, and menopause. The reason for this difference is not well understood but may involve differences in sex steroids as well as the higher incidence of depression and anxiety disorders in women.[65] The course of insomnia is often chronic, with high rates of relapse after treatment.

Risk factors for insomnia include age; female gender; comorbid medical, psychiatric, and substance abuse disorders; shift work; unemployment; and low socioeconomic status. Common medical conditions that can cause insomnia include sleep-disordered breathing, heart failure, diabetes, chronic obstructive pulmonary disease, and gastroesophageal reflux. Patients with pain and psychiatric conditions have insomnia rates estimated as high as 50% to 75%.[64,66–68]

Evaluation and Management

A thorough evaluation of sleep problems should focus on specific insomnia complaints, presleep conditions, sleep-wake patterns, and daytime consequences as well as medical and psychiatric history. Standardized questionnaires, such as the Epworth Sleepiness Scale, help establish a baseline level of symptoms and monitor for changes during treatment. The American Academy of Sleep Medicine guidelines suggest that patients keep a log for a minimum of 2 weeks prior to and during treatment.[68] Polysomnography may be indicated when breathing or movement disorders are suspected.

Goals of treatment include improving sleep quality and quantity and minimizing daytime related impairments. It is essential to treat comorbid medical and psychiatric conditions.

Nonpharmacologic Interventions

Behavioral approaches for insomnia have been shown as effective as medication treatment, to provide greater protection from relapse long term, and to be free from problematic medication side effects.[69,70] Sleep hygiene education is helpful but rarely adequate for treatment of more severe and chronic insomnia.[71] **Table 2** is an overview of behavioral approaches for insomnia.

Pharmacologic Treatments

In selecting medication treatment of insomnia, the American Academy of Sleep Medicine recommends considering symptom patterns, treatment goals, past treatment responses, patient preference, cost, availability of other treatments, comorbid conditions, contraindications, concurrent medication interactions, and side effects to help guide choice of agent.[68] **Table 3** summarizes the major pharmacologic treatment of insomnia. Additionally, a recent review article on insomnia was also published in the *New England Journal of Medicine* in October 2015[72] and is a helpful resource for clinical management.

Insomnia and the Female Reproductive Life Cycle

Menstrual cycle

There have been inconsistent results in studies looking at the relationship between the menstrual cycle and sleep difficulties despite subjective reports of insomnia or hypersomnia from women. Some studies have shown a higher incidence of sleep disruption related to premenstrual symptoms and PMDD, but consistent evidence is lacking.[73]

Perinatal

Prevalence rates for sleep disruptions in pregnancy range from 15% to 80% depending on criteria and trimester.[74] Seriously disrupted sleep during pregnancy is

Table 2	
Behavioral therapies for insomnia	
Treatment	**Description**
Stimulus control therapy	Instructions to reassociate the bed/bedroom with sleep and to establish a consistent sleep-wake schedule
Sleep restriction therapy	Method limits time in bed to the actual sleep time, consolidated and more efficient sleep
Relaxation training	Reduces somatic tension interfering with sleep
Cognitive therapy	Psychotherapy changing cognitions about sleep and insomnia and its consequences
Sleep hygiene education	Guidelines about the environment (light noise, and temperature) that may promote or disrupt sleep

Adapted from Kryger MH, Roth T, Dement WC, editors. Principles and practice of sleep medicine. 4th edition. Philadelphia: Saunders; 2005.

Table 3
Pharmacologic treatment of insomnia

Medication Class	Examples	Indication	Side Effects
Nonbenzodiazepine receptor agonists	• Zaleplon • Eszopiclone • Zolpidem	• First-line pharmacologic treatment • *May* have less tolerance and rebound than benzodiazepines	• Amnesia, • Hallucinations • Fugue states
Benzodiazepine receptor agonists	• Triazolam • Estazolam • Quazepam • Temazepam • Flurazepam	First-line pharmacologic treatment	• Dependence • Discontinuation syndrome • Cognitive side effects
Melatonin receptor agonist	Ramelteon	May be preferable to benzodiazepine receptor agonists, especially in patients with substance abuse	Dizziness
Sedating antidepressants	• Trazodone • Mirtazapine • Doxepin • Amitriptyline	• Second-line treatment • Most appropriate for patients with comorbid depression • Lower doses used for sleep	Various side effects according to medication class

associated with higher rates of caesarian delivery and increased risk of postpartum mood and anxiety disorders.[75] Most women report increased fatigue, daytime sleepiness, and night awakenings during the first trimester, with some relief and more daytime energy in the second trimester.[76] Sleep is typically poorest during the third trimester, largely due to physical discomfort, heartburn, and restless legs syndrome.[77] Rates of sleep apnea increase in the second half of pregnancy, related to weight gain, mucosal edema, and changes in respiratory physiology.[76] Because of a paucity of data, there is no recommended treatment algorithm for treatment of insomnia in pregnancy. When possible, nonpharmacological interventions should be tried first. A recent review of sleep medications in pregnancy, including benzodiazepines, did not find evidence of increased risk for congenital malformations, although there were possible effects on other pregnancy outcomes.[78] The investigators point out that the small number of studies prohibits any definitive conclusions about safety of these medications in pregnancy. Clinicians must weigh the available data against the risks of continued poor sleep, for example, in women at high risk for mood disorders in the perinatal period.

In the postpartum period women develop lower sleep efficiency, shorter latency to rapid-eye-movement sleep (characteristic of depression), and reduction in total sleep time. These are due not only to the demands of newborn nursing and care but also to a result of an abrupt drop in hormones and melatonin levels immediately after delivery. Postpartum sleep disturbance is linked to higher rates of mood disorders.[76]

Menopause and perimenopause
Disturbed sleep, night sweats, and daytime fatigue are common complaints of women during the menopausal transition and up to 60% of menopausal women complain of insomnia[74]; 50% of menopausal women with sleep complaints were found to have a primary sleep disorder, including sleep apnea, restless leg syndrome, or both.[79] Both

serotonergic medications and hormone therapy have been shown to be helpful for treatment of sleep and hot flashes.[80]

REFERENCES

1. Kessler RCR. Lifetime and 12-month prevalence of DSM-III-R psychiatric disorders in the United States. Results from the National Comorbidity Survey. Arch Gen Psychiatry 1994;51(1):8.
2. Centers for Disease Control and Prevention (CDC). Current depression among adults—United States, 2006 and 2008. MMWR Morb Mortal Wkly Rep 2010; 59(38):1229.
3. Wharton WW. Neurobiological underpinnings of the estrogen - mood relationship. Curr Psychiatry Rev 2012;8(3):247–56.
4. Gillies GE. Estrogen actions in the brain and the basis for differential action in men and women: a case for sex-specific medicines. Pharmacol Rev 2010; 62(2):155–98.
5. Joinson CC. Timing of menarche and depressive symptoms in adolescent girls from a UK cohort. Br J Psychiatry 2011;198(1):17–23.
6. Munk-Olsen TT. New parents and mental disorders: a population-based register study. JAMA 2006;296(21):2582.
7. Freeman EW. Associations of hormones and menopausal status with depressed mood in women with no history of depression. Arch Gen Psychiatry 2006;63(4):375.
8. Scholle SH. Trends in women's health services by type of physician seen: data from the 1985 and 1997-98 NAMCS. Womens Health Issues 2002;12(4):165.
9. Bentley SM. Major depression. Med Clin North Am 2014;98(5):981–1005.
10. McHugh RK. Epidemiology of substance use in reproductive-age women. Obstet Gynecol Clin North Am 2014;41(2):177–89.
11. Cosci FF. Mood and anxiety disorders as early manifestations of medical illness: a systematic review. Psychother Psychosom 2015;84(1):22–9.
12. Trevillion KK. Experiences of domestic violence and mental disorders: a systematic review and meta-analysis. PLoS One 2012;7(12):e51740.
13. Okuda MM. Mental health of victims of intimate partner violence: results from a national epidemiologic survey. Psychiatr Serv 2011;62(8):959.
14. Leading causes of death by age group, all females-United States, 2013. Available at: http://www.cdc.gov/women/lcod/2013/WomenAll_2013.pdf. Accessed September 26, 2015.
15. Kim JJ. Suicide risk among perinatal women who report thoughts of self-harm on depression screens. Obstet Gynecol 2015;125(4):885–93.
16. McDowell AK. Practical suicide-risk management for the busy primary care physician. Mayo Clin Proc 2011;86(8):792–800.
17. Kessler RC. Sex and depression in the national comorbidity survey. I: lifetime prevalence, chronicity and recurrence. J Affect Disord 1993;29(2–3):85.
18. Spitzer RL. Validity and utility of the PRIME-MD patient health questionnaire in assessment of 3000 obstetric-gynecologic patients: the PRIME-MD Patient Health Questionnaire Obstetrics-Gynecology Study. Am J Obstet Gynecol 2000;183(3):759.
19. Cerimele JM. Presenting symptoms of women with depression in an obstetrics and gynecology setting. Obstet Gynecol 2013;122(2):313–8.
20. Deneke DE. Screening for depression in the primary care population. Psychiatr Clin North Am 2015;38(1):23–43.

21. American Psychiatric Association (APA). Practice guideline for the treatment of patients with major depressive disorder. 3rd edition. Arlington (VA): American Psychiatric Association (APA); 2010.

22. American Psychiatric Association. Practice guideline for the treatment of patients with bipolar disorder (revision). Am J Psychiatry 2002;159(4 Suppl):1.

23. Cameron CC. Optimizing the management of depression: primary care experience. Psychiatry Res 2014;220(Suppl 1):S45–57.

24. Thronson LR. Psychopharmacology. Med Clin North Am 2014;98(5):927–58.

25. Haley CL. The clinical relevance of self-reported premenstrual worsening of depressive symptoms in the management of depressed outpatients: a STAR*D report. J Womens Health (Larchmt) 2013;22(3):219–29.

26. Deligiannidis KM. Complementary and alternative medicine for the treatment of depressive disorders in women. Psychiatr Clin North Am 2010;33(2):441–63.

27. Cohen LS. Relapse of major depression during pregnancy in women who maintain or discontinue antidepressant treatment. JAMA 2006;295(5):499.

28. ACOG Committee on Practice Bulletins–Obstetrics. ACOG practice bulletin: clinical management guidelines for obstetrician-gynecologists number 92, April 2008 (replaces practice bulletin number 87, November 2007). Use of psychiatric medications during pregnancy and lactation. Obstet Gynecol 2008;111(4):1001.

29. Yonkers KA. The management of depression during pregnancy: a report from the American Psychiatric Association and the American College of Obstetricians and Gynecologists. Gen Hosp Psychiatry 2009;31(5):403–13.

30. Freeman EW. Longitudinal pattern of depressive symptoms around natural menopause. JAMA Psychiatry 2014;71(1):36.

31. Parry BL. Perimenopausal depression. Am J Psychiatry 2008;165(1):23–7.

32. Brenner CJ. Diagnosis and management of bipolar disorder in primary care: a DSM-5 update. Med Clin North Am 2014;98(5):1025–48.

33. Cerimele JM. The prevalence of bipolar disorder in primary care patients with depression or other psychiatric complaints: a systematic review. Psychosomatics 2013;54(6):515–24.

34. Miller LJ. Bipolar disorder in women. Health Care Women Int 2015;36(4):475–98.

35. Hirschfeld RM. Development and validation of a screening instrument for bipolar spectrum disorder: the mood disorder questionnaire. Am J Psychiatry 2000; 157(11):1873.

36. Manning JS. Bipolar disorder, bipolar depression and comorbid illness. J Fam Pract 2015;64(6 Suppl):S10.

37. Geddes JR. Treatment of bipolar disorder. Lancet 2013;381(9878):1672–82.

38. Pompili MM. Electroconvulsive treatment during pregnancy: a systematic review. Expert Rev Neurother 2014;14(12):1377–90.

39. Sit DD. Light therapy for bipolar disorder: a case series in women. Bipolar Disord 2007;9(8):918–27.

40. Payne JL. Reproductive cycle-associated mood symptoms in women with major depression and bipolar disorder. J Affect Disord 2007;99(1–3):221–9.

41. Marengo EE. Unplanned pregnancies and reproductive health among women with bipolar disorder. J Affect Disord 2015;178:201–5.

42. Viguera ACA. Risk of recurrence of bipolar disorder in pregnant and nonpregnant women after discontinuing lithium maintenance. Am J Psychiatry 2000; 157(2):179.

43. Viguera AC. Risk of recurrence in women with bipolar disorder during pregnancy: prospective study of mood stabilizer discontinuation. Am J Psychiatry 2007; 164(12):1817–24.

44. Jones II. Bipolar disorder, affective psychosis, and schizophrenia in pregnancy and the post-partum period. Lancet 2014;384(9956):1789–99.
45. Munk-Olsen TT. Psychiatric disorders with postpartum onset: possible early manifestations of bipolar affective disorders. Arch Gen Psychiatry 2012;69(4):428.
46. Spinelli MG. Postpartum psychosis: detection of risk and management. Am J Psychiatry 2009;166(4):405–8.
47. Marsh WK. Symptom severity of bipolar disorder during the menopausal transition. Int J Bipolar Disord 2015;3(1):35.
48. Carter RMR. One-year prevalence of subthreshold and threshold DSM-IV generalized anxiety disorder in a nationally representative sample. Depress Anxiety 2001;13(2):78.
49. Kennedy BLB. Utilization of medical specialists by anxiety disorder patients. Psychosomatics 1997;38(2):109–12.
50. Kessler RC. Lifetime prevalence and age-of-onset distributions of DSM-IV disorders in the national comorbidity survey replication. Arch Gen Psychiatry 2005; 62(6):593.
51. Simon NM. The implications of medical and psychiatric comorbidity with panic disorder. J Clin Psychiatry 2005;66(Suppl 4):8.
52. Hamilton MM. The assessment of anxiety states by rating. Br J Med Psychol 1959;32(1):50.
53. Beck ATA. An inventory for measuring clinical anxiety: psychometric properties. J Consult Clin Psychol 1988;56(6):893.
54. Locke AB. Diagnosis and management of generalized anxiety disorder and panic disorder in adults. Am Fam Physician 2015;91(9):617.
55. Davidson JRJ, Zhang W, Connor KM, et al. A psychopharmacological treatment algorithm for generalised anxiety disorder (GAD). J Psychopharmacol 2010; 24(1):3–26.
56. Schweizer EE. Strategies for treatment of generalized anxiety in the primary care setting. J Clin Psychiatry 1997;58(Suppl 3):27.
57. Altemus MM. Sex differences in anxiety and depression clinical perspectives. Front Neuroendocrinol 2014;35(3):320–30.
58. Goodman JH. Anxiety disorders during pregnancy: a systematic review. J Clin Psychiatry 2014;75(10):e1153–84.
59. Levine RE. Anxiety disorders during pregnancy and postpartum. Am J Perinatol 2003;20(5):239–48.
60. Sichel DAD. Postpartum obsessive compulsive disorder: a case series. J Clin Psychiatry 1993;54(4):156.
61. Wijma KK. Posttraumatic stress disorder after childbirth: a cross sectional study. J Anxiety Disord 1997;11(6):587.
62. Bellantuono CC. Benzodiazepine exposure in pregnancy and risk of major malformations: a critical overview. Gen Hosp Psychiatry 2013;35(1):3–8.
63. Hickey MM. Evaluation and management of depressive and anxiety symptoms in midlife. Climacteric 2012;15(1):3–9.
64. Ohayon MM. Epidemiology of insomnia: what we know and what we still need to learn. Sleep Med Rev 2002;6(2):97.
65. Lindberg EE. Sleep disturbances in a young adult population: can gender differences be explained by differences in psychological status? Sleep 1997; 20(6):381.
66. Taylor DJ. Comorbidity of chronic insomnia with medical problems. Sleep 2007; 30(2):213.

67. Benca RM. Special considerations in insomnia diagnosis and management: depressed, elderly, and chronic pain populations. J Clin Psychiatry 2004; 65(Suppl 8):26.
68. Schutte-Rodin SS. Clinical guideline for the evaluation and management of chronic insomnia in adults. J Clin Sleep Med 2008;4(5):487.
69. Wang MY. Cognitive behavioural therapy for primary insomnia: a systematic review. J Adv Nurs 2005;50(5):553–64.
70. Morgenthaler TT. Practice parameters for the psychological and behavioral treatment of insomnia: an update. An american academy of sleep medicine report. Sleep 2006;29(11):1415.
71. Morin CMC. Nonpharmacological interventions for insomnia: a meta-analysis of treatment efficacy. Am J Psychiatry 1994;151(8):1172.
72. Winkelman JW. Insomnia disorder. N Engl J Med 2015;373(15):1437–44.
73. Mauri MM. Sleep in the premenstrual phase: a self-report study of PMS patients and normal controls. Acta Psychiatr Scand 1988;78(1):82.
74. Soares CN. Sleep disorders in women: clinical evidence and treatment strategies. Psychiatr Clin North Am 2006;29(4):1095–113.
75. Lee KA. Sleep in late pregnancy predicts length of labor and type of delivery. Am J Obstet Gynecol 2004;191(6):2041–6.
76. Kryger MH, Roth T, Dement WC, editors. Principles and practice of sleep medicine. 5th edition. Philadelphia: Saunders/Elsevier; 2011.
77. Driver HSH. A longitudinal study of sleep stages in young women during pregnancy and postpartum. Sleep 1992;15(5):449.
78. Okun ML. A review of sleep-promoting medications used in pregnancy. Am J Obstet Gynecol 2015;212(4):428–41.
79. Freedman RR. Sleep disturbance in menopause. Menopause 2007;14(5):826–9.
80. Ensrud KE. Effects of estradiol and venlafaxine on insomnia symptoms and sleep quality in women with hot flashes. Sleep 2015;38(1):97.
81. Vigod SN, Gomes T, Wilton AS, et al. Antipsychotic drug use in pregnancy: high dimensional, propensity matched, population based cohort study. BMJ 2015;350:h2298.
82. Coughlin CG, Blackwell KA, Bartley C, et al. Obstetric and neonatal outcomes after antipsychotic medication exposure in pregnancy. Obstet Gynecol 2015; 125(5):1224–35.
83. Baker GA, Bromley RL, Briggs M, et al, Liverpool and Manchester Neurodevelopment Group. IQ at 6 years after in utero exposure to antiepileptic drugs: a controlled cohort study. Neurology 2015;84(4):382–90.
84. Gerrett D, Lamont T, Paton C, et al. Prescribing and monitoring lithium therapy: summary of a safety report from the National Patient Safety Agency. BMJ 2010; 341:c6258.
85. Thase ME. Bipolar disorder maintenance treatment: monitoring effectiveness and safety. J Clin Psychiatry 2012;73(4):e15.

Evaluation of Anemia

Jody L. Kujovich, MD

KEYWORDS

- Anemia • Iron deficiency • Hemolysis • Thalassemia • Vitamin B_{12} • Macrocytosis

KEY POINTS

- The degree of macrocytosis may simplify the differential diagnosis of macrocytic anemia. An MCV >110 is characteristic of vitamin B_{12} and folate deficiency, myelodysplasia, and certain medications.
- The evaluation of macrocytic anemia should include testing for vitamin B_{12} and folate deficiency. An elevated methylmalonic acid level is the most specific test for B_{12} deficiency. Homocysteine levels are high in B_{12} and folate deficiency.
- Iron deficiency (low ferritin) precedes the development of anemia. A normal hemoglobin excludes anemia but does not rule out iron deficiency.
- Thalassemia trait is associated with mild or no anemia and more marked microcytosis than iron deficiency, which does not result in microcytosis until the Hb fall to less than 10 g/dL.
- Laboratory evidence of hemolysis includes an increased reticulocyte count, LDH, indirect bilirubin, and low haptoglobin level. The combination of an elevated LDH and low haptoglobin level is highly sensitive for hemolysis.

GENERAL CONSIDERATIONS

Anemia is a common problem encountered in primary care, occasionally discovered on routine testing. In clinical practice, anemia is defined as a reduction in hemoglobin (Hb) or hematocrit (Hct) obtained as part of a complete blood count (CBC). In general, red blood cell (RBC) associated measurements are lower in women compared with men. Anemia is often defined as Hb values that are more than 2 SD below the mean[1,2]: men, Hb less than 13.4 g/dL; and women, Hb less than 12 g/dL. These definitions have several limitations. Normal Hb levels vary not only with sex but also with ethnicity.[1] Because the normal range is defined as the mean $\pm$ 2 SD, then 2.5% of normal adults have values greater than 2 SD below the normal range and are diagnosed with anemia. An individual's Hb or Hct may also decline substantially from prior baseline values without falling below the normal reference range.

Disclosure: The author has no conflicts to disclose.
Department of Pediatric Hematology/Oncology, The Hemophilia Center, Oregon Health & Science University, 707 Southwest Gaines Street, Portland, OR 97239, USA
E-mail address: kujovich@ohsu.edu

Obstet Gynecol Clin N Am 43 (2016) 247–264
http://dx.doi.org/10.1016/j.ogc.2016.01.009   obgyn.theclinics.com

It is also important to recognize that Hb, Hct, and RBC counts are concentrations that depend on RBC mass and plasma volume. Hb and Hct values decline when plasma volume increases (hemodilution) and are higher if plasma volume decreases (hemoconcentration). For example, patients with anemia who are volume depleted may have near normal Hb and Hct values on initial testing because of hemoconcentration. The underlying anemia becomes apparent only after normal volume status is restored.

Automated cell counters also measure the mean cell volume (MCV) and the red cell distribution width (RDW), an estimate of the variation in cell size. A normal RBC has a volume of 80 to 96 fL and is approximately the size of a nucleus of a small lymphocyte on a peripheral blood smear. An increased RDW indicates a substantial variation in RBC size but is not diagnostic of a particular disorder.

The MCV is a key parameter for classification of anemia. The first step in the evaluation of anemia is to classify it as macrocytic (MCV >100 fL), microcytic (MCV <80 fL), or normocytic (MCV 80–100 fL). This narrows the differential diagnosis of possible causes and directs further evaluation. The next step is to determine if the anemia is new or a long-standing problem. Recently diagnosed anemia is usually an acquired disorder, whereas a lifelong history of anemia is more likely to be an inherited disorder, especially if accompanied by a family history. Review of the electronic medical record may determine when the Hb began to fall and when the RBC indices began to change.

MACROCYTIC ANEMIA

Macrocytic anemias are characterized by an MCV greater than 100 (**Box 1**). The severity of the macrocytosis may simplify the differential diagnosis. A marked macrocytosis (MCV >110 fL) is characteristic of vitamin B_{12} and folate deficiency, primary bone marrow disorders (myelodysplasia), and the use of certain medications. In contrast, a mild macrocytosis (MCV 100–110 fL) is more characteristic of alcohol abuse, liver disease, marked reticulocytosis, and hypothyroidism.

Box 1
Causes of macrocytic anemia MCV >100

- Vitamin B_{12} deficiency
- Folate deficiency
- Medications
  - Hydroxyurea
  - Methotrexate
  - Imatinib
  - Anticonvulsants
  - Azathioprine
  - Nitrous oxide
- Primary bone marrow disorder
  - Myelodysplasia
  - Aplastic anemia
- Alcohol abuse
- Reticulocytosis
- Hypothyroidism

Causes

Megaloblastic anemia

Deficiencies of vitamin B_{12} and/or folate result in megaloblastic anemia defined by distinctive peripheral blood smear findings including oval-shaped macrocytes (macro-ovalocytes) and hypersegmented neutrophils. Hypersegmentation is defined as 1% of neutrophils with six nuclear lobes or at least 5% with five or more lobes. Vitamin B_{12} and folate deficiency should be confirmed or excluded because both are correctable disorders that can lead to serious complications if untreated.

When vitamin B_{12} or folate deficiency is diagnosed, the next step is to determine the cause. Folate deficiency develops less frequently in the United States since the introduction of mandatory folic acid fortification of grain products. It is most common in elderly individuals with a poor diet, alcoholics, and patients with malabsorption or an increased folate requirement (hemolytic anemia, psoriasis). People with alcoholism typically have inadequate dietary intake of folate. Alcohol also interferes with folate absorption and metabolism.[3] Folate stores are limited and can be depleted within weeks to a few months in contrast to vitamin B_{12} stores, which may last for years after cessation of vitamin B_{12} intake or absorption.

Dietary vitamin B_{12} deficiency is uncommon in adults but can develop in those with an exclusively vegan diet. Most cases are caused by impaired absorption. If vitamin B_{12} deficiency is confirmed in an individual with adequate vitamin B_{12} intake, then malabsorption must be present. Vitamin B_{12} absorption in the distal ileum requires intrinsic factor (IF), synthesized by gastric parietal cells. Pernicious anemia is an autoimmune gastritis resulting from the destruction of gastric parietal cells and is the most common cause of severe vitamin B_{12} deficiency.[4] Destruction of gastric parietal cells results in a lack of IF to bind ingested vitamin B_{12}. Chronic atrophic gastritis with hypochlorhydria and the inability to release dietary protein-bound vitamin B_{12} affects 20% of older adults.[4] Patients who have undergone bariatric surgery are also at risk for developing vitamin B_{12} and folate deficiency. Other causes of vitamin B_{12} deficiency include pancreatic insufficiency, blind loop syndrome (bacterial absorption of vitamin B_{12}–IF complexes), partial gastrectomy, and surgical resection or disease of the terminal ileum.

Medications

A variety of drugs that interfere with DNA synthesis, absorption, metabolism, or processing of folate and/or vitamin B_{12} may cause macrocytosis and megaloblastic anemia. These include anticonvulsants, hydroxyurea, metformin, chemotherapy, and nitrous oxide.

Myelodysplastic disorders

Myelodysplastic disorders are a group of clonal primary bone marrow disorders that present with macrocytic anemia often associated with other cytopenias and dysplastic cell morphology on the peripheral blood smear. The diagnosis should be considered after exclusion of vitamin B_{12} and folate deficiency, especially in older individuals. Bone marrow biopsy is required to confirm or exclude the diagnosis.

Alcohol abuse

Alcohol abuse is often associated with alcoholic liver disease, and poor nutrition resulting in folate deficiency. However, macrocytosis develops with chronic alcohol use even in the absence of these other causes and before the development of anemia. Macrocytosis usually resolves within 2 to 4 months of abstinence from alcohol.[3]

Liver disease

Up to two-thirds of patients with chronic liver disease develop a macrocytosis. In contrast to megaloblastic anemia, the RDW is normal because the macrocytic RBCs are uniformly round. Target cells are commonly seen in the peripheral blood smear.

Reticulocytosis

Because a reticulocyte is almost twice as large as a mature RBC, marked reticulocytosis may increase the MCV. A rough rule of thumb is that each 1% increase in the percentage of reticulocytes results in a corresponding 1-fL increase in the MCV.[5] Macrocytic anemia with reticulocytosis indicates increased RBC turnover, which may reflect hemolysis or a response to blood loss or replacement of iron, vitamin B_{12}, and/or folate in deficient patients.

Hypothyroidism

Hypothyroidism may be associated with a normocytic or, less commonly, a mildly macrocytic anemia.

Spurious macrocytosis

A markedly increased MCV can occur as an artifact when cold agglutinins are present. Cold agglutinins cause RBC to clump and RBC doublets and triplets are counted as larger RBC by automated instruments. In these cases, warming the specimen and reagents to body temperature should result in a normal MCV.

Evaluation

In addition to a CBC, the evaluation of macrocytic anemia should include a reticulocyte count; liver function tests; vitamin B_{12}, folate, and lactate dehydrogenase (LDH) levels; and review of the peripheral blood smear. Laboratory testing in megaloblastic anemia reflects the biochemical consequences of ineffective erythropoiesis. The RDW is usually markedly elevated reflecting the effects of vitamin B_{12} and/or folate deficiencies on RBC production; serum levels of LDH, indirect bilirubin, and aspartate aminotransferase are increased; and the haptoglobin level may be low.

Vitamin B_{12} levels less than 200 pg/mL strongly suggest vitamin B_{12} deficiency and vitamin B_{12} levels greater than 400 pg/mL usually exclude a deficiency. However, false-negative and false-positive values are common when the lower limit of normal reference range is used as the threshold for a deficiency.[4] Vitamin B_{12} levels fall during pregnancy in most healthy women. Vitamin B_{12} levels below the normal range are found in 35% to 50% of pregnant women but do not indicate a total body deficit in most cases.[6–8] Because vitamin B_{12} levels may be above the lower end of the laboratory reference range in patients with clinical vitamin B_{12} deficiency, metabolite levels (homocysteine and methylmalonic acid [MMA]) are used to confirm or exclude a tissue deficiency. The levels of both homocysteine and MMA are markedly elevated in most (>98%) patients with clinical vitamin B_{12} deficiency.[4,9] An elevated MMA is the most sensitive and specific test for vitamin B_{12} deficiency. A high homocysteine level is less specific because it is also increased in folate deficiency and renal failure. Normal MMA and homocysteine levels strongly suggest normal vitamin B_{12} status.

A low serum folate level (<4 ng/mL) indicates folate deficiency. Homocysteine levels are increased in folate and vitamin B_{12} deficiency and thus cannot be used to distinguish between the two deficiencies. There is some evidence that borderline folate levels (4–8 ng/mL) associated with high homocysteine levels may reflect a tissue deficiency.[10]

IF antibody testing has a high specificity (100%) but a low sensitivity (50%–70%) for the diagnosis of pernicious anemia.[11] Antiparietal cell antibodies are more sensitive (80%) but less specific. Elevated serum gastrin levels and low pepsinogen I levels are highly sensitive for the diagnosis of pernicious anemia (90%–92%) but both tests lack specificity. Chronic atrophic gastritis can also be diagnosed by elevated serum gastrin and low serum pepsinogen I levels.

MICROCYTIC ANEMIA

Microcytic anemias are characterized by the production of smaller than normal RBC (MCV <80 fL). Impaired RBC production results from a deficiency of either heme or globin chains and is associated with hypochromic (low mean corpuscular hemoglobin [MCH]) and microcytic (low MCV) RBC on the peripheral blood smear.

Causes

The three most common causes of microcytic anemia in clinical practice are iron deficiency; α- or β-thalassemia trait; and, less often, anemia of inflammation (also called anemia of chronic disease).

Iron deficiency anemia

Iron deficiency refers to the reduction of iron stores and is reflected by a low ferritin level. Iron deficiency anemia occurs when depleted iron stores result in anemia (low Hb/Hct). It is important to recognize that iron deficiency precedes the development of anemia. When iron losses exceed iron intake, reserve iron (reflected by the ferritin level) is gradually depleted. At this stage, iron present in the labile iron pool from daily RBC turnover is still enough to maintain normal Hb synthesis (low ferritin normal Hb). Continued iron loss eventually impairs Hb synthesis resulting in a mild normocytic anemia (normal MCV). At this stage, serum iron may be low with an increased total iron-binding capacity (TIBC) and low transferrin saturation. Untreated iron deficiency eventually results in a more severe microcytic anemia (**Table 1**).

When iron deficiency anemia is diagnosed, it is imperative to determine the cause. Women are at high risk for iron deficiency and anemia because of the monthly loss of iron with menstrual bleeding. Heavy menstrual bleeding is the most common cause of iron deficiency. In one study, 33% of women with heavy menstrual bleeding had iron deficiency (ferritin <10) and 27% also had anemia (Hb <12).[12] Pregnancy also increases iron requirements. Iron deficiency develops in approximately 38% of pregnant women, and iron deficiency anemia in at least 21%.[13–16]

Table 1 **Stages in iron deficiency**			
Test	**Iron Deficiency No Anemia**	**Iron Deficiency Mild Anemia**	**Severe Iron Deficiency Anemia**
Serum iron	nl	↓	↓↓
TIBC	nl/↑	↑	↑↑
Transferrin saturation	nl	↓	↓↓
Ferritin	<40	<20	<10
Hb	nl	9–12	6–7
MCV	nl	nl	↓
RBC morph	nl	+/− Slightly hypochromic	Microcytic hypochromic

Abbreviations: nl, normal.

Several other populations are at increased risk for iron deficiency. Surgical procedures that bypass the duodenum, the primary site of iron absorption, result in iron deficiency without iron supplementation. Bariatric surgery (laparoscopic Roux-en-Y gastric bypass) is an emerging cause of iron deficiency and anemia because the procedure removes a site for iron absorption and increases gastric pH. Iron deficiency develops in up to 45% of these patients, particularly women.[13,17]

Obesity per se may be associated with mild iron deficiency because of subclinical inflammation associated with increased hepcidin levels, which impair iron absorption.[14] Individuals who donate blood regularly are at risk for iron deficiency.

Iron deficiency anemia is one of the most common extraintestinal manifestations of celiac disease. Celiac disease is responsible for a 5% to 6% of cases of unexplained iron deficiency anemia and is a known cause of refractory iron deficiency.[15] *Helicobacter pylori* infection impairs iron absorption because the bacteria compete for available iron and reduce the bioavailability of vitamin C. *H pylori* may also cause gastric microerosions that cause bleeding.[18] Iron deficiency anemia in endurance athletes may also be multifactorial: exercise-induced hemolysis resulting in urinary iron loss, impaired iron absorption caused by training-induced inflammation, and occult gastrointestinal tract blood loss may all be involved.[19] In postmenopausal women and other patients without an obvious source of blood loss evaluation of the gastrointestinal tract is mandatory because a high percentage of patients have an identifiable source of blood loss.[20]

Because iron deficiency is the most common cause of microcytic anemia, the initial step is the determination of serum ferritin. A low serum ferritin (<30 g/dL) is diagnostic of iron deficiency. It is important to recognize that a normal Hb/Hct excludes anemia but does not rule out iron deficiency. Other iron studies (serum iron, TIBC, transferrin saturation) do not reliably distinguish iron deficiency anemia from anemia of inflammation and have limited value in the evaluation of anemia. Serum iron is low in both iron deficiency and anemia of inflammation and increases after recent oral iron intake. An elevated TIBC is specific for iron deficiency but has a low sensitivity because it is lowered by inflammation, poor nutrition, and aging. Transferrin saturation is calculated as the serum iron divided by TIBC multiplied by 100 (TF sat = serum iron/TIBC $\times$ 100). Low transferrin saturation indicates an iron supply insufficient to support normal erythropoiesis, but the value is low in both iron deficiency and anemia of inflammation (**Table 2**). Although ferritin is an acute-phase protein that is elevated by inflammation, a ferritin level greater than or equal to 100 excludes iron deficiency. In equivocal cases, a response to a limited therapeutic trial of iron therapy confirms the diagnosis.

Table 2
Laboratory tests in microcytic anemias

Test	Iron Deficiency Anemia	Anemia of Inflammation	α- or β-Thalassemia Trait
MCV	↓	nl or ↓ (>70)	↓↓ (65–75)
RDW	↑↑	nl or sl ↑	nl or sl ↑
RBC	↓	↓	↑ or nl
Serum iron	↓	↓	nl or ↑
TIBC	↑	nl or ↓	nl or ↓
Transferrin saturation	↓	↓	nl
Ferritin	↓↓	nl or ↑	nl or ↑
Soluble transferrin receptor	↑	nl	↑

Abbreviations: nl, normal; sl, slightly.

An increase in the absolute reticulocyte count at 1 week and/or an increase in Hb level after 2 weeks is diagnostic of iron deficiency anemia.[21] Severe iron deficiency anemia is associated with the classic peripheral smear findings of anisocytosis (variation in RBC size), poikilocytosis (variation in cell shape), microcytosis, and hypochromia, paralleling the corresponding RBC indices (high RDW, low MCV, low MCH).

Thalassemia

Thalassemia is a disorder of Hb (hemoglobinopathy) characterized by reduced or absent production of either α globin (α-thalassemia) or β globin (β-thalassemia). Disruption of the normally tightly regulated and balanced production of α and non-α globin results in microcytosis and ineffective erythropoiesis.

Adults with thalassemia encountered in a primary care setting are usually heterozygous for the α and β forms of the disorder (α- or β-thalassemia trait or minor) and have at most a mild anemia. The diagnosis is suggested by a pre-existing mild microcytic anemia in a patient with normal or increased iron stores. A family history of anemia not responsive to iron supplements is common.

β-Thalassemia β-Thalassemia trait results from the inheritance of one abnormal β globin allele. Affected individuals have a mild clinical course and most are asymptomatic. Women with β-thalassemia trait may develop a more severe anemia during pregnancy because of their limited ability to increase red cell mass in response to the increase in plasma volume.[22]

β-Thalassemia trait may be misdiagnosed as iron deficiency anemia because both disorders are characterized by a low MCV and hypochromic and microcytic RBC on a peripheral blood smear. However, in β-thalassemia trait, peripheral smear findings also include target cells and basophilic stippling, and the microcytosis is more pronounced with only a mild anemia. Patients with β-thalassemia trait typically have Hct greater than or equal to 30% (Hb 10–13 g/dL) and MCV less than or equal to 75 (MCV 65–75). In contrast, iron deficiency does not result in microcytosis until the Hct falls below 30%. An increased total RBC count despite a mild anemia is characteristic of β-thalassemia trait reflecting the increased number of smaller RBC. The RDW is normal or near normal because the RBCs are uniformly microcytic. In iron deficiency anemia, the total RBC count falls in parallel with the severity of the anemia with a markedly increased RDW, reflecting the heterogeneity in RBC size (see **Table 2**).

Levels of serum iron and ferritin are increased and transferrin (TIBC) levels are normal or reduced in patients with β-thalassemia trait. The diagnosis is usually confirmed by Hb electrophoresis: a mildly increased Hb A_2 (α_2/δ_2) (3.5%–7%) level is the most important marker of β-thalassemia trait. Hb F levels are increased in approximately 50% of patients. The combination of a mild microcytic hypochromic anemia with normal iron stores and a mildly increased Hb A_2 level is strong presumptive evidence for a diagnosis of β-thalassemia trait. Coexisting iron deficiency and thalassemia complicates the diagnosis. Although concurrent iron deficiency may blunt the expected increase in Hb A_2 levels, recent evidence suggests Hb A_2 levels remain greater than 3.5%.[23,24] However, because rare forms of β-thalassemia trait are not associated with an increased Hb A_2 level, a normal level does not exclude the diagnosis. Definitive diagnosis requires molecular testing.

α-Thalassemia Normal individuals have four functional α globin genes, two on each chromosome 16 ($\alpha\alpha/\alpha\alpha$). The four α-thalassemia disorders result from the deletion or inactivation of one, two, three, or all four α globin genes. Most patients with α-thalassemia have deletions of α globin genes, but nondeletion mutations also occur.

Deletion of one of the four α globin genes (αα/α-) does not cause anemia or microcytosis (silent carrier). α-Thalassemia trait is caused by the loss of two α globin genes, but can occur in two different ways: loss of both α globin genes in cis (from the same chromosome) (–/αα) is a common genotype in southeast Asian populations. Loss of two genes in trans (one from each chromosome) (α-/α-) is more common in African and Mediterranean populations. The two different α-thalassemia genotypes are clinically very similar but have different implications for genetic counseling.[25]

Deletion or inactivation of three of the four α globin genes (α-/–) results in Hb H disease, a chronic microcytic hemolytic anemia of varying severity. The excess β chains that accumulate form tetramers (Hb H) that precipitate as the RBC ages causing membrane damage and hemolysis. Deletion of all four α globin genes results in Hb Bart's (γ globin tetramer) and hydrops fetalis.

Evaluation

The diagnosis should be considered in ethnic groups with a high prevalence of α-thalassemia. α-Thalassemia trait resembles mild β-thalassemia trait. Adults have mild or no anemia with hypochromic microcytic RBC and target cells on the peripheral blood smear. The RBC count is usually increased and the RDW is normal or near normal. Routine laboratory tests (CBC, RBC indices, iron studies) usually differentiate α- and β-thalassemia trait from iron deficiency anemia (see **Table 2**). Hb A_2 levels are not increased in α-thalassemia trait in contrast to β-thalassemia trait. In clinical practice, a presumptive diagnosis is based on the combination of microcytosis, mild or no anemia, normal iron stores, and Hb electrophoresis. Definitive diagnosis and determination of α globin genotype require genetic testing. Targeted mutation analysis detects common deletion mutations and differentiates between deletions occurring in cis (αα/–) or in trans (α-/α-). DNA sequence analysis is used to detect point mutations if a deletional mutation is not identified and the suspicion of α-thalassemia is high.[25] Women diagnosed with α- or β-thalassemia trait who are considering pregnancy should receive genetic counseling on the implications of the diagnosis.

Anemia of Inflammation

Acquired microcytic anemia that is not caused by iron deficiency may reflect an underlying systemic disorder. Anemia of inflammation is the second most common cause of anemia after iron deficiency. The symptoms are usually those of the underlying disease. Although frequently associated with infection, inflammatory conditions, and malignancy, anemia may also accompany other acute and chronic disorders with an inflammatory component (eg, diabetes, heart failure).[26]

The pathophysiology of anemia of inflammation is multifactorial and involves dysregulation of iron metabolism caused by cytokine-induced upregulation of hepcidin, the central regulator of iron homeostasis. Elevated hepcidin levels impair the release of storage iron from the reticuloendothelial system and inhibit intestinal absorption of iron, both reducing the availability of iron for erythropoiesis.[27,28] A relative decrease in the production of and response to erythropoietin also contributes to the hypoproliferative anemia.

Evaluation

Anemia of inflammation should be suspected in a patient with a normocytic or mildly microcytic hypoproliferative anemia and acute or chronic infection or an inflammatory disorder. Most patients have a mild to moderately severe normocytic normochromic anemia. The anemia is microcytic and hypochromic in less than 25% and the MCV is rarely less than 70.[28] There is no single laboratory test that reliably confirms the diagnosis. Instead, it is a diagnosis of exclusion based on a characteristic pattern of laboratory abnormalities (see **Table 2**). The reticulocyte count is inappropriately low for the degree of anemia reflecting decreased RBC production. Serum iron, TIBC, and transferrin saturation are low and the ferritin level is normal or increased. A low TIBC and high ferritin level distinguish anemia of inflammation from iron deficiency anemia (see **Table 2**). Increased inflammatory markers (C-reactive protein, erythrocyte sedimentation rate), an inappropriately decreased erythropoietin level (with normal renal function), and the absence of other causes of anemia support the diagnosis. The soluble transferrin receptor is a truncated fragment of the membrane receptor. The soluble transferrin receptor level is normal in anemia of inflammation and increased in iron deficiency.[26] Measurement of the soluble transferrin receptor may be useful to distinguish between these two causes of anemia, although a high level is not specific for iron deficiency.

Other Causes

Other causes of microcytic anemia are much less common. Chronic lead poisoning impairs heme synthesis resulting in a microcytic anemia associated with basophilic stippling on the peripheral smear. Inherited disorders of iron metabolism (eg, iron refractory iron deficiency anemia) and defects in heme (sideroblastic anemias) are rare and require specialized testing.[16,29] Hematology consultation is recommended in cases of unexplained microcytic anemia.

NORMOCYTIC ANEMIA

Normocytic anemia, characterized by a normal MCV (80–96 fL), is the most frequently encountered type of anemia. The causes include (1) reduced production of normal size RBC (anemia of inflammation, primary bone marrow disorders), (2) RBC loss or destruction (bleeding, hemolysis), and (3) a disproportionate increase in plasma volume relative to red cell mass (pregnancy, fluid overload). Concurrent disorders causing microcytic and macrocytic anemias (eg, combined iron and vitamin B_{12} deficiency) may also present with a normal MCV.

Decreased Red Blood Cell Production

Anemia of inflammation is the most common normocytic anemia and is discussed previously. It is important to recognize that nearly all anemias are normocytic during the early stages. Thus, mild or partially treated iron, vitamin B_{12}, or folate deficiencies are possible causes of a normocytic anemia. Endocrine deficiencies (hypothyroidism, adrenal or pituitary insufficiency) are often associated with a hypoproliferative anemia. Anemia accompanies acute and chronic renal failure and is characterized by inappropriately low erythropoietin levels. A variety of primary bone marrow disorders (aplastic anemia, pure red cell aplasia, myeloproliferative and infiltrative disorders) are also on the differential diagnosis.

Pregnancy

During normal pregnancy plasma volume expands by nearly 50% in the third trimester, but the red cell mass increases by only 25%, resulting in a reduction in Hb and Hct. This disproportionate increase in plasma volume relative to red cell mass is responsible for the physiologic anemia of pregnancy.[30] The MCV increases approximately 4 fL in healthy pregnant women but usually remains within the normal reference range.

Bleeding

Acute or recent bleeding results in a normocytic anemia. The Hb and Hct are initially normal and do not reflect the amount of blood loss until the volume deficit is replaced by movement of fluid from the extravascular into the intravascular space, usually 36 to 48 hours after an acute bleeding episode.

HEMOLYTIC ANEMIA

The normal RBC is comprised of Hb, specialized cell membrane proteins, and metabolic machinery essential to maintain its deformability, oxygen transport ability, and protection against oxidant damage. An inherited or acquired defect in any of these components may impair the integrity of the RBC and shorten its survival in the circulation. Hemolytic anemias are usually normocytic but may be macrocytic if accompanied by a brisk reticulocytosis. Hemolytic anemias can be categorized as hereditary (intrinsic) or acquired (**Box 2**).

Hereditary Red Cell Defects

Hereditary hemolytic anemias caused by intrinsic RBC defects include hemoglobinopathies (sickle cell disease, unstable Hb disease), RBC membrane disorders, and enzyme deficiencies.

Hereditary Spherocytosis

Hereditary spherocytosis is the most common hemolytic anemia caused by an RBC membrane defect. It is caused by mutations involving five genes that encode proteins involved in the coupling of the membrane cytoskeleton to the lipid bilayer. The membrane defects result in decreased surface/volume ratio (spherocytes), dehydration (increased MCH concentration), reduced RBC deformability, and splenic destruction (extravascular hemolysis). Spherocytes are osmotically fragile and are selectively removed by the spleen.[31] Patents with hereditary spherocytosis usually present with moderate hemolytic anemia, jaundice, splenomegaly, and often pigment gallstones. However, the clinical severity varies from asymptomatic compensated hemolysis (normal Hb, increased reticulocyte count) to severe cases requiring transfusion.

Box 2
Hemolytic anemias

Intrinsic red cell defects
   Membrane defects: hereditary spherocytosis/elliptocytosis
   Enzyme deficiencies: glucose 6-phosphate dehydrogenase, pyruvate kinase
   Hemoglobinopathies: unstable Hb, sickle cell disorders

Immune
   Autoimmune hemolytic anemia (warm antibody)
   Cold agglutinin
   Drug induced

Nonimmune
   Hypersplenism
   Infection: malaria, babesiosis, clostridial sepsis
   Paroxysmal nocturnal hemoglobinuria
   Prosthetic valves
   Microangiopathic: thrombotic thrombocytopenic purpura, hemolytic uremic syndrome, HELLP
   Wilson's disease

Although severe cases present in childhood, milder cases may be diagnosed at any age. Diagnosis is usually based on typical clinical features (splenomegaly, sphero-cytes, increased MCH concentration, reticulocytosis) in a patient with a family history. Several screening tests are available for equivocal cases. Biochemical assay of membrane proteins and genetic testing may be required in rare cases.[31]

Glucose 6-Phosphate Dehydrogenase Deficiency

Glucose 6-phosphate dehydrogenase (G6PD) deficiency is the most common RBC enzyme defect and is transmitted as an X-linked trait. Because the G6PD gene is located on the X chromosome, males have only one allele. In a male with a G6PD deficiency variant, all RBC are deficient. Females with G6PD deficiency may be heterozygous or homozygous for a variant gene. Homozygous females are rare except in regions where G6PD deficiency is prevalent. Homozygous females are as severely affected as hemizygous males, because all of their RBC are G6PD deficient. Heterozygous females have a dual population of normal and G6PD-deficient RBC as a result of X chromosome inactivation (lyonization). Although the average ratio is 50:50, the spectrum ranges from a majority of normal RBC to a predominance of G6PD-deficient cells. Heterozygous females with a large excess of G6PD-deficient RBC may develop a hemolytic anemia as severe as G6PD-deficient males.[32] At least 187 G6PD variants have been identified associated with variable severity of hemolysis depending on the level of residual enzymatic activity.[32] Most pathogenic variants predispose to acute hemolysis under conditions of increased oxidative stress induced by infection, drugs, or food. A G6PD variant common in the Mediterranean region and Middle East is associated with chronic hemolysis. The diagnosis should be suspected in patients of African, Mediterranean, or Asian origin with a history of acute hemolysis triggered by infection or a known oxidative drug. The peripheral smear may show "bite cells" reflecting oxidant injury to Hb. Supravital staining of the peripheral blood smear may reveal denatured Hb as Heinz bodies during hemolytic episodes. G6PD deficiency is confirmed by demonstrating decreased enzyme activity in RBC, and several screening tests are available.[32] G6PD enzymatic activity declines as the cell ages; the youngest RBC (reticulocytes) have the highest enzyme activity. G6PD activity may be transiently normal immediately following an acute hemolytic episode and the selective destruction of older more deficient RBC. Testing should be repeated several months after the hemolytic episode if a false-negative result is suspected.

Acquired Hemolytic Anemias

Acquired hemolytic anemias include autoimmune hemolytic anemia (AIHA) and disorders associated with nonimmune hemolysis.

Autoimmune hemolytic anemia

AIHA is caused by autoantibodies directed against membrane RBC antigens. It is classified into warm, cold, and mixed forms based on the direct antiglobulin test (DAT) (Coomb test) and thermal characteristics of the autoantibody. Warm autoantibodies are usually IgG and react at 37°C. Cold agglutinins are typically IgM and react optimally at 0°C to 5°C. AIHA is primary (idiopathic) or secondary to an underlying disorder.

At least 50% of cases of warm antibody AIHA are idiopathic and females are more commonly affected than males. Secondary AIHA occurs in association with underlying autoimmune (lupus), infectious (human immunodeficiency virus), and lymphoproliferative (chronic lymphocytic leukemia) disorders, and drugs. The diagnosis is suspected in cases of new-onset hemolytic anemia with characteristic microspherocytes on a peripheral blood smear. Spherocytes reflect the reduced surface/volume ratio caused by phagocytosis of the IgG-coated RBC membrane in the spleen. The reticulocyte count is usually increased, but may be low in 20% because of autoantibody reactivity against bone marrow RBC precursors.[33] The diagnosis is confirmed by identification of an RBC autoantibody with the DAT. In warm antibody AIHA the DAT is positive for RBC bound IgG ± C3. Although a positive DAT is suggestive of AIHA, it occurs in the absence of clinical hemolysis in 0.1% of healthy blood donors and up to 8% of hospitalized patients.[34,35] DAT-negative AIHA occurs rarely, and may reflect low titer or low-affinity antibodies or an IgA or IgM isotype.[36] Diagnosis of DAT-negative AIHA requires specialized testing or a response to empiric immunosuppressive therapy.

Cold agglutinins are autoantibodies that bind to RBC antigens at low temperatures causing agglutination and complement-mediated hemolysis. Acute cold agglutinin-induced hemolysis occurs with certain infections (eg, mycoplasma, Epstein-Barr virus). Chronic cold agglutinin disease is caused by a clonal lymphoproliferative disorder. Cooling of blood during flow through acral parts of the circulation facilitates binding to the RBC and causes agglutination.[37] Approximately 90% of patients experience cold-induced acrocyanosis and/or Raynaud symptoms.[37] IgM antibodies bound to the RBC membrane bind complement and activate the classical complement pathway resulting in hemolysis. When IgM-coated RBCs return to the warmer (37°C) central parts of the body, the antibodies detach but C3 remains bound. This pathophysiology is reflected by the DAT, which is usually strongly positive for C3 but negative for bound IgG. The diagnosis is confirmed by a DAT positive for C3 and an elevated cold agglutin titer (>64).[38] In the most cases the cold agglutinin is a monoclonal IgM kappa.[37]

Nonimmune hemolysis

Causes of nonimmune hemolysis include fragmentation (mechanical valves) and microangiopathic destruction (thrombotic microangiopathy). Mechanical trauma to RBC in these disorders results from high-velocity jets (malfunctioning cardiac valves) or intravascular fibrin strands that shear RBC (thrombotic thrombocytopenic purpura, hemolytic uremic syndrome, disseminated intravascular coagulation). Mild compensated hemolysis associated with mechanical cardiac valves is now less common because of improvements in valve design. Severe hemolysis primarily occurs in the setting of paravalvular leak.[39] Evidence of hemolysis should increase suspicion of structural valve deterioration, which is usually evident on echocardiogram. Laboratory findings include reticulocytosis, high LDH and indirect bilirubin, low haptoglobin, and fragmented RBC on peripheral smear. In contrast to thrombotic microangiopathies, the platelet count is normal.

Other causes of nonimmune hemolysis include destruction of the RBC by pathogens (malaria, babesiosis), hypersplenism, paroxysmal nocturnal hemoglobinuria (PNH), and Wilson's disease.[40] Anemia associated with hypersplenism is primarily caused by trapping and destruction of RBC in an enlarged spleen. PNH, a rare acquired clonal disorder of bone marrow stem cells, results from an acquired somatic mutation in the PIG-A gene that prevents glycosylphosphatidylinositol-anchored proteins from binding to cell membranes. Several glycosylphosphatidylinositol-linked proteins protect the RBC from complement-mediated lysis. RBCs derived from the PNH clone lack this protective shield and are highly sensitive to complement-mediated cell lysis. PNH may be associated with iron deficiency because of chronic or recurrent hemoglobinuria. The diagnosis is confirmed by flow cytometry for PIG-linked proteins on leukocytes and RBC.

Wilson's disease is an autosomal-recessive disease characterized by progressive accumulation of copper. Hemolytic anemia may be the initial manifestation and precede symptomatic liver disease. Hemolysis results from oxidant effects of copper on Hb, direct membrane damage, and inhibition of glycolytic enzymes.[40,41]

Evaluation

The evaluation of normocytic anemia requires additional testing, which should include a reticulocyte count; renal and liver function tests; and assessment of iron, vitamin B_{12}, and folate status. The rate of fall in Hb and Hct often provides diagnostic clues. A history of acute-onset anemia suggests hemolysis, especially when the fall in Hb occurs more rapidly than is explained by decreased red cell production. A rapid fall in Hb excludes bone marrow suppression as the sole cause and indicates blood loss and/or

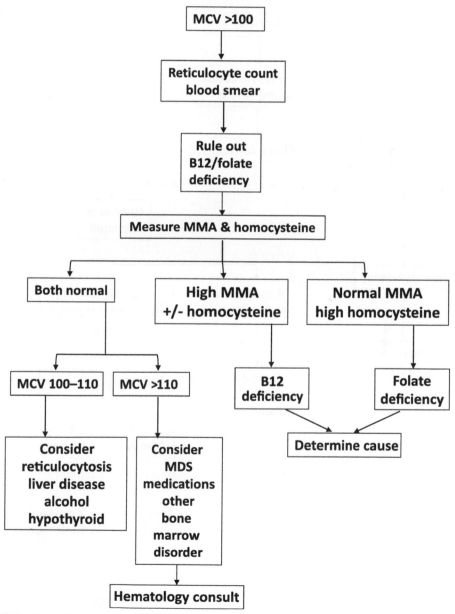

Fig. 1. Evaluation of macrocytic anemia. MDS, myelodysplasia.

increased RBC destruction must also be present. The presence of spherocytes, red cell fragments (schistocytes), and polychromasia on the peripheral blood smear suggest hemolysis. The reticulocyte count is increased in most patients with hemolysis, but is not specific for hemolysis because a reticulocytosis also occurs after acute blood loss and correction of nutritional deficiencies. The reticulocyte response may be blunted by concurrent bone marrow suppression, destruction of erythroid precursors, nutritional depletion (especially folate), renal failure, or infection.

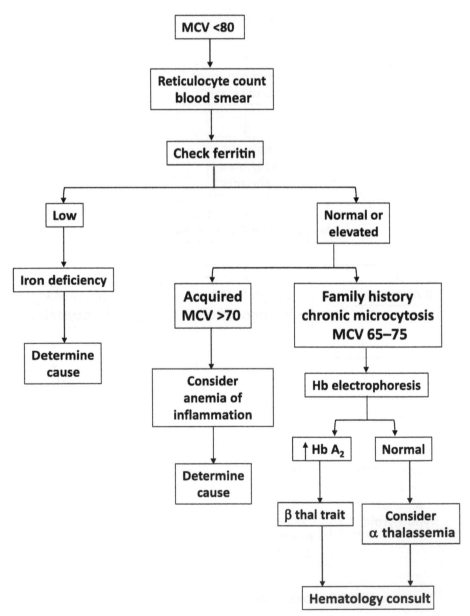

Fig. 2. Evaluation of microcytic anemia.

Laboratory evidence of hemolysis includes an elevated LDH and indirect bilirubin and low haptoglobin. However, LDH is a nonspecific marker of tissue damage and high levels occur in other disorders (eg, myocardial and renal infarction). Haptoglobin binds irreversibly to free Hb released during hemolysis and the complexes are rapidly cleared by the reticuloendotheial system. Haptoglobin levels are low or undetectable in hemolytic anemia. A higher level may reflect a milder degree of hemolysis or concurrent inflammation because haptoglobin is an acute-phase protein. Although no single

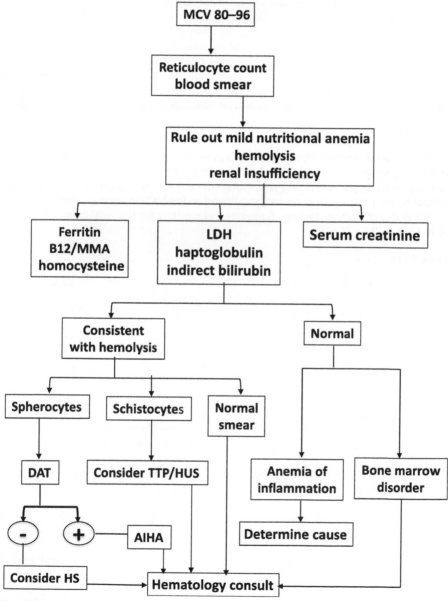

Fig. 3. Evaluation of normocytic anemia. HS, hereditary spherocytosis; HUS, hemolytic uremic syndrome; TTP, thrombotic thrombocytopenic purpura.

test is specific for hemolysis, one study found that the combination of an elevated LDH and low haptoglobin level had 90% sensitivity for a diagnosis of hemolysis. The combination of a normal LDH and haptoglobin greater than 25 mg/dL was 92% sensitive for excluding hemolysis.[42,43]

An increased serum concentration of indirect bilirubin results from the catabolism of Hb heme within phagocytic cells. Hb released into the circulation may be filtered by the kidneys and taken up by rental tubular cells where iron is deposited as hemosiderin. When the renal tubular cells are sloughed, iron is detected by Prussian blue staining of the urine sediment. More specific tests may be required to confirm the cause of hemolysis (DAT, cold agglutin titer, G6PD level, flow cytometry for PNH).

The differential diagnosis of a normocytic anemia that is not caused by bleeding, nutritional deficiency, renal insufficiency, or hemolysis is likely anemia of inflammation, or a primary bone marrow disorder. The presence of multiple cytopenias, immature myeloid cells, hyposegmented neutrophils, nucleated RBC, or teardrop-shaped RBC suggests a primary bone marrow disorder or infiltrative process. A bone marrow biopsy may be required for diagnosis and hematology consultation is recommended.

SUMMARY

The evaluation of anemia often begins in a primary care setting. The initial approach requires correlation of information from the history and physical examination with the CBC, reticulocyte count, and peripheral smear findings. Classification of anemias as macrocytic, microcytic, or normocytic based on the MCV limits the differential diagnosis and directs further testing. Suggested algorithms for the evaluation of anemia are in **Figs. 1–3**.

REFERENCES

1. Cappellini MD, Motta I. Anemia in clinical practice-definition and classification: does hemoglobin change with aging? Semin Hematol 2015;52(4):261–9.
2. Beutler E, Waalen J. The definition of anemia: what is the lower limit of normal of the blood hemoglobin concentration? Blood 2006;107(5):1747–50.
3. Ballard HS. The hematological complications of alcoholism. Alcohol Health Res World 1997;21(1):42–52.
4. Stabler SP. Clinical practice. Vitamin B12 deficiency. N Engl J Med 2013;368(2): 149–60.
5. Green R, Dwyre DM. Evaluation of macrocytic anemias. Semin Hematol 2015; 52(4):279–86.
6. Shields RC, Caric V, Hair M, et al. Pregnancy-specific reference ranges for haematological variables in a Scottish population. J Obstet Gynaecol 2011;31(4): 286–9.
7. Zamorano AF, Arnalich F, Sanchez Casas E, et al. Levels of iron, vitamin B12, folic acid and their binding proteins during pregnancy. Acta Haematol 1985;74(2): 92–6.
8. Metz J, McGrath K, Bennett M, et al. Biochemical indices of vitamin B12 nutrition in pregnant patients with subnormal serum vitamin B12 levels. Am J Hematol 1995;48(4):251–5.
9. Savage DG, Lindenbaum J, Stabler SP, et al. Sensitivity of serum methylmalonic acid and total homocysteine determinations for diagnosing cobalamin and folate deficiencies. Am J Med 1994;96(3):239–46.
10. De Bruyn E, Gulbis B, Cotton F. Serum and red blood cell folate testing for folate deficiency: new features? Eur J Haematol 2014;92(4):354–9,

11. Carmel R. How I treat cobalamin (vitamin B12) deficiency. Blood 2008;112(6): 2214–21.
12. Muse K, Mabey RG, Waldbaum A, et al. Tranexamic acid increases hemoglobin and ferritin levels in women with heavy menstrual bleeding. J Womens Health (Larchmt) 2012;21(7):756–61.
13. Obinwanne KM, Fredrickson KA, Mathiason MA, et al. Incidence, treatment, and outcomes of iron deficiency after laparoscopic Roux-en-Y gastric bypass: a 10-year analysis. J Am Coll Surg 2014;218(2):246–52.
14. Aigner E, Feldman A, Datz C. Obesity as an emerging risk factor for iron deficiency. Nutrients 2014;6(9):3587–600.
15. Hershko C, Camaschella C. How I treat unexplained refractory iron deficiency anemia. Blood 2014;123(3):326–33.
16. Camaschella C. Iron-deficiency anemia. N Engl J Med 2015;372(19):1832–43.
17. Stein J, Stier C, Raab H, et al. Review article: the nutritional and pharmacological consequences of obesity surgery. Aliment Pharmacol Ther 2014;40(6):582–609.
18. Franceschi F, Zuccala G, Roccarina D, et al. Clinical effects of Helicobacter pylori outside the stomach. Nat Rev Gastroenterol Hepatol 2014;11(4):234–42.
19. Peeling P, Dawson B, Goodman C, et al. Athletic induced iron deficiency: new insights into the role of inflammation, cytokines and hormones. Eur J Appl Physiol 2008;103(4):381–91.
20. Zhu A, Kaneshiro M, Kaunitz JD. Evaluation and treatment of iron deficiency anemia: a gastroenterological perspective. Dig Dis Sci 2010;55(3):548–59.
21. Friedman AJ, Shander A, Martin SR, et al. Iron deficiency anemia in women: a practical guide to detection, diagnosis, and treatment. Obstet Gynecol Surv 2015;70(5):342–53.
22. Leung TY, Lao TT. Thalassaemia in pregnancy. Best Pract Res Clin Obstet Gynaecol 2012;26(1):37–51.
23. Verhovsek M, So CC, O'Shea T, et al. Is HbA2 level a reliable diagnostic measurement for beta-thalassemia trait in people with iron deficiency? Am J Hematol 2012;87(1):114–6.
24. Passarello C, Giambona A, Cannata M, et al. Iron deficiency does not compromise the diagnosis of high HbA(2) beta thalassemia trait. Haematologica 2012; 97(3):472–3.
25. Origa R, Moi P, Galanello R, et al. Alpha-thalassemia. In: Pagon RA, Adam MP, Ardinger HH, et al, editors. GeneReviews(R). Seattle (WA): 1993.
26. Weiss G, Goodnough LT. Anemia of chronic disease. N Engl J Med 2005;352(10): 1011–23.
27. Weiss G. Anemia of chronic disorders: new diagnostic tools and new treatment strategies. Semin Hematol 2015;52(4):313–20.
28. Gangat N, Wolanskyj AP. Anemia of chronic disease. Semin Hematol 2013;50(3): 232–8.
29. Bruno M, De Falco L, Iolascon A. How I diagnose non-thalassemic microcytic anemias. Semin Hematol 2015;52(4):270–8.
30. Horowitz KM, Ingardia CJ, Borgida AF. Anemia in pregnancy. Clin Lab Med 2013; 33(2):281–91.
31. Bolton-Maggs PH, Langer JC, Iolascon A, et al, General Haematology Task Force of the British Committee for Standards in Haematology. Guidelines for the diagnosis and management of hereditary spherocytosis—2011 update. Br J Haematol 2012;156(1):37–49.
32. Luzzatto L, Seneca E. G6PD deficiency: a classic example of pharmacogenetics with on-going clinical implications. Br J Haematol 2014;164(4):469–80.

33. Barcellini W, Fattizzo B, Zaninoni A, et al. Clinical heterogeneity and predictors of outcome in primary autoimmune hemolytic anemia: a GIMEMA study of 308 patients. Blood 2014;124(19):2930–6.
34. Lau P, Haesler WE, Wurzel HA. Positive direct antiglobulin reaction in a patient population. Am J Clin Pathol 1976;65(3):368–75.
35. Judd WJ, Barnes BA, Steiner EA, et al. The evaluation of a positive direct antiglobulin test (autocontrol) in pretransfusion testing revisited. Transfusion 1986; 26(3):220–4.
36. Naik R. Warm autoimmune hemolytic anemia. Hematol Oncol Clin North Am 2015; 29(3):445–53.
37. Berentsen S, Ulvestad E, Langholm R, et al. Primary chronic cold agglutinin disease: a population based clinical study of 86 patients. Haematologica 2006; 91(4):460–6.
38. Berentsen S, Tjonnfjord GE. Diagnosis and treatment of cold agglutinin mediated autoimmune hemolytic anemia. Blood Rev 2012;26(3):107–15.
39. Shapira Y, Vaturi M, Sagie A. Hemolysis associated with prosthetic heart valves: a review. Cardiol Rev 2009;17(3):121–4.
40. Beris P, Picard V. Non-immune hemolysis: diagnostic considerations. Semin Hematol 2015;52(4):287–303.
41. Liapis K, Charitaki E, Delimpasi S. Hemolysis in Wilson's disease. Ann Hematol 2011;90(4):477–8.
42. Marchand A, Galen RS, Van Lente F. The predictive value of serum haptoglobin in hemolytic disease. JAMA 1980;243(19):1909–11.
43. Galen RS. Application of the predictive value model in the analysis of test effectiveness. Clin Lab Med 1982;2(4):685–99.

Cardiovascular Disease in Women

Primary and Secondary Cardiovascular Disease Prevention

Monika Sanghavi, MD[a], Martha Gulati, MD, MS, FACC, FAHA[b],*

KEYWORDS

- Women • Cardiovascular disease • Primary prevention • Secondary prevention

KEY POINTS

- Primary and secondary prevention of cardiovascular disease will require involvement of an extended health care team. Obstetricians and gynecologists are uniquely positioned within the system because they are the primary or only contact women have with the system.
- A large portion of risk associated with cardiovascular disease is attributable to modifiable lifestyle changes and risk factor management.
- The broad application of studied and proven risk reduction strategies may help improve the burden of disease.

INTRODUCTION

Cardiovascular disease (CVD) remains the leading cause of death in the United States.[1] Despite advances in medical therapy, CVD claims the life of a woman every minute.[1] Although urgent and emergent cardiovascular issues require specialty training, the primary and secondary prevention of CVD is a large undertaking that requires involvement of an extended health care team.

Obstetricians and gynecologists are uniquely positioned within the health care system to improve cardiovascular health because they are often the only point of contact for women across the age spectrum. It is critical that obstetricians and gynecologists seize the opportunity to enhance primary and secondary CVD prevention by using the team approach.

Disclosures: There are no relevant conflicts of interest of any of the authors to disclose.
[a] Cardiology, Department of Medicine, University of Texas Southwestern Medical Center, 5323 Harry Hines Boulevard, Dallas, TX 75390-9047, USA; [b] Division of Cardiology, University of Arizona-Phoenix, 1300 North 12th Street, Suite 407, Phoenix, AZ 85006, USA
* Corresponding author. University of Arizona College of Medicine, 550 East Van Buren Street, Phoenix, AZ 85004-2230.
E-mail address: marthagulati@email.arizona.edu

Obstet Gynecol Clin N Am 43 (2016) 265–285
http://dx.doi.org/10.1016/j.ogc.2016.01.001
0889-8545/16/$ – see front matter © 2016 Elsevier Inc. All rights reserved.

CVD is an umbrella term, which encompasses coronary heart disease (CHD), peripheral vascular disease (PVD), and cerebrovascular (CV) disease. Although these disease processes have distinct clinical manifestations with unique treatments involving different specialties, including cardiologists/cardiovascular surgeons, vascular surgeons, and neurologists, respectively, all 3 are characterized by atherosclerosis caused by common risk factors.

Among CVDs, CHD makes up most events for both men and women less than the age of 75.[1] The incidence of CHD in women lags behind men by 10 years, suggesting a protective effect in women that is lost with age, specifically after the onset of menopause and cessation of endogenous estrogen production by the ovaries. However, it is important to recognize that young women are still affected, and quick, accurate diagnosis requires a high index of suspicion by all health care providers. In addition, it is never too early to initiate preventive measures.

This article focuses on CHD prevention (primary and secondary) with additional comments when needed regarding PVD and CV disease.

PRIMARY PREVENTION

Primary prevention involves the management of currently present risk factors to prevent the onset of CVD. Currently identified traditional risk factors, as discussed later, may account for up to 90% of population-attributable risk of heart disease.[2] This is in contrast to primordial prevention, which is the prevention of the onset of risk factors. The absence of traditional cardiac risk factors in midlife is associated with a low lifetime risk of heart disease.[3] Therefore, primordial prevention is the most definitive form of prevention but requires education and adoption of lifestyle changes at a very young age. Unfortunately, by the age of 55, most women have at least one major cardiac risk factor putting them at increased lifetime risk of CVD and making primary prevention of significant clinical relevance.

Traditional risk factors can be divided into nonmodifiable (age, sex, race, family history) and modifiable risk factors (smoking, blood pressure, cholesterol levels, physical activity, weight, diabetes mellitus, and diet). New, sex-specific risk factors have been identified for women and are reviewed (**Table 1**). Every clinic visit is an opportunity to help women understand and modify their risk factors.

Nonmodifiable Risk Factors

Age
Age is one of the most powerful predictors of CVD. The prevalence of CVD increases with age in both men and women.[4]

Table 1
Risk factors for cardiovascular disease

Traditional Nonmodifiable	Traditional Modifiable	Sex-Specific
Age	Smoking	Gestational hypertension
Sex	Physical inactivity	Gestational diabetes
Family history	Diet	Pre-eclampsia
Race	Weight	PCOS
	Diabetes mellitus	Breast cancer
	Hypertension	—
	High cholesterol	

Race

There are racial/ethnic differences in risk factors and CVD risk. Black adults have higher death rates at all ages compared with whites. Asian/Pacific Islanders may have lower heart disease death rates in all age groups, but higher stroke death rates at younger ages.[5] These differences may be explained by differences in risk factors. Black women have higher rates of hypertension compared with other races.[5] Hypercholesterolemia is generally high among Mexican American and white women.[5]

Family history

A premature family history of heart disease, defined as a first-degree relative with CHD before the age of 65 for women and 55 for men,[6,7] imparts an increased risk of heart disease. A parental history of premature CVD is associated with a multivariable adjusted odds ratio of 2 in men and 1.7 in women for the development of CVD compared with those without a premature family history.[8] The 2010 American College of Cardiology Foundation/American Heart Association (ACCF/AHA) Guideline for Assessment of Cardiovascular Risk in Asymptomatic Adults recommends that family history of atherothrombotic CVD should be obtained for cardiovascular risk assessment in all asymptomatic adults.[9]

Modifiable Cardiovascular Disease Risk Factors

Smoking

There is a strong and clearly established causal relationship between smoking and CVD. There is a lower prevalence of smoking among women than men (15.9% vs 20.5%)[1]; however, smoking is a stronger risk factor for CVD in women than men. There is a 25% higher relative risk of heart disease in women smokers compared with men smokers.[10]

Smoking reduction does not confer the same benefits as smoking cessation; therefore, smoking cessation is preferred. Smoking cessation is an important lifestyle modification that can reduce CV events and all-cause mortality.[11] The reduction in all-cause mortality is at least one-third in a *Cochran Review* of 20 studies.[11] In addition, the avoidance of passive environmental exposure is beneficial and highlights the need for smoking cessation to be a family-level intervention to ensure success for the patient.

The combination of counseling and pharmacotherapy provides higher rates of successful smoking cessation than either intervention alone.[12] When counseling a patient on smoking cessation, remember the 5A's (assess, advise, assist, arrange, and avoid) (**Box 1**).[13]

Of note, it is important to know that weight gain averages 2.3-4.5 kg after smoking cessation; this is especially a concern for women who are contemplating quitting. However, weight gain does not negate the benefits of smoking cessation.[14] One study demonstrated that vigorous exercise added to smoking cessation reduced the weight gain and increased the chance of abstinence.[12]

Hypertension

Women have a higher prevalence of hypertension compared with men after the age of 65.[15] Incremental increases in blood pressure have a strong linear association with cardiovascular and overall mortality starting at blood pressures of at least 115/75 if not lower.[16]

Screening is recommended for patients aged 18 or older by the US Preventive Service Task Force (USPSTF) and screening should continue at intervals of 2 years for normotensive individuals and annually for those classified as prehypertensive. Blood pressure should be measured when the patient is relaxed and seated with the arm

---

Box 1
5 A's of smoking cessation

1. Every tobacco user should be ADVISED at every visit to quit.
2. The tobacco user's willingness to quit should be ASSESSED at every visit.
3. Patients should be ASSISTED by counseling and by development of a plan for quitting that may include pharmacotherapy and/or referral to a smoking cessation program.
4. ARRANGEMENT for follow-up is recommended.
5. All patients should be advised at every office visit to AVOID exposure to environmental tobacco smoke at work, home, and public places.

From Sanghavi M, Khera A. Secondary prevention guidelines. In: Wong ND, Amsterdam EA, Blumenthal RS, editors. ASPC manual of preventive cardiology. 1st edition. New York: Demos Medical Publishing; 2015. p. 208; with permission.

---

outstretched and supported. Initial blood pressure measurements should be measured in both arms with the higher reading used for longitudinal monitoring. If there is greater than or equal to 20 mm Hg difference between the 2 arms, the patient should be referred for evaluation for possible vascular stenosis.

Diagnosis of hypertension is made when the blood pressure is greater than or equal to 140/90 on at least 2 separate occasions (**Table 2**). Recent USPSTF (US Preventive Services task Force) guideline updates recommend confirmation of hypertension diagnosis with ambulatory or home blood pressure monitoring.[17] Medication-induced increases in blood pressure (eg, nonsteroidal anti-inflammatory drug use, oral contraceptive pill use, steroids) should be excluded before confirming diagnosis and pursuing treatment options.

Once definitively diagnosed, maintaining good blood pressure control is an important aspect of risk reduction in these individuals. Of note, based on the 1999 to 2004 NHANES (National Health and Nutrition Examination Survey), hypertensive women were more likely to be treated than men, but are less like to achieve adequate blood pressure control.[18]

In general, a goal of less than 140/90 in those with hypertension is reasonable. There is some controversy regarding stricter versus more lenient blood pressure control, especially in older individuals after the latest JNC (Joint National Committee) 8 Panel guidelines.[19] A recently published trial, the SPRINT (Systolic Blood Pressure Intervention Trial), suggests certain patient populations may benefit from tighter control with a blood pressure target of less than 120/80.[20] A patient's individual target should be based on a discussion between provider and patient regarding risks and benefits.

Table 2
Classification of blood pressure

Classification	Systolic Blood Pressure	Diastolic Blood Pressure
Normal	<120	<80
Prehypertension	120–139	80–89
Stage I hypertension	140–159	90–99
Stage II hypertension	≥160	≥100

Adapted From Chobanian AV, Bakris GL, Black HR, et al. The Seventh Report of the Joint National Committee on prevention, detection, evaluation, and treatment of high blood pressure: the JNC 7 report. JAMA 2003;289(19):2561.

Blood pressure reduction should be a multipronged approach through dietary changes, weight loss, and increasing physical activity, as adjuncts to pharmacotherapy. These lifestyle changes can have a modest effect on blood pressure similar in magnitude to some blood pressure medications (**Table 3**). Multiple algorithms for blood pressure management exist.[21,22] The key is having a clear, algorithm that is simple to follow and implement and is applied consistently at every visit.

Diabetes mellitus

Diabetics have a 2- to 4-fold higher risk of CVD mortality compared with people without diabetes mellitus. Many studies suggest that diabetes conveys higher risk for CVD mortality in women compared with men.[23–25] Even type I diabetes has recently been shown to have twice the excess risk of fatal and nonfatal vascular events in women when compared with men.[26]

Screening at regular intervals should be considered for adults of all ages who are overweight (body mass index [BMI] $\geq$ 25 kg/m^2) or obese (BMI $\geq$ 30 kg/m^2) and have at least one other risk factor (including but not limited to women with polycystic ovarian syndrome [PCOS], history of gestational diabetes, women delivering babies >9 lb, and physical inactivity) according to the American Diabetes Association (ADA) 2015 guidelines.[27] The BMI cutoff for being overweight in Asian Americans has decreased to 23 kg/m^2 to reflect the increased risk in this population at lower BMI levels.[27] Screening is recommended to start at the age of 45 in the absence of risk factors with repeat testing at 3-year intervals.

Diabetes is diagnosed when either fasting blood glucose is greater than or equal to 126 mg/dL or glycated hemoglobin (HgbA1c) is greater than or equal to 6.5%, and prediabetes, or impaired fasting glucose, is diagnosed when fasting blood sugar is 100 mg/dL to 125 mg/dL and HgbA1c 5.7% to 6.4% (**Table 4**). Oral glucose tolerance tests can also be done but are not generally part of routine clinical practice. There is good evidence to suggest that intervention (lifestyle or medication) when patients have prediabetes can prevent or delay the onset of diabetes[28]; this is also true for women with a history of gestational diabetes.[29]

Table 3
Effect of lifestyle modifications on blood pressure

Modification	Recommendation	Average Systolic Blood Pressure Reduction Range
Weight reduction	Maintain normal body weight (BMI 18.5–24.9 kg/m^2)	5–20 mm Hg/10 kg
DASH eating plan	Adopt a diet rich in fruits, vegetables, and low-fat dairy products with reduced content of saturated and total fat	8–14 mm Hg
Dietary sodium restriction	Reduced dietary sodium intake to $\leq$100 mmol per day (2.4 g sodium or 6 g sodium chloride)	2–8 mm Hg
Aerobic physical activity	Regular aerobic physical activity (eg, brisk walking) at least 30 minutes per day, most days of the week	4–9 mm Hg
Moderation alcohol consumption	Women: limit to $\leq$1 drink per day	2–4 mm Hg

Adapted From Chobanian AV, Bakris GL, Black HR, et al. The Seventh Report of the Joint National Committee on prevention, detection, evaluation, and treatment of high blood pressure: the JNC 7 report. JAMA 2003;289(19):2561.

Table 4
Diagnosis of prediabetes and diabetes

Method for Diagnosis	Prediabetes	Diabetes
HbA1c	5.7%–6.4%	≥6.5%
Fasting plasma glucose[a]	100–125 mg/dL	≥126 mg/dL
2-h Oral glucose tolerance test[b]	140–199 mg/dL	≥200 mg/dL
Random plasma glucose[c]	—	≥200 mg/dL

[a] No caloric intake for 8 h.
[b] Glucose load of 75 g anhydrous glucose dissolved in water.
[c] In a patient with classic symptoms of hyperglycemia or hyperglycemic crisis.
Adapted from American Diabetes Association. (4) Foundations of care: education, nutrition, physical activity, smoking cessation, psychosocial care, and immunization. Diabetes Care 2015;38 Suppl:S20–30.

In those diagnosed with diabetes, lifestyle changes and metformin should be considered the first line of treatment and should be initiated in all individuals without a contraindication (hypersensitivity to metformin or renal dysfunction [creatinine ≥1.5 mg/dL in men and ≥1.4 mg/dL in women]). In addition, it should be used with caution in patients with impaired liver function. The goal hemoglobin A1c (HbA1c) in the general diabetic population is less than 7%. Lower or higher goals can be individualized based on duration of disease, comorbidities, and risk of hypoglycemia.

If an individual does not reach his or her HbA1c goal by 3 months, expert consultation should be considered so they can be started on an additional agent based on the risk-benefit profile of the other antihyperglycemics.[30]

Elevated body mass index
Almost two-thirds of Americans are considered overweight or obese, defined as a BMI greater than or equal to 25 kg/m[2].[31] BMI is a measurement of weight calibrated to a person's height. It is a tool by which practitioners can discuss weight loss goals with their patients. A normal BMI is considered to be between 18.5 and 24.9 kg/m[2]. There is good evidence from randomized trials that a 5% to 10% weight reduction can reduce the risk of CVD risk factors.[32]

Weight loss drugs can be considered in patients with a BMI greater than or equal to 30 kg/m[2] with no related comorbidities or in patients with a BMI greater than or equal to 27 kg/m[2] with comorbidities.[33] Referral for bariatric surgery can be considered in patients with severe obesity (BMI ≥ 40 kg/m[2] or BMI ≥35 kg/m[2] with comorbid conditions) when less invasive methods have failed.[33]

Some argue that BMI is not the best way to assess obesity because it does not take into account body composition and fat distribution. Getting a waist circumference (measured on the bare abdomen at the level of the iliac crest) is a simple way to assess abdominal adiposity and objectively monitor the effect of lifestyle changes. The normal value, according to the US Department of Health and Human Services, is less than or equal to 35 inches in women (the World Health Organization suggests lower cutoffs for specific ethnic populations). More advanced techniques to assess fat distribution are being used in research to help fine-tune risk assessment, but have not translated into general clinical practice.

Pregnancy is a time of significant weight gain, and 2 studies have shown that weight gain and retention at 1 year postpartum can result in an abnormal cardiometabolic profile[34] and is a predictor of being overweight in the future.[35] There is an opportunity for obstetricians to make an impact in a woman's cardiometabolic health by encouraging weight loss and healthy lifestyle changes as part of the postpartum visit.

Physical inactivity

Physical inactivity has a strong association with CHD with the lowest risk in those with the highest level of activity.[36] A recent study found that after the age of 30, the population risk of heart disease attributable to physical inactivity outweighed all other risk factors in women.[37] The AHA recommends at least 150 minutes of moderate intensity physical activity or 75 minutes of vigorous intensity activity per week, or an equivalent combination of moderate and vigorous intensity activity at least 3 days a week to target low-density lipoprotein cholesterol (LDL-C), non-high-density lipoprotein cholesterol (non-HDL-C), and blood pressure lowering.[38] Exercise does not have to be consecutive and can be divided up to help incorporate it into a busy schedule.

Simply monitoring physical activity can help increase it.[39] Use of pedometers and other activity trackers can help individuals track their activity and reach the recommended goal of at least 10,000 steps a day.

Diet

Diet can have a significant impact on CVD through weight, lipids, as well as blood pressure. There is little consensus regarding the optimal diet and dietary composition of macronutrients (carbohydrates, proteins, and fats). However, common characteristics of healthful dietary patterns include an emphasis on fruits, vegetables, beans and nuts, and in some, whole grains and fish.

The Dietary Approaches to Stop Hypertension (DASH) Dietary pattern, which is rich in fruits, vegetables, whole grains, and low fat dairy foods, is recommended for patients with hypertension or prehypertension and its adoption is associated a modest blood pressure reduction.[40] Blood pressure reduction is greatest when the DASH diet is combined with reduced sodium intake.[40]

The Mediterranean dietary pattern, which is rich in fruits, vegetables, legumes, nuts, fish, and low fat dairy with moderate consumption of olive oil as the primary source of fat, has an established role in the primary prevention of CVD from the results of the Prevención con Dieta Mediterránea (PREDIMED) trial. This study demonstrated a reduction in cardiovascular events with this diet, including a significant reduction in the risk of acute myocardial infarction (MI), stroke, and death from cardiovascular causes.[41]

The AHA recommends a diet low in saturated fats and high in fruits, vegetables, fish, whole grains, and high-fiber foods.[38]

There are many dietary options for individuals, and there is no clear consensus on which one is recommended. However, the overall goal of a diet is to reduce dietary intake to match energy expenditure when trying to maintain weight and maintaining a negative overall energy balance when trying to lose weight.

Alcohol Epidemiologic studies have demonstrated a nonlinear relationship between alcohol consumption and CHD events, with the lowest risk in light to moderate drinkers and higher risk at the 2 ends of the spectrum.[42] Recommendations for alcohol consumption depend on the individual's current consumption pattern. For women, heavy drinking is considered an average of more than 2 drinks per day. In general, light to moderate drinkers do not need to change their drinking habit and may enjoy a cardiovascular protective benefit. Heavy drinkers should be advised to reduce alcohol consumption to improve overall health risk. Those who abstain from alcohol should not be advised to drink for cardiovascular health benefit due to concern for progression to heavier drinking and alcohol dependence.

Vitamins Currently, there is insufficient evidence to recommend generalized use of multivitamins, antioxidants, B vitamins, vitamin E, and β-carotene in the prevention of CVD. There is some suggestion that calcium supplementation may do harm, but should not be withheld in women at risk of osteoporosis based on current data. Low vitamin D levels have been associated with cardiovascular risk[43]; however, it is unclear if the low level is a target for therapy or just a marker of risk. Trials with vitamin D supplementation have not demonstrated definitive benefit.[44] A large randomized trial of vitamin D and ω-3 is underway and, it is hoped, will help shed light on this question.[45]

Risk prediction models

Risk prediction models are tools that integrate multiple risk factors into a single risk score to help patients quantify and understand their overall risk. A personalized risk assessment can help to serve as a platform for discussion of lifestyle changes and pharmacotherapy as well as a motivational instrument. The AHA/American College of Cardiology (ACC) in 2013 introduced the Atherosclerotic Cardiovascular Disease (ASCVD) risk prediction system to help assess 10-year risk of fatal or nonfatal stroke, coronary death, and nonfatal MI, but also provides an assessment of lifetime risk that can be helpful in individuals with multiple risk factors but low short-term risk due to age or sex[46] (**Fig. 1**). This new scoring system has largely replaced the Framingham risk score for clinical risk assessment. The advantage of the new scoring system is that it also helps provide assessment of risk for stroke, which was not included in the Framingham score. In addition, the estimates of risk are based on data from multiple community-based populations and are applicable to African American and non-Hispanic white men and women.[47]

Other scoring systems used include the Reynold's score for women (which incorporates additional information such as high-sensitivity C-reactive protein [HsCRP] and family history), which has recently been shown to calibrate well in overall risk assessment.[48] However, the routine measurement of HsCRP is not recommended.

All individuals without diabetes, not on statins, and with LDL-C levels between 70 and 189 mg/dL should have their ASCVD score estimated. A risk score of greater than or equal to 7.5% suggests high risk, and treatment with statins should be considered. Previously, a cutoff of greater than 20% Framingham risk score was used as a threshold to initiate treatment. Some guidelines also recommend using a scoring system such as these to determine whether a patient should be on aspirin (see later discussion).

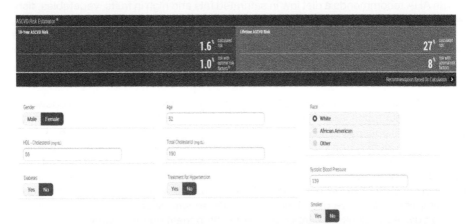

Fig. 1. ASCVD risk estimator. [a] Intended for use if there is not ASCVD and the LDL-cholesterol is <190 mg/dL. [b] Optimal risk factors include: total cholesterol of 170 mg/dL, HDL-cholesterol of 50 mg/dL, systolic BP of 110 mm Hg, not taking medications for hypertension, not a diabetic, not a smoker. (*From* American College of Cardiology. ASCVD risk estimator. Available at: http://tools.acc.org/ASCVD-Risk-Estimator/. Accessed February 26, 2016.)

A limitation of all of these models is that age and sex are such strong drivers of risk that young adults and women often have low short-term risk based on these algorithms, which is why the lifetime risk assessment by the ASCVD scoring system is beneficial for counseling. In addition, most risk calculators do not include nontraditional risk factors or sex-specific risk factors.

Cholesterol/statin therapy

Cholesterol levels have consistently been shown to be associated with cardiovascular risk. Increased levels of total cholesterol, LDL-C, and triglycerides imply higher risk, and conversely, lower levels of HDL-C are associated with higher risk. However, lowering of triglyceride and increasing HDL levels by pharmaceutical means have not demonstrated consistent CVD benefits. This finding is in contrast to LDL-C. Lowering LDL-C has consistently demonstrated a reduction in cardiovascular events. Although multiple medications have demonstrated a favorable improvement in cholesterol profiles, until recently, statins were the only pharmacologic therapy to demonstrate CV event reduction. Now ezetimibe, added to moderate intensity statin, has also demonstrated a reduction in CV events in those with established CHD.[49]

Recently, the guidelines have moved away from treatment to specific LDL-C targets and instead match treatment potency with calculated risk.[46]

The ACC/AHA Cholesterol Guidelines recommend statin therapy for 4 specific groups.[46] These groups include the following:

- Individuals over the age of 21 with established clinical ASCVD
- Individuals with a primary elevation of LDL-C levels greater than or equal to 190 mg/dL
- Diabetics aged 40 to 75 years old with LDL-C levels between 70 and 189 mg/dL
- Individuals without evidence of ASCVD or diabetes but with LDL-C levels between 70 and 189 mg/dL and a 10-year risk of ASCVD greater than or equal to 7.5%

Aspirin

Multiple guidelines have been released with no clear consensus on recommendations for treatment with aspirin for primary prevention.[7,50,51] However, most agree that the risk of bleeding must be weighed against the benefit of CVD risk reduction either by calculating the risk of bleeding and CVD events or by ensuring the risk of CVD events is higher than a certain threshold. In addition, aspirin's CVD benefit in women may be predominantly through the reduction of ischemic strokes rather than reduction of MIs. The 3 most commonly cited guideline recommendations for aspirin treatment are listed in **Table 5**.

Table 5
Guideline-based recommendations for aspirin use in primary prevention

Guideline	Recommendations for Aspirin Use in Primary Prevention
1. USPSTF (2009)[50]	Women, 55–79 y old, if stroke benefit[a] > bleeding risk[b]
2. ACCF/AHA (2009)[51]	Women, if 10-y CHD risk ≥20%[c]
3. AHA Guidelines for Prevention of CVD in Women (2011)[7]	Women ≥65 y old, if blood pressure is controlled and benefits of ischemic stroke and MI prevention > bleeding risk Women <65, aspirin is reasonable for ischemic stroke prevention

[a] Stroke risk can be calculated using tools such as the Western Stroke Calculator.
[b] Bleeding risk is based on the USPSTF table.
[c] Based on the Framingham Risk Score. Not based on the ASCVD risk score.
Data from Refs.[7,50,51]

Hormonal therapy

Although hormone replacement therapy after menopause makes physiologic sense (because estrogen has known favorable effects on lipid profiles and vascular endothelial function, and observational studies demonstrated significant benefit), hormonal replacement therapy (HRT) in postmenopausal women has been demonstrated to increase the risk of CHD and stroke events in women on estrogen and progestin. The Women's Health Initiative also showed an increased risk of stroke with no difference in CHD events in women on estrogen alone.[52] As a result, hormone replacement therapy is not recommended for the primary prevention of CHD.

The "timing hypothesis" questions whether there may be benefit of HRT in younger women, less than 10 years out from menopause based on subgroup analysis of the data. However, more studies are needed to definitively answer this age and timing hypothesis.

CEREBROVASCULAR DISEASE

The lifetime risk of stroke is greater in women compared with men, likely due to the fact that the risk of stroke substantially increases with age, and women, in general, have a longer life expectancy.[53,54]

The risk of stroke caused by atherosclerotic disease can be reduced by risk factor modifications as discussed above for CHD. Of all of the risk factors, hypertension is one of the most important modifiable risk factors for stroke. Women presenting with strokes are more likely to have a history of hypertension than men.[55] Pharmacologic treatment of hypertension can reduce the risk of a primary stroke by one-third.

Atrial fibrillation, an abnormal, irregular, heart rhythm arising from the upper chambers of the heart, is also a significant cause of ischemic strokes, usually through thromboembolism from thrombi in the left atrial appendage. Women with atrial fibrillation are at higher risk for ischemic stroke than men.[56] When diagnosed, the risk of stroke can be significantly reduced by initiation of anticoagulation therapy when appropriate. Women with a history of atrial fibrillation or those with undetermined causes of palpitations, dizziness, or shortness of breath should be referred for expert consultation for diagnostic and treatment purposes.

Recently released guidelines for prevention of stroke in women recognize the increased risk of stroke associated with pregnancy-related complications, such as pre-eclampsia and gestational hypertension. These guidelines recommend treating woman at high risk of pre-eclampsia with low-dose aspirin after 12 weeks' gestation and calcium in those with a low-calcium diet.[57]

PERIPHERAL VASCULAR DISEASE

Although most PVD risk factors are similar to those described for CVD, for patients with PVD, smoking is the most important risk factor and has the strongest correlation with developing peripheral arterial disease (PAD). Smoking cessation reduces the risk of disease progression, as evidenced by lower rates of amputations and lower incidence of rest ischemia in patients who quit. In addition, it reduces the risk of MI and death from other vascular causes as discussed above.

The USPSTF found insufficient evidence to recommend routine screening for PAD.[58] However, there may be a role for screening in certain high-risk populations. The ADA recommends ankle-brachial index screening in patients with diabetes 50 years of age or older, with repeat screening at 5-year intervals if normal. In addition, screening can be considered in those less than 50 years of age with risk factors.

The AHA recommends screening in those 65 years of age or older, or in those 50 or younger with a history of diabetes, smoking, exertional leg pain symptoms, or a non-healing ulcer.[59]

SEX-SPECIFIC RISK FACTORS
Gestational Hypertension and Pre-Eclampsia

A large cohort study in Finland found that any elevation of blood pressure in pregnancy is associated with an increased future risk of developing CVD, chronic kidney disease, and diabetes mellitus.[60] More specifically, women who experience pre-eclampsia have a 3.6- to 6.1-fold greater risk of developing hypertension, and a 3.1- to 3.7-fold higher risk of developing diabetes, depending on the severity of disease,[61] and are at increased risk of ischemic stroke.[62]

Gestational Diabetes

A history of gestational diabetes doubles the risk of diabetes postpartum and increases a woman's lifetime risk for developing diabetes.[63] Studies have also showed at least 1.5 times greater risk of CVD in women with a history of gestational diabetes compared with women without gestational diabetes.[64] These women need lifelong therapeutic lifestyle modifications[7] and diabetes screening at regular intervals.

Other Pregnancy-Related Risk Factors

Many other pregnancy-related risk factors, including preterm birth,[65] low gestational weight,[65] and number of live births, have associations with future risk of CVD[66,67] but need further investigation. Most recently, glycosuria and hemoglobin drop have also been associated with increased risk of CVD death.[68]

Polycystic Ovary Syndrome

PCOS is associated with many of the features of metabolic syndrome as well as insulin resistance.[69] In addition, studies have shown higher incidence of cardiovascular events in women with PCOS.[70] It remains unclear if PCOS is an independent risk factor for premature CVD in women. However, recent data suggest PCOS is associated with an elevated risk, independent of traditional risk factors in older postmenopausal women.[70]

Functional Hypothalamic Amenorrhea

It is estimated that up to 10% of premenopausal women have documented ovarian dysfunction and an even larger proportion has subclinical hormonal dysfunction that may result in an increased risk of CVD. In a large cohort study, women with menstrual irregularities had a 50% increased risk of nonfatal and fatal CHD compared with women with regular menstrual cycling. Additional data indicate that functional hypothalamic amenorrhea is associated with premature coronary atherosclerosis in women undergoing coronary angiography[71] and that use of oral contraceptive therapy may be protective.[72] Although these findings suggest that amenorrhea and cycling irregularity may be a risk factor for CVD in women, further work is still needed.

Breast Cancer Therapy

Recent advancements in breast cancer treatment have led to improved survival but increase a woman's future risk of CVD.[73] There is a linear relationship between the dose of ionizing radiation exposure during breast cancer radiotherapy and the risk of major coronary events in women.[74] The risk of CHD begins within a few years after exposure and appears to continue for at least 20 years, with the highest risk of CHD in those women with pre-existing CVD risk factors.[74]

In addition, commonly used chemotherapeutic agents, such as anthracycline and trastuzumab, increase the risk of heart failure and cardiomyopathy. Although it is unclear whether breast cancer itself, or specific therapies for breast cancer, increase the risk for CVD, this is an increasingly important issue in the management of women surviving breast cancer.

Risk assessment with sex-specific risk factors

Currently, there is no risk assessment tool that takes into account sex-specific risk factors or incorporates these nontraditional risk factors into the current risk assessment algorithm. Clinicians often do a personalized risk adjustment based on these factors and monitor women at regular intervals to assess and manage risk factors. Nonetheless, it is important to assess for these sex-specific risk factors and help women understand that they warrant more aggressive traditional risk factor modification and monitoring for CVD (see summary of recommendations in **Table 6**).

DISEASE MANAGEMENT AND SECONDARY PREVENTION
Coronary Heart Disease

Once a woman suffers an MI, she has a roughly 20% chance of having a heart attack or dying from CHD in the next 5 years. Although there is a lower prevalence of CVD in younger women (less than the age of 50), the consequences of premature CHD are more fatal for women compared with men, with a 2-fold increase in mortality after acute MI in women less than the age of 50 years.[75] The goal of secondary prevention is to slow the progression of disease once it is established and reduce the risk of future cardiovascular events. There is an expanding body of literature demonstrating that risk factor management through pharmacologic agents and lifestyle changes (see **Fig. 1**) can improve survival, reduce risk of recurrent events, and enhance quality of life in these patients.[13]

Table 6
Interval screening of risk factors

	Normal Risk Women	Women at Increased Risk	History of Pre-Eclampsia[a]
Diabetes[b]	Age ≥45, repeat every 3 years if normal	Any age if overweight with risk factors, repeat at regular intervals	Yearly blood pressure, lipids, fasting blood glucose, and BMI screening
Lipids[c]	Age ≥45, repeat every 5 years if normal	Women ≥20 who are at increased risk	
Blood pressure[c]	Age ≥18, repeat ever 3–5 years if normal	Annual screening for • Overweight • Prehypertension • African Americans • Age ≥40	
BMI[c]	All adults at regular intervals (consider evaluation at every visit)		

[a] Women with history of pre-eclampsia delivered at less than 37 weeks gestation or with recurrent pre-eclampsia. American College of Gynecology recommendations if benefits outweigh cost/risks.
[b] American Diabetes Association 2015 Guidelines.
[c] US Preventive Task Force recommendations.
Adapted from American Diabetes Association. (4) Foundations of care: education, nutrition, physical activity, smoking cessation, psychosocial care, and immunization. Diabetes Care 2015;38 Suppl:S20–30.

The risk factor modification strategy detailed above (with the exception of risk prediction models, which are not used once the presence of disease has been established) applies to secondary prevention of disease. However, there are additional disease-specific recommendations that need to be considered (**Fig. 2**).

Medications
Antiplatelet agents Aspirin 75 to 162 mg is recommended in all patients with CHD unless contraindicated. Clopidogrel 75 mg daily is an alternative for those who are intolerant or allergic to aspirin. The addition of P2Y12 receptor antagonists (clopidogrel, prasugrel, and ticagrelor) and duration of treatment are recommended based on the clinical presentation and intervention strategy.[13] Expert consultation is recommended regarding initiation and discontinuation of these agents.

Renin-angiotensin-aldosterone blockers Angiotensin-converting enzyme inhibitors (ACE-I) should be started and continued indefinitely in all patients with left ventricular ejection fraction 40% or lower and in those with hypertension, diabetes, or chronic kidney disease, unless contraindicated.[76] The most common side effect with ACE-I is a persistent, dry cough. Angiotensin receptor blockers can be substituted in those who are ACE-I intolerant.

β-blockers β-Blockers (carvedilol and Toprol XL) should be used indefinitely in all patients with left ventricular systolic dysfunction and for 3 years after an acute coronary

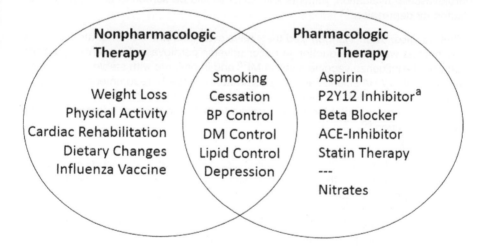

Nonpharmacologic Therapy
Weight Loss
Physical Activity
Cardiac Rehabilitation
Dietary Changes
Influenza Vaccine

Smoking Cessation
BP Control
DM Control
Lipid Control
Depression

Pharmacologic Therapy
Aspirin
P2Y12 Inhibitor[a]
Beta Blocker
ACE-Inhibitor
Statin Therapy

Nitrates

Indications for urgent cardiology consultation
- New or worsening chest pain
- New heart failure symptoms
- Worsening LV systolic function (ejection fraction)
- Difficult to control BP or lipids despite treatment or intolerance to medications

Fig. 2. Secondary prevention of coronary artery disease. [a]Only a short-term treatment after acute coronary syndrome or ACS, whereas the others are used long term. BP, blood pressure; DM, diabetes mellitus; LV, left ventricular.

syndrome.[11] Otherwise, β-blockers should be considered as an antianginal medication in patients with chronic angina and for therapy in patients with underlying hypertension or other tachyarrhythmias wherein chronic β-blocker use may be indicated.

Nitrates Nitrates can be used as antianginal medications in the oral form or as acute treatment of chest pain in the sublingual form.

Other considerations
Cardiac rehabilitation The use of cardiac rehabilitation in the secondary prevention of CHD is well established and supported. A recent meta-analysis supports 20% to 25% lower all-cause mortality and cardiac mortality in those undergoing exercise-based cardiac rehabilitation when compared with usual medical care.[77] Cardiac rehabilitation is recommended for all patients after acute coronary syndrome or coronary intervention (percutaneous coronary intervention or coronary artery bypass grafting) as well as for patients with chronic angina or PAD. Clinic visits are an opportunity to confirm awareness of this recommendation and encourage compliance.

Depression screening Depression has a 3-fold higher prevalence in patients with CHD than in the general population. Psychosocial factors such as depression are considered pathogenic because they often promote unhealthy behaviors and inhibit adherence to treatment recommendations. Therefore, as part of a comprehensive cardiovascular evaluation, patients with CHD should be screened and appropriately treated for depression.[13]

Influenza vaccination Randomized trials have evaluated and demonstrated a mortality benefit as well as a reduction in major adverse cardiovascular events in patients receiving the influenza vaccine after an MI[78] and in patients with stable coronary disease.[79] An ACC/AHA science advisory committee released a recommendation in 2006 commenting that "influenza vaccination is now recommend with the same enthusiasm as control of cholesterol, blood pressure, and other modifiable risk factors" for secondary prevention.[80]

Hormonal therapy
Oral contraceptives The 2006 American College of Obstetricians and Gynecologists guidelines suggests that the use of progestin-only contraceptives may be safer than combination oral, transdermal, or vaginal ring contraceptives in women with CHD, CV disease, hypertension with vascular disease, or age greater than 35 years, and tobacco use or obesity with age greater than 35.[81] An intrauterine device may also be an appropriate contraceptive choice in these women.[81]

Hormonal replacement therapy Based on the results of the Heart and Estrogen/progestin Replacement Study (HERS) I and HERS II trial,[82,83] HRT is not recommended for the secondary prevention of CHD in women. In general, women with underlying CVD or high risk of CVD should not be placed on HRT. Women with severe vasomotor symptoms requiring treatment should be offered other, nonhormonal treatment options.

Cerebrovascular Disease

A cornerstone of secondary stroke prevention due to atherosclerotic disease is antiplatelet therapy. Options include aspirin (81 mg daily is considered sufficient), dipyridamole, or clopidogrel. In addition, statin therapy is indicated for secondary stroke prevention.

Carotid endartectomy is important in the secondary prevention of stroke if done at the right time for patients with significant obstructive carotid artery disease.

Peripheral Vascular Disease

The presence of PVD is considered a CHD equivalent, and risk factors should be managed as such. The initiation of antiplatelet therapy with either 75 to 325 mg of

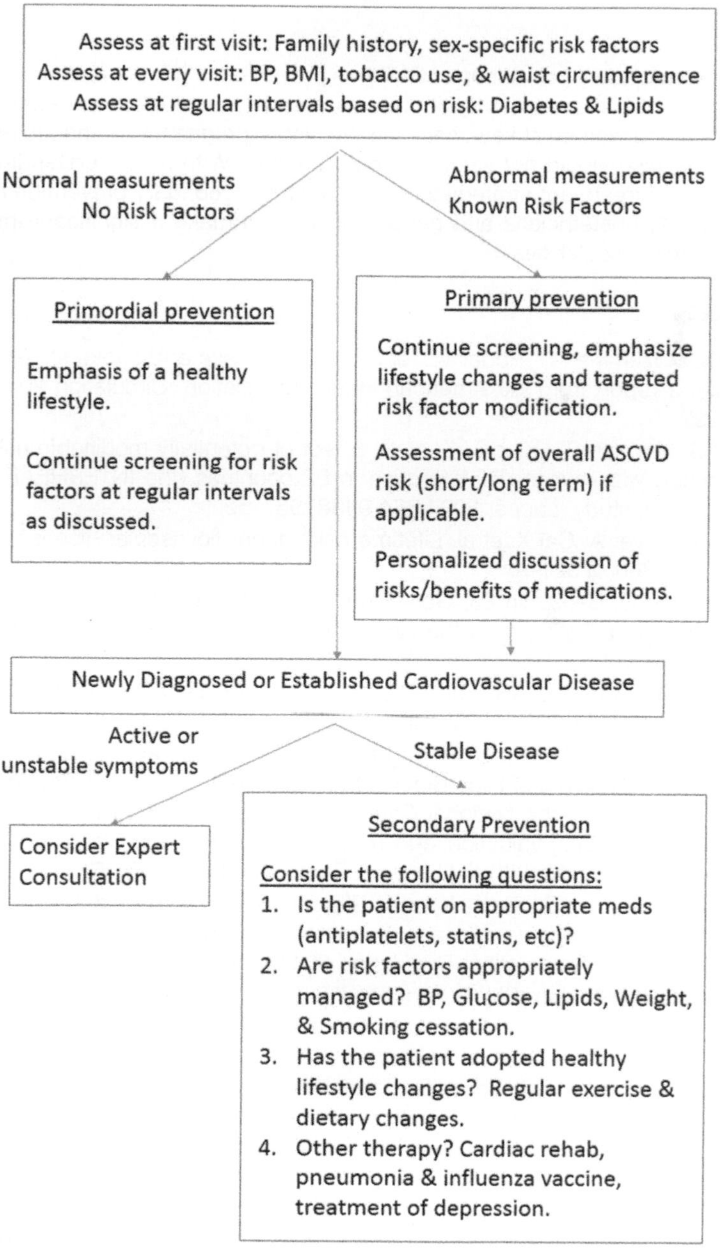

Fig. 3. Comprehensive cardiovascular evaluation in women.

aspirin or 75 mg of clopidogrel daily is considered standard of care in order to help reduce the risk of vascular death and MI.

A formal exercise program is the most effective treatment for PAD and can help improve symptoms and function in patients with claudication. Based on a meta-analysis, this intervention has been shown to be as effective as percutaneous angio-plasty in improving walking distance and quality of life in patients with intermitted claudication.[84]

SUMMARY

Primary and secondary prevention of CVD has proven benefit in preventing future CVD in women. Efforts in these areas by obstetricians and gynecologists can allow for additional outreach to women at key phases in their lives (pregnancy, menopause, and so on) who otherwise would not seek medical attention. With an understanding of the goals and basic treatment strategies for primary and secondary prevention (summarized in **Fig. 3**), obstetricians and gynecologists can make a significant impact on women's cardiovascular health.

REFERENCES

1. Go AS, Mozaffarian D, Roger VL, et al. Heart disease and stroke statistics–2014 update: a report from the American Heart Association. Circulation 2014;129(3): e28–292.
2. Yusuf S, Hawken S, Ounpuu S, et al. Effect of potentially modifiable risk factors associated with myocardial infarction in 52 countries (the INTERHEART study): case-control study. Lancet 2004;364(9438):937–52.
3. Berry JD, Dyer A, Cai X, et al. Lifetime risks of cardiovascular disease. N Engl J Med 2012;366(4):321–9.
4. Mozaffarian D, Benjamin EJ, Go AS, et al. Heart disease and stroke statistics–2015 update: a report from the American Heart Association. Circulation 2015; 131(4):e29–322.
5. Mensah GA, Mokdad AH, Ford ES, et al. State of disparities in cardiovascular health in the United States. Circulation 2005;111(10):1233–41.
6. National Cholesterol Education Program (NCEP) Expert Panel on Detection, Evaluation, and Treatment of High Blood Cholesterol in Adults (Adult Treatment Panel III). Third report of the National Cholesterol Education Program (NCEP) Expert Panel on Detection, Evaluation, and Treatment of High Blood Cholesterol in Adults (Adult Treatment Panel III) final report. Circulation 2002;106(25):3143–421.
7. Mosca L, Benjamin EJ, Berra K, et al. Effectiveness-based guidelines for the prevention of cardiovascular disease in women–2011 update: a guideline from the American Heart Association. Circulation 2011;123:1243–62.
8. Lloyd-Jones DM, Nam BH, D'Agostino RB Sr, et al. Parental cardiovascular disease as a risk factor for cardiovascular disease in middle-aged adults: a prospective study of parents and offspring. JAMA 2004;291(18):2204–11.
9. Greenland P, Alpert JS, Beller GA, et al. 2010 ACCF/AHA guideline for assessment of cardiovascular risk in asymptomatic adults: a report of the American College of Cardiology Foundation/American Heart Association Task Force on Practice Guidelines. Circulation 2010;122(25):e584–636.
10. Huxley RR, Woodward M. Cigarette smoking as a risk factor for coronary heart disease in women compared with men: a systematic review and meta-analysis of prospective cohort studies. Lancet 2011;378(9799):1297–305.

11. Critchley JA, Capewell S. Mortality risk reduction associated with smoking cessa-tion in patients with coronary heart disease: a systematic review. JAMA 2003; 290(1):86–97.

12. Rigotti NA. Treatment of tobacco use and dependence. New Engl J Med 2002; 346(7):506–12.

13. Smith SC Jr, Benjamin EJ, Bonow RO, et al. AHA/ACCF secondary prevention and risk reduction therapy for patients with coronary and other atherosclerotic vascular disease: 2011 update: a guideline from the American Heart Association and American College of Cardiology Foundation. Circulation 2011;124(22): 2458–73.

14. Williamson DF, Madans J, Anda RF, et al. Smoking cessation and severity of weight gain in a national cohort. New Engl J Med 1991;324(11):739–45.

15. National Centre for Health Statistics. Health, United States, 2009: with special feature on medical technology. Hyattsville (MD); 2010. Available at: http://www.cdc.gov/nchs/data/hus/hus09.pdf. Accessed February 16, 2016.

16. Lewington S, Clarke R, Qizilbash N, et al. Age-specific relevance of usual blood pressure to vascular mortality: a meta-analysis of individual data for one million adults in 61 prospective studies. Lancet 2002;360(9349):1903–13.

17. Screening for high blood pressure in adults: U.S. Preventive Services Task Force recommendation statement. Ann Intern Med 2015;163(10):778–86.

18. Gu Q, Burt VL, Paulose-Ram R, et al. Gender differences in hypertension treat-ment, drug utilization patterns, and blood pressure control among US adults with hypertension: data from the National Health and Nutrition Examination Sur-vey 1999-2004. Am J Hypertens 2008;21(7):789–98.

19. James PA, Oparil S, Carter BL, et al. 2014 evidence-based guideline for the man-agement of high blood pressure in adults: report from the panel members ap-pointed to the Eighth Joint National Committee (JNC 8). JAMA 2014;311(5): 507–20.

20. Wright JT Jr, Williamson JD, Whelton PK, et al. A randomized trial of intensive versus standard blood-pressure control. N Engl J Med 2015;373(22):2103–16.

21. Jaffe MG, Lee GA, Young JD, et al. Improved blood pressure control associated with a large-scale hypertension program. JAMA 2013;310(7):699 705.

22. Go AS, Bauman MA, Coleman King SM, et al. An effective approach to high blood pressure control: a science advisory from the American Heart Association, the American College of Cardiology, and the Centers for Disease Control and Pre-vention. Hypertension 2014;63(4):878–85.

23. Natarajan S, Liao Y, Cao G, et al. Sex differences in risk for coronary heart dis-ease mortality associated with diabetes and established coronary heart disease. Arch Intern Med 2003;163(14):1735–40.

24. Juutilainen A, Kortelainen S, Lehto S, et al. Gender difference in the impact of type 2 diabetes on coronary heart disease risk. Diabetes Care 2004;27(12): 2898–904.

25. Huxley R, Barzi F, Woodward M. Excess risk of fatal coronary heart disease asso-ciated with diabetes in men and women: meta-analysis of 37 prospective cohort studies. BMJ 2006;332(7533):73–8.

26. Huxley RR, Peters SA, Mishra GD, et al. Risk of all-cause mortality and vascular events in women versus men with type 1 diabetes: a systematic review and meta-analysis. Lancet Diabetes Endocrinol 2015;3(3):198–206.

27. Standards of medical care in diabetes–2015: summary of revisions. Diabetes Care 2015;38(Suppl):S4.

28. Gillies CL, Abrams KR, Lambert PC, et al. Pharmacological and lifestyle interventions to prevent or delay type 2 diabetes in people with impaired glucose tolerance: systematic review and meta-analysis. BMJ 2007;334(7588):299.
29. Aroda VR, Christophi CA, Edelstein SL, et al. The effect of lifestyle intervention and metformin on preventing or delaying diabetes among women with and without gestational diabetes: the Diabetes Prevention Program outcomes study 10-year follow-up. J Clin Endocrinol Metab 2015;100(4):1646–53.
30. American Diabetes Association. Standards of medical care in diabetes—2015 abridged for primary care providers. Clin Diabetes 2015;33(2):97–111.
31. Flegal KM, Carroll MD, Ogden CL, et al. Prevalence and trends in obesity among US adults, 1999-2008. JAMA 2010;303(3):235–41.
32. Rosenzweig JL, Ferrannini E, Grundy SM, et al. Primary prevention of cardiovascular disease and type 2 diabetes in patients at metabolic risk: an Endocrine Society clinical practice guideline. J Clin Endocrinol Metab 2008;93(10):3671–89.
33. Clinical guidelines on the identification, evaluation, and treatment of overweight and obesity in adults–the evidence report. National Institutes of Health. Obes Res 1998;6(Suppl 2):51S–209S.
34. Kew S, Ye C, Hanley AJ, et al. Cardiometabolic implications of postpartum weight changes in the first year after delivery. Diabetes Care 2014;37(7):1998–2006.
35. Linne Y, Dye L, Barkeling B, et al. Long-term weight development in women: a 15-year follow-up of the effects of pregnancy. Obes Res 2004;12(7):1166–78.
36. Oguma Y, Shinoda-Tagawa T. Physical activity decreases cardiovascular disease risk in women: review and meta-analysis. Am J Prev Med 2004;26(5):407–18.
37. Brown WJ, Pavey T, Bauman AE. Comparing population attributable risks for heart disease across the adult lifespan in women. Br J Sports Med 2015; 49(16):1069–76.
38. Eckel RH, Jakicic JM, Ard JD, et al. 2013 AHA/ACC guideline on lifestyle management to reduce cardiovascular risk: a report of the American College of Cardiology/American Heart Association Task Force on Practice Guidelines. Circulation 2014;129(25 Suppl 2):S76–99.
39. Bravata DM, Smith-Spangler C, Sundaram V, et al. Using pedometers to increase physical activity and improve health: a systematic review. JAMA 2007;298(19): 2296–304.
40. Sacks FM, Svetkey LP, Vollmer WM, et al. Effects on blood pressure of reduced dietary sodium and the Dietary Approaches to Stop Hypertension (DASH) diet. New Engl J Med 2001;344(1):3–10.
41. Estruch R, Ros E, Salas-Salvado J, et al. Primary prevention of cardiovascular disease with a Mediterranean diet. New Engl J Med 2013;368(14):1279–90.
42. Gaziano JM, Gaziano TA, Glynn RJ, et al. Light-to-moderate alcohol consumption and mortality in the Physicians' Health Study enrollment cohort. J Am Coll Cardiol 2000;35(1):96–105.
43. Wang TJ, Pencina MJ, Booth SL, et al. Vitamin D deficiency and risk of cardiovascular disease. Circulation 2008;117(4):503–11.
44. Autier P, Gandini S. Vitamin D supplementation and total mortality: a meta-analysis of randomized controlled trials. Arch Intern Med 2007;167(16):1730–7.
45. Manson JE, Bassuk SS, Lee IM, et al. The VITamin D and OmegA-3 TriaL (VITAL): rationale and design of a large randomized controlled trial of vitamin D and marine omega-3 fatty acid supplements for the primary prevention of cancer and cardiovascular disease. Contemp Clin Trials 2012;33(1):159–71.
46. Stone NJ, Robinson JG, Lichtenstein AH, et al. 2013 ACC/AHA guideline on the treatment of blood cholesterol to reduce atherosclerotic cardiovascular risk in

adults: a report of the American College of Cardiology/American Heart Association Task Force on Practice Guidelines. Circulation 2014;129(25 Suppl 2):S1–45.

47. Goff DC Jr, Lloyd-Jones DM, Bennett G, et al. 2013 ACC/AHA guideline on the assessment of cardiovascular risk: a report of the American College of Cardiology/American Heart Association Task Force on Practice Guidelines. Circulation 2014;129(25 Suppl 2):S49–73.

48. Cook NR, Paynter NP, Eaton CB, et al. Comparison of the Framingham and Reynolds Risk scores for global cardiovascular risk prediction in the multiethnic Women's Health Initiative. Circulation 2012;125(14):1748–56. S1-11.

49. Cannon CP, Blazing MA, Giugliano RP, et al. Ezetimibe added to statin therapy after acute coronary syndromes. New Engl J Med 2015;372(25):2387–97.

50. Aspirin for the prevention of cardiovascular disease. U.S. Preventive Services Task Force recommendation statement. Ann Intern Med 2009;150(6):396–404.

51. Redberg RF, Benjamin EJ, Bittner V, et al. AHA/ACCF [corrected] 2009 performance measures for primary prevention of cardiovascular disease in adults: a report of the American College of Cardiology Foundation/American Heart Association task force on performance measures (writing committee to develop performance measures for primary prevention of cardiovascular disease): developed in collaboration with the American Academy of Family Physicians; American Association of Cardiovascular and Pulmonary Rehabilitation; and Preventive Cardiovascular Nurses Association: endorsed by the American College of Preventive Medicine, American College of Sports Medicine, and Society for Women's Health Research. Circulation 2009;120(13):1296–336.

52. Writing Group for the Women's Health Initiative Investigators, Rossouw JE, Anderson GL, et al. Risks and benefits of estrogen plus progestin in healthy postmenopausal women: principal results from the women's health initiative randomized controlled trial. JAMA 2002;288(3):321–33.

53. Reeves MJ, Bushnell CD, Howard G, et al. Sex differences in stroke: epidemiology, clinical presentation, medical care, and outcomes. Lancet Neurol 2008; 7(10):915–26.

54. Petrea RE, Beiser AS, Seshadri S, et al. Gender differences in stroke incidence and poststroke disability in the Framingham heart study. Stroke 2009;40(4): 1032–7.

55. Roquer J, Campello AR, Gomis M. Sex differences in first-ever acute stroke. Stroke 2003;34(7):1581–5.

56. Fang MC, Singer DE, Chang Y, et al. Gender differences in the risk of ischemic stroke and peripheral embolism in atrial fibrillation: the AnTicoagulation and Risk factors In Atrial fibrillation (ATRIA) study. Circulation 2005;112(12):1687–91.

57. Bushnell C, McCullough LD, Awad IA, et al. Guidelines for the prevention of stroke in women: a statement for healthcare professionals from the American Heart Association/American Stroke Association. Stroke 2014;45(5):1545–88.

58. Moyer VA. Screening for peripheral artery disease and cardiovascular disease risk assessment with the ankle-brachial index in adults: U.S. Preventive Services Task Force recommendation statement. Ann Intern Med 2013;159(5):342–8.

59. Creager MA, Belkin M, Bluth EI, et al. 2012 ACCF/AHA/ACR/SCAI/SIR/STS/SVM/SVN/SVS key data elements and definitions for peripheral atherosclerotic vascular disease: a report of the American College of Cardiology Foundation/American Heart Association Task Force on Clinical Data Standards (Writing Committee to Develop Clinical Data Standards for Peripheral Atherosclerotic Vascular Disease). Circulation 2012;125(2):395–467.

60. Mannisto T, Mendola P, Vaarasmaki M, et al. Elevated blood pressure in pregnancy and subsequent chronic disease risk. Circulation 2013;127(6):681–90.
61. Lykke JA, Langhoff-Roos J, Sibai BM, et al. Hypertensive pregnancy disorders and subsequent cardiovascular morbidity and type 2 diabetes mellitus in the mother. Hypertension 2009;53(6):944–51.
62. Brown DW, Dueker N, Jamieson DJ, et al. Preeclampsia and the risk of ischemic stroke among young women: results from the Stroke Prevention in Young Women Study. Stroke 2006;37(4):1055–9.
63. Ratner RE. Prevention of type 2 diabetes in women with previous gestational diabetes. Diabetes Care 2007;30(Suppl 2):S242–5.
64. Rich-Edwards JW, Fraser A, Lawlor DA, et al. Pregnancy characteristics and women's future cardiovascular health: an underused opportunity to improve women's health? Epidemiol Rev 2014;36:57–70.
65. Smith GC, Pell JP, Walsh D. Pregnancy complications and maternal risk of ischaemic heart disease: a retrospective cohort study of 129,290 births. Lancet 2001; 357(9273):2002–6.
66. Sanghavi M, Kulinski J, Ayers CR, et al. Association between number of live births and markers of subclinical atherosclerosis: the Dallas Heart Study. Eur J Prev Cardiol 2015;23:391–9.
67. Parikh NI, Cnattingius S, Dickman PW, et al. Parity and risk of later-life maternal cardiovascular disease. Am Heart J 2010;159(2):215–21.e6.
68. Cirillo PM, Cohn BA. Pregnancy complications and cardiovascular disease death: 50-year follow-up of the child health and development studies pregnancy cohort. Circulation 2015;132(13):1234–42.
69. Moran LJ, Misso ML, Wild RA, et al. Impaired glucose tolerance, type 2 diabetes and metabolic syndrome in polycystic ovary syndrome: a systematic review and meta-analysis. Hum Reprod Update 2010;16(4):347–63.
70. Shaw LJ, Bairey Merz CN, Azziz R, et al. Postmenopausal women with a history of irregular menses and elevated androgen measurements at high risk for worsening cardiovascular event-free survival: results from the National Institutes of Health–National Heart, Lung, and Blood Institute sponsored Women's Ischemia Syndrome Evaluation. J Clin Endocrinol Metab 2008;93(4):1276–84.
71. Bairey Merz CN, Johnson BD, Sharaf BL, et al. Hypoestrogenemia of hypothalamic origin and coronary artery disease in premenopausal women: a report from the NHLBI-sponsored WISE study. J Am Coll Cardiol 2003;41(3):413–9.
72. Merz CN, Johnson BD, Berga S, et al. Past oral contraceptive use and angiographic coronary artery disease in postmenopausal women: data from the National Heart, Lung, and Blood Institute-sponsored Women's Ischemia Syndrome Evaluation. Fertil Steril 2006;85(5):1425–31.
73. Jones LW, Haykowsky MJ, Swartz JJ, et al. Early breast cancer therapy and cardiovascular injury. J Am Coll Cardiol 2007;50(15):1435–41.
74. Darby SC, Ewertz M, McGale P, et al. Risk of ischemic heart disease in women after radiotherapy for breast cancer. N Engl J Med 2013;368(11):987–98.
75. Vaccarino V, Parsons L, Every NR, et al. Sex-based differences in early mortality after myocardial infarction. National Registry of Myocardial Infarction 2 participants. New Engl J Med 1999;341(4):217–25.
76. Shaw LJ, Bugiardini R, Merz CN. Women and ischemic heart disease: evolving knowledge. J Am Coll Cardiol 2009;54(17):1561–75.
77. Taylor RS, Brown A, Ebrahim S, et al. Exercise-based rehabilitation for patients with coronary heart disease: systematic review and meta-analysis of randomized controlled trials. Am J Med 2004;116(10):682–92.

78. Gurfinkel EP, Leon de la Fuente R, Mendiz O, et al. Flu vaccination in acute coronary syndromes and planned percutaneous coronary interventions (FLUVACS) Study. Eur Heart J 2004;25(1):25–31.
79. Ciszewski A, Bilinska ZT, Brydak LB, et al. Influenza vaccination in secondary prevention from coronary ischaemic events in coronary artery disease: FLUCAD study. Eur Heart J 2008;29(11):1350–8.
80. Davis MM, Taubert K, Benin AL, et al. Influenza vaccination as secondary prevention for cardiovascular disease: a science advisory from the American Heart Association/American College of Cardiology. Circulation 2006;114(14):1549–53.
81. ACOG Committee on Practice Bulletins-Gynecology. ACOG practice bulletin. No. 73: use of hormonal contraception in women with coexisting medical conditions. Obstet Gynecol 2006;107(6):1453–72.
82. Hulley S, Grady D, Bush T, et al. Randomized trial of estrogen plus progestin for secondary prevention of coronary heart disease in postmenopausal women. Heart and Estrogen/progestin Replacement Study (HERS) Research Group. JAMA 1998;280(7):605–13.
83. Hulley S, Furberg C, Barrett-Connor E, et al. Noncardiovascular disease outcomes during 6.8 years of hormone therapy: Heart and Estrogen/progestin Replacement Study follow-up (HERS II). JAMA 2002;288(1):58–66.
84. Frans FA, Bipat S, Reekers JA, et al. Systematic review of exercise training or percutaneous transluminal angioplasty for intermittent claudication. Br J Surg 2012;99(1):16–28.

Hypertension in Women
Evaluation and Management

George W. Weyer, MD[a], Beth Dunlap, MD[b,1], Sachin D. Shah, MD[a,*]

KEYWORDS

- Hypertension • Women's health • Cardiovascular disease • Diagnosis • Treatment

KEY POINTS

- Hypertension is a leading cause of cardiovascular morbidity and mortality for women.
- Special considerations in women include the relationship of menopause to onset of hypertension, the impact of hormone replacement therapy on cardiovascular risk, and blood pressure effects of combined oral contraceptives and treatment of blood pressure in women of reproductive age.
- Diagnosis and appropriate staging of hypertension require sequential high-quality blood pressure measurements in the office setting, corroborated, when possible, with home- or ambulatory-based measurements.
- Treatment of elevated blood pressure or hypertension of any stage should include extensive and ongoing efforts to encourage lifestyle modifications.
- Choice of pharmacologic therapy, when initiated, should be individualized and should include medications with the best evidence for reducing cardiovascular morbidity and mortality.

INTRODUCTION

Hypertension is the most commonly encountered chronic medical condition in primary care and one of the most significant modifiable cardiovascular risk factors for women and men. The prevalence and severity of hypertension increase considerably with advancing age in women to the point that a higher proportion of women than men are hypertensive after age 65.[1] Timely diagnosis and evidence-based management offer an important opportunity to reduce the risk of hypertension-related morbidity and mortality, including cardiovascular events, end-stage renal disease (ESRD), and heart failure. High-quality clinical trials have repeatedly shown significant

Disclosure Statement: The authors have nothing to disclose.
[a] Department of Medicine, University of Chicago, 5841 South Maryland Avenue, MC 3051, Chicago, IL 60637, USA; [b] Department of Family and Community Medicine, Northwestern University, Abbott Hall, 4th Floor, 710 North Lake Shore Drive, Chicago, IL, USA
[1] Present address: 2323 Grand Avenue, Waukegan, IL 60085.
* Corresponding author.
E-mail address: sdshah@uchicago.edu

Obstet Gynecol Clin N Am 43 (2016) 287–306
http://dx.doi.org/10.1016/j.ogc.2016.01.002
0889-8545/16/$ – see front matter © 2016 Elsevier Inc. All rights reserved.

improvements in patient-oriented outcomes when hypertension is well controlled, yet many hypertensive patients remain undiagnosed, uncontrolled, or managed with inappropriate pharmacotherapy.

In this article, the initial diagnosis, evaluation, and management of hypertension in nonpregnant women are discussed, with a focus on topics of relevance for obstetrician-gynecologists (OB/GYNs) and other women's health providers. Hypertension management during pregnancy is not discussed, because this is outside of the area of expertise and the intended scope of this article.

HYPERTENSION AND CARDIOVASCULAR RISK IN WOMEN

OB/GYNs are well positioned to both diagnose and treat uncomplicated hypertension as well as recognize when referral is appropriate.[2] OB/GYNs frequently provide primary care to women; according to a recently published analysis of the National Ambulatory Medical Care Survey, primary care visits comprised 17.1% of all visits to OB/GYN providers in 2010.[3] Although the average age of women receiving primary care within OB/GYN practices is younger than those seen by generalists (38.3 years vs 55.4 years), 83.2% of these visits included office-based blood pressure (BP) assessment. In this setting, the reported frequency of a hypertension diagnosis was 8.6%.[3] This percentage approximates the 7.7% hypertension prevalence reported for reproductive-aged women in a recently published analysis of the National Health and Nutrition Examination Survey (NHANES) 1999 to 2008.[4]

In the US population as a whole, an estimated 32.6% of adults and 41.7 million adult women had a diagnosis of high BP in 2012.[1] Although fewer women than men less than age 45 have hypertension, the genders share a similar prevalence between ages 45 to 64, and, older than the age of 64, the prevalence of hypertension in women surpasses that of men (**Fig. 1**).[1]

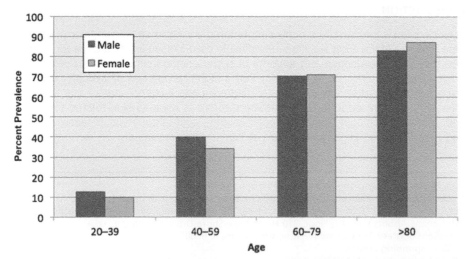

Fig. 1. Prevalence of high BP in adults by age and sex 2007 to 2010. (*From* National Institutes of Health and National Heart, Lung, Blood Institute. NHLBI Fact Book for Fiscal Year 2012. Disease statistics. 2013. Available at: http://www.nhlbi.nih.gov/about/documents/factbook/2012/chapter4. Accessed September 4, 2015.)

Although the prevalence of hypertension is lower for reproductive-aged women, younger patients are also less likely to be aware of their hypertension diagnosis, receive treatment, or have their hypertension controlled. Considering that only about 50% of the general population has adequately controlled hypertension, this is a particularly concerning finding.[5]

Cardiovascular disease is the leading cause of mortality in both women and men.[1] Among US women, cardiovascular disease was estimated to cause approximately 1 death per minute in 2007.[6] Despite reductions in incidence, it is estimated that annually 55,000 more women than men have strokes, with women aged 55 to 74 having a 1 in 5 lifetime risk versus 1 in 6 for men.[1,7] Although incidence and death rates for coronary heart disease (CHD) have also declined significantly for all populations in recent years (mortalities declined 39% between 2001 and 2009) and remain lower in women than men, this diagnosis continues to affect 5% of US women overall.

The relative contribution of hypertension to overall cardiovascular disease–related morbidity and mortality, particularly for women, is significant. Recent population-based studies have estimated the risk attributable to hypertension for overall cardiovascular disease is greater than other traditional risk factors (smoking, hyperlipidemia, obesity, and diabetes), accounting for one-third of cardiovascular disease incidence in women compared with one-fifth in men.[8,9]

In addition, hypertension is a major cause of ESRD and heart failure. The prevalence of heart failure with preserved ejection fraction, which is strongly linked to chronic, uncontrolled hypertension, has been sharply increasing, particularly in older women.[10]

Identification and treatment of hypertension are also important areas of focus to reduce health disparities related to cardiovascular disease. Non-Hispanic black race/ethnicity is a strong, nonmodifiable patient characteristic associated with increased hypertension risk; in addition to its higher prevalence, hypertension is also diagnosed at younger ages and is more difficult to control in this group.[4,11,12] Hypertension contributes in part to the large disparities in rates of cardiovascular disease between whites and blacks in the United States,[13] including a CHD attributable death rate of 88/100,000 in white women compared to with 99/100,000 in African American women in 2011.[1]

Improving rates of BP control in women improve cardiovascular outcomes. Clinical trials demonstrate significant reductions in cardiovascular disease risk in patients adequately treated for hypertension; reductions of 10 mm Hg in systolic BP or 5 mm Hg in diastolic BP result in a 41% decline in stroke rates and 22% decline in CHD, benefits that are consistent between women and men.[1,14,15]

SPECIAL CONSIDERATIONS FOR WOMEN

Although many of the risk factors for the development of hypertension in women are nonmodifiable, recent analyses of large population-based studies suggest that large proportions of hypertension incidence can be attributed to modifiable health risks.

Role of Obesity

A recent analysis of women of reproductive age using data from the NHANES revealed that advancing age (even within the premenopausal cohort), race/ethnicity, diabetes, chronic kidney disease, and obesity were all independent risk factors for hypertension. Of these, obesity, which is present in more than 30% of women of reproductive age, is the most significant modifiable risk factor.[4] Women with body mass index (BMI) of 30 to 35 kg/m^2 had a 4-fold increased likelihood of hypertension, whereas women with BMI greater than 35 kg/m^2 had a 6-fold increased likelihood.[4]

The importance of obesity as a risk factor for hypertension in women was also noted in the Nurses' Health Study II, a prospective cohort study started in 1991 that enrolled and followed 83,882 healthy women aged 25 to 41 for 14 years.[16] This study identified 6 modifiable risk factors for the development of hypertension, the most significant of which was obesity. An estimated 40% (95% confidence interval [CI], 38%–41%) of new cases of hypertension in this population was attributable to overweight or obesity (defined as BMI >25.0).[16] The other 6 modifiable risk factors, while statistically significant, accounted for smaller proportions of new cases. In order of diminishing population attributable risk, they are routine nonnarcotic analgesic use, not following the Dietary Approaches to Stop Hypertension (DASH) style diet, not engaging in daily vigorous exercise, no or excessive alcohol consumption, and supplemental folic acid use lower than 400 μg/d.[16]

Hypertension and Combined Oral Contraceptives

Combined oral contraceptives (COC) are widely prescribed for birth control and off-label purposes, with approximately 80% of American women using them at some time during the reproductive years. However, the development of hypertension secondary to COC therapy is also common[17] and requires physicians to balance the risks and benefits of this therapy in women.

The original Nurses' Health Study, which prospectively evaluated nearly 70,000 female nurses aged 25 to 42, showed that women taking COC have a significantly higher risk of hypertension compared with those who had never used COC. The relative risk (RR) was 1.8 for current COC users, and 1.2 for previous COC users, although the absolute risk was small, with only 41.5 cases of hypertension per 10,000 person-years attributable to COC use.[18] In early studies with high-dose estrogen (at least 50 μg) and a progestin dose of 1 to 4 mg, roughly 5% of women developed overt hypertension.[19] Current COC formulations contain as little as 20% of the estrogen and progestin as previous preparations, but hypertension seems to be associated with even these low-dose (30 μg) preparations. A 2015 meta-analysis showed, however, that there is no significant association between ever use of COC and all-cause mortality.[20]

Risk factors for the development of hypertension while on COC include a personal history of pregnancy-induced hypertension, family history of hypertension, occult renal disease, age greater than 35 years, and duration of COC use. The BP elevation due to COC is reversible, and discontinuation of use typically leads to a return to prior baseline BP within weeks.[21] If a patient remains hypertensive at 4 weeks after cessation of COC, the patient should be evaluated for chronic hypertension.

In patients with pre-existing chronic hypertension who desire contraception, COC are generally contraindicated, based on the risk for vascular complications, particularly in women who are older than 35 and smoke.[22] In one prospective cohort study of reproductive-aged women, only a small number had true contraindications to COC; however, hypertension was the most commonly encountered contraindication in this cohort.[23] A 2015 Cochrane meta-analysis looking at the risk of arterial thrombotic complications in women on COC showed that the risk was only increased with estrogen doses greater than 50 μg, and low-dose estrogen combined with levonorgestrel was the safest choice.[24]

Hypertension and Polycystic Ovarian Syndrome

In women with polycystic ovarian syndrome (PCOS), the hallmarks of which include androgen excess, infertility, and irregular menses, COC are first line for initial and ongoing treatment.[25] Although this therapy is highly effective for preventing endometrial cancer and mitigating some of the most bothersome side effects of androgen excess, these patients also often have comorbid cardiovascular risk factors. In US women with PCOS, about 30% exhibit symptoms of metabolic syndrome, which include hyperglycemia, insulin resistance, increased abdominal circumference, hypertension, and dyslipidemia.[26] Although the benefits of COC outweigh the risks in many of these patients, there must be careful ongoing monitoring for hypertension, smoking, and other metabolic parameters that may increase risk.[27]

Role of Menopause

The strongest nonmodifiable risk factor for hypertension in women is age.[1,4] Although postmenopausal women undeniably have a higher incidence of hypertension than reproductive-aged women, the independent role menopause plays on the incidence of hypertension is controversial.[28]

Age-related declines in estrogen may contribute to an increase in BP via activation of the renin-angiotensin system.[29] However, other potentially confounding risk factors also known to worsen with age, such as obesity and salt sensitivity, make it difficult to statistically distinguish the specific role of menopause.[28]

Clinically, the connection between menopause and hypertension is appropriately overshadowed by the question of whether the use of hormone replacement therapy (HRT) can ameliorate the increased risks of stroke and coronary artery disease associated with the menopause transition. In 2015, the Cochrane Collaboration reviewed and updated their meta-analysis of trials examining the utility of HRT for either primary or secondary prevention of cardiovascular disease and examined the hypothesis that the timing of HRT initiation relative to the onset of menopause may modify the impact on cardiovascular disease.[30]

The *Cochrane Review*'s subgroup analysis demonstrated lower overall mortality (RR 0.70, 95% CI 0.52–0.95) and CHD (death from cardiovascular causes and nonfatal myocardial infarction; RR 0.52, 95% CI 0.29–0.96) in the HRT group for those who started less than 10 years after menopause. However, there remained an increased risk for venous thromboembolism (VTE; RR 1.74, 95% CI 1.11–2.73) in the early HRT group. For women who started HRT more than 10 years after menopause, there was high-quality evidence that it had little effect on death or CHD, but significantly increased risk of stroke and VTE. The investigators caution, however, that definitive studies assessing the timing hypothesis with patient-centered endpoints would require larger populations with longer follow-up periods.[24]

Current guidance from major specialty societies suggests use of HRT for control of menopausal symptoms, while increasing the risks for VTE and breast cancer, generally carries an acceptable risk profile in recently postmenopausal women without significant comorbidities. However, they do not support the use of HRT for prevention of hypertension or cardiovascular disease.[31,32]

DIAGNOSIS OF HYPERTENSION

The office-based diagnosis of hypertension is made after at least 3 office BP measurements, taken with proper technique and on separate visits, are noted to be in the hypertensive range. See **Box 1** for the components of proper technique and **Box 2** for diagnostic definitions. BPs that are elevated before potentially anxiety-provoking examinations or procedures should be repeated afterward or at another encounter. Although proper technique may be challenging in everyday practice, it remains essential for accurate diagnosis.

Given the risks associated with overdiagnosis or underdiagnosis and potential for harm with overtreatment, particularly in the elderly, a physician diagnosing or treating

---

Box 1
Components of proper blood pressure measurement technique

- Seated for 3 to 5 minutes with back and both feet supported
- Proper sized blood pressure cuff placed over a bare arm
- No recent vigorous physical activity
- Calibrated machine or other device with appropriately trained clinical staff
- Arm supported at the level of the heart
- Quiet room with no conversation
- Free from pain or anxiety
- Empty bladder
- No smoking in past 30 minutes
- Patient free from stimulant medications (albuterol, over-the-counter decongestants, caffeine, illicits)

---

hypertension is obligated to either personally recheck the BP or ensure that his or her clinic has a reliable, high-quality BP measurement process in triage.[33]

White Coat Hypertension

White coat hypertension (WCHT) is a common clinical entity characterized by elevated (greater than 140/90) BP in the office, but normotensive measurements otherwise. WCHT is a common phenomenon with an approximate prevalence of 15%. Although seen in all types of patients, some guidelines cite women, particularly older women and pregnant women, as having a higher prevalence.[34] In addition, many studies show WCHT to be persistent across many separate visits with the same provider. The pathophysiology, although incompletely understood, is likely related to an exaggerated sympathetic response to the clinical environment.[35] Given the risks of overdiagnosis and treatment, particularly in older patients or in young women desiring children, it is important to remain aware of WCHT as a possible diagnosis.

The true clinical significance of WCHT is a matter of debate, because studies have shown inconsistent results. However, increasing evidence suggests WCHT is not a completely benign phenomenon. One study found patients with WCHT had an odds ratio of 4.6 for developing chronic hypertension compared with normotensive controls, over an 11-year follow-up period.[36] Other studies have shown an association between WCHT and signs of metabolic dysregulation, including dyslipidemia and impaired

---

Box 2
Diagnosis of hypertension

At least 3 separate visits with office-based blood pressure measurements 140/90 or higher
    A strong preference should be given for corroboration of elevated office-based
    measurements with either ambulatory or home-based measurements

or

One office visit with confirmed blood pressure measurement of 180/110 or higher
    This qualifies as either Hypertensive Urgency or Emergency and should be managed as such
    without waiting for subsequent visits. If a clear inciting cause is not identified, blood
    pressures at this level can be assumed to represent underlying chronic hypertension.

---

glucose tolerance.[37] Patients with WCHT will likely benefit from close follow-up, which should include global cardiovascular risk reduction counseling and lifestyle modifications as appropriate.

Ambulatory and Home Blood Pressure Monitoring

Given the complexities and potential confounding issues associated with office BP readings to both accurately diagnose and assess treatment of BP, home (HBPM) and 24-hour ambulatory BP monitoring (ABPM) are increasingly in use. According to the American Heart Association (AHA), home BP readings are better predictors of true cardiovascular risk and should be used in the evaluation and follow-up of patients with suspected or established hypertension. Home monitoring may be of particular value in special populations, including older women (who often have significant variability in pressures), pregnant women, and people with chronic kidney disease and diabetes, wherein BP control is of particular importance.

In the October 2015 update of their hypertension screening guideline, the United States Preventive Services Task Force (USPSTF) explicitly recommended obtaining ambulatory or home measurements before diagnosing hypertension.[38] This recommendation followed similar recommendations by the 2015 Canadian Hypertension Education Guidelines and the 2013 European Society of Hypertension and Society of Cardiology Guidelines, which both provide extensive guidance recommending home measurements particularly for patients with mild elevations on office measurement or in those without signs of end-organ damage and low overall cardiovascular risk.[34,39–41] Issues of cost and availability may limit ABPM and HBPM, but ABPM is becoming more widely reimbursed, and these readings should be used when possible, particularly in special populations such as the elderly and pregnant women.[42]

INITIAL EVALUATION OF HYPERTENSION
History and Physical Examination

There are several key historical elements that must be obtained from each patient with newly diagnosed hypertension. Assessment of pre-existing cardiovascular risk factors and other medical conditions, presence of target organ damage, and past antihypertensive therapy are essential. A comprehensive social and lifestyle history, which assesses dietary habits (including salt intake), alcohol consumption, tobacco use, stress levels, social support, and physical activity, provides additional valuable insight. The clinician should also inquire about any family history of hypertension, renal disease, early cardiovascular disease, stroke, or diabetes. See **Box 3** for a list of cardiovascular risk factors in women.

In the parous patient, a history of pre-eclampsia is an important marker of increased cardiovascular risk. Not only does a history of pre-eclampsia confer a higher risk for developing hypertension and diabetes, it doubles the risk of future coronary and cerebrovascular events.[6] Onset of pre-eclampsia before 32 weeks is even more concerning, placing women at 5 times higher risk for subsequent vascular disease. The AHA 2014 Guidelines for the Prevention of Stroke in Women suggest that women's cardiovascular risk should be evaluated as soon as 6 months postpartum after a pregnancy complicated by pre-eclampsia.[43]

Although OB/GYNs are significantly more likely than their internal medicine colleagues to take a pregnancy history and appreciate its importance on future cardiovascular risk, they are less likely to do follow-up evaluation for other cardiovascular risk factors.[44] The follow-up evaluation for other cardiovascular risk factors is an important next step to mitigating the excess risk.

Box 3
Cardiovascular risk factors in women

- Personal history of ASCVD or pre-eclampsia
- Dyslipidemia (high low-density lipoprotein and/or low high-density lipoprotein)
- Diabetes mellitus
- Hypertension
- Smoking
- Age greater than 55
- Family history of early CHD (first-degree male relative <55 or female <65)
- Obesity and/or metabolic syndrome
- Sedentary lifestyle
- Excess alcohol consumption

ASCVD, Atherosclerotic cardiovascular disease; includes acute coronary syndromes, history of myocardial infarction, stable or unstable angina, coronary or other arterial revascularization, stroke, transient ischemic attack, and peripheral arterial disease.

Current medications, including over-the-counter drugs and herbal supplements, should be reviewed in detail. Oral contraceptives, corticosteroids, sympathomimetics, and antimigraine drugs can cause elevations in BP. Nonsteroidal anti-inflammatory drugs besides aspirin can mitigate the effects of antihypertensive drugs and may cause some degree of BP elevations themselves.[45]

Physical examination should look for signs of secondary causes of hypertension and target organ damage as a consequence of hypertension (**Box 4**).

Box 4
Physical examination in patients with hypertension

- General appearance, BMI, skin
  - Evaluate for metabolic syndrome (abdominal obesity)
  - Evaluate for skin changes that may suggest rare secondary causes (eg, striae in Cushing syndrome)
- Funduscopy
  - Evaluate for retinal changes, such as hemorrhages, exudates, and papilledema
- Neck examination
  - Assess for thyromegaly and carotid bruits
- Cardiopulmonary examination
  - Crackles, jugular venous distension, or S3 gallop may indicate heart failure
- Abdominal examination
  - Palpable kidneys suggest polycystic kidney disease
  - Abdominal bruits may suggest renal vascular disease
- Neurologic examination
  - Evaluate mental status for changes suggestive of hypertensive encephalopathy
  - Evaluate for deficits suggestive of acute or previous stroke
- Vascular examination
  - Difference of >10mmHg in BP between arms may suggest subclavian stenosis or peripheral arterial disease
  - Reduced leg pulses or lower extremity BP suggest coarctation of aorta

All patients newly diagnosed with hypertension should undergo measurement of hemoglobin or hematocrit, serum electrolytes, serum creatinine, diabetes screening, and fasting lipid levels, urinalysis with microscopy, and 12-lead electrocardiography.[41] Additional testing may be indicated on the basis of history, clinical findings, suspicion for secondary causes (**Table 1**), or anticipated therapy.

Table 1
Secondary causes of hypertension

Secondary Cause	Prevalence	Symptoms	Testing	Treatment
Obstructive sleep apnea	Most common	Snoring Daytime sleepiness Morning headache Witnessed apneas	Polysomnography	CPAP
Primary aldosteronism	Common	Hypokalemia	Serum aldosterone, plasma renin activity	Spironolactone, eplerenone, surgery
Renal artery stenosis (fibromuscular dysplasia)	Common	Renal bruit Renal injury	Duplex Doppler ultrasonography, CT angiography, MR angiography	Revascularization in selected patients
Renal parenchymal disease	Uncommon	Abnormal GFR Proteinuria	Serum creatinine, spot protein-creatinine ratio or 24-h, renal US, possible biopsy	Treat underlying cause if possible
Drug-induced or heavy EtOH use	Uncommon	Drug specific	History	Cessation
Thyroid disorder	Uncommon	Hot or cold intolerant Constipation or diarrhea Irregular menstrual cycle	TSH, free thyroxine	Treat underlying disorder
Cushing syndrome	Rare	Buffalo hump Central obesity Moon facies Striae	Dexamethasone suppression test, 24-h urinary free cortisol, adrenal CT	Cause-dependent, often surgery
Pheochromoocytoma	Very rare	Headaches Diaphoresis Palpitations Labile BP	Plasma catecholamines or metanephrines; complex work-up; seek specialty assistance	Surgical

Abbreviations: CPAP, continuous positive airway pressure; CT, computed tomography; GFR, glomerular filtration rate; MR, magnetic resonance; TSH, thyroid-stimulating hormone; US, ultrasound.

Data from Weir MR. Hypertension. Ann Intern Med 2014. http://dx.doi.org/10.1001/jama.201; and Viera AJ, Neutze DM. Diagnosis of secondary hypertension: an age-based approach. Am Fam Physician 2010;82(12):1471–8.

Initial decision-making and triaging of hypertensive patients rely on the appropriate staging of hypertension (see *Hypertension management algorithms in* **Figs. 2** and **3**). For example, although patients with stage 1 hypertension may be offered an 8-week or longer trial of lifestyle modifications before initiation of pharmacotherapy, stage 2 hypertension should be addressed immediately with pharmacotherapy in addition to lifestyle changes.

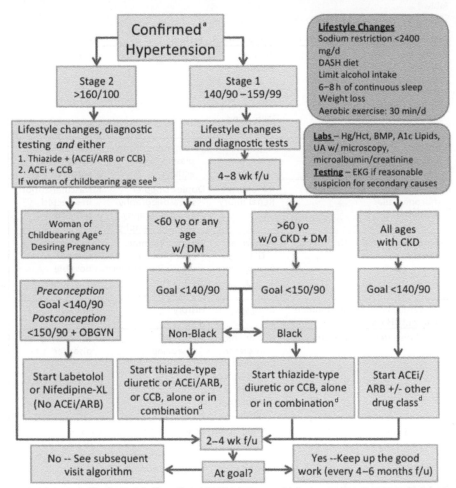

Fig. 2. Initial treatment approach for confirmed hypertension. [a] Unless BP is >180/110, a minimum of 3 separate office measurements is recommended with a preference for including ambulatory or home-based monitoring used to confirm the diagnosis. [b] If woman with stage 2 hypertension desires pregnancy, use Labetolol or Nifedipine XL with more liberal BP goal (<150/90). If not desiring pregnancy, then strongly consider long-acting reversible contraception (LARC) or progesterone-only oral contraception and treat as if non-childbearing. [c] If not desiring pregnancy, then strongly recommend an LARC, see CDC Medical Eligibility for Contraception Eligibility. [d] See the table of agents and compelling indications for specific drug classes. A1c, glycated hemoglobin; ACEi, angiotensin-converting enzyme inhibitor; BMP, basic metabolic panel; CCB, calcium channel blocker; CKD, chronic kidney disease; DM, diabetes mellitus; EKG, electrocardiogram; f/u, follow-up; Hg/Hct, hemoglobin/hematocrit; UA, urinalysis.

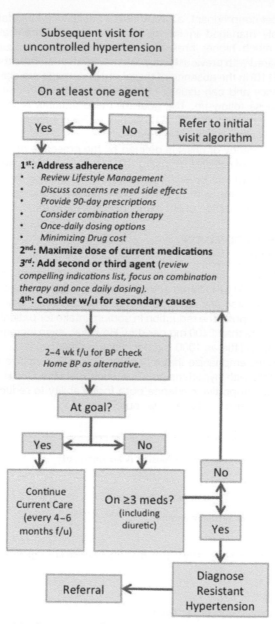

Fig. 3. Subsequent visits for uncontrolled hypertension.

Patients with severe hypertension ($\geq$180/110) require a careful analysis of risks for short-term complications and the presence of target organ damage. In a pregnant patient, severe hypertension may evolve over hours or days and is often associated with rapidly progressive target organ damage and fetal distress. For these women, sustained BPs of $\geq$160/110 qualify as a hypertensive emergency and require immediate inpatient evaluation and management to prevent adverse maternal-fetal outcomes.[46]

By contrast, most nonpregnant, asymptomatic adults with longstanding hypertension can be safely managed in the outpatient setting. Chronically hypertensive patients tolerate much higher pressures without developing acute target organ dysfunction compared with previously normotensive patients. Patients with severe hypertension ($\geq$180/110) in the absence of target organ damage are classified as having hypertensive urgency and can usually be managed safely with oral medications as outpatients with close follow-up. The goal for these patients is to reduce BP over days. Emergency evaluation and rapid reduction of BP in patients with hypertensive urgency are not indicated and may be harmful.[47]

Hypertensive emergency or crisis is defined by the presence of target organ damage as a consequence of rapidly increasing BP, irrespective of the absolute BP value. Clinical scenarios in which severe hypertension constitutes an emergency are included in **Box 5**. Patients with hypertensive emergency require admission to an intensive care unit for reduction of BP within minutes to hours.[47]

MANAGEMENT OF HYPERTENSION
Lifestyle Interventions

Lifestyle interventions are appropriate for every patient with hypertension. These lifestyle interventions should be initiated at the first visit in patients presenting with known or suspected hypertension and addressed at each subsequent visit.[48]

Strong evidence supports the reduction in sodium intake for patients with hypertension, ideally to no more than 2400 mg per day. However, even incremental reductions in sodium intake by as little as 1000 mg per day are effective.

The AHA guidelines emphasize that a healthy, culturally sensitive eating pattern is essential for patients with hypertension. One such diet, the DASH diet, outlined in **Table 2**, has strong supportive evidence both for its ability to reduce BP and for its ability to reduce long-term cardiovascular outcomes.[49]

Box 5
Clinical scenarios in which severe hypertension is an emergency

Cardiovascular
- Acute left ventricular failure with pulmonary edema
- Myocardial infarction or unstable angina
- Aortic dissection
- Postoperative from coronary artery bypass grafting or vascular surgery

Neurologic
- Hypertensive encephalopathy
- Subarachnoid or intracranial hemorrhage
- Thrombotic stroke
- Papilledema/retinal hemorrhage

Other
- Acute or worsening renal insufficiency
- Eclampsia
- Adrenergic crisis (catecholamine excess)
- Acute microangiopathic hemolytic anemia

Table 2
Dietary Advances to Stop Hypertension diet

Food Group	Servings (2000 Kcal/d)	Serving Size
Fresh vegetables	4–5	1 cup raw 1/2 cup cut-up or cooked
Fresh fruits	4–5	1 medium fruit ½ cup fresh ¼ cup dried
Whole-grain, high-fiber grains	6–8	1 slice of bread ½ cup cooked grain
Low-fat or fat-free dairy	2–3	1 cup milk or yogurt 1 1/2 oz cheese
Lean meats, poultry, or fish[a]	6 or less	1 oz cooked 1 egg
Fats and oils (plant-based preferred)	2–3	1 tsp
Nuts, seeds, legumes	3–4 per week	1 1/2 oz nuts 2 Tbsp or 1/2 oz seeds
Sodium	<2400 mg (<1500 mg offers more benefit)	
Sweets	<5 per week	1 Tbsp sugar

Patient Education Materials from the National Health Lung Blood Institute (NHLBI):
(1) Your guide to lowering your blood pressure with DASH. https://www.nhlbi.nih.gov/files/docs/public/heart/dash_brief.pdf.
(2) DASH recipes for heart health. http://www.nhlbi.nih.gov/health/resources/heart/hbp-dash-recipes-html.
[a] Oily fish most beneficial and lowest in mercury. Note that pregnant women or those planning pregnancy should avoid eating fish with the potential for the highest level of mercury contamination (eg, tuna, shark, swordfish, king mackerel, marlin, or tile fish).

Maintenance of a Healthy Body Weight

As described above, obesity is the leading modifiable risk factor for the development of hypertension, particularly in younger women. Women should maintain a healthy body weight (goal BMI of ≤ 25 kg/m^2 in US women) through a combination of appropriate levels of physical activity and dietary calorie intake.

Unfortunately, for obese or morbidly obese women, there is little evidence to suggest that standard medical management offers a clinically relevant probability of achieving a healthy body weight.[50] For morbidly obese women with appropriate risk profiles, bariatric surgery may result in larger and more durable reductions in body weight and more significant improvements in BP.[51]

Physical Activity

Women should be counseled to get at least 150 minutes per week of moderate aerobic exercise, 75 minutes per week of vigorous aerobic exercise, or an equivalent combination preferably performed in at least 10-minute episodes spread throughout the week. Women needing to lose weight or sustain weight loss should be counseled to target 60 to 90 minutes of at least moderate intensity activity (eg, brisk walking) on most, if not all, days of the week.[6]

Cigarette Smoke Exposure

Patients who smoke should be counseled on cessation; additional support may include pharmacotherapy if indicated and referral to intensive cessation programs.

Pharmacotherapy

General principles

Once the diagnosis of hypertension is made, pharmacotherapy, in conjunction with lifestyle modification, should be initiated if BP remains elevated at 140/90 mm Hg or higher. For most stage 1 patients, an 8-week trial of lifestyle modifications is reasonable before starting medications.

The initial choice of medication depends on many factors, including cost, patient age, comorbidities, race/ethnicity, other medication use, and potential side effects. In women of reproductive age, selection of therapy must be informed by an understanding of which medications are contraindicated during pregnancy or while breastfeeding.

Individualized treatment plan

Recommended treatment is summarized in the displayed algorithms (see **Figs. 2** and **3**).

Although there is ongoing controversy surrounding BP goals, recent guidelines suggest targeting less than 140/90 for most patients, including those with diabetes and chronic kidney disease at any age, and less than 150/90 for patients over the age of 60 with no history of those comorbidities.[40] Once the goal is established, choice of initial antihypertensive therapy is also individualized, although thiazide diuretics should be part of the drug regimen for most patients unless contraindicated or superseded by compelling indications for other agents in specific vascular diseases (summarized in **Table 3**).

In pregnant women with exposure to angiotensin-converting enzyme (ACE) inhibitors or angiotensin receptor blocker (ARBs), severe fetopathy has been well documented. Fetal effects associated with perinatal exposure to these classes include death, ESRD, intrauterine growth restriction, oligohydramnios, and severe cerebral and pulmonary complications. Both of these drug classes are contraindicated in reproductive-age women in the absence of effective contraception.[52,53]

Ongoing Management Considerations

Generally, agents from the 3 first-line drug classes (diuretics, ACE inhibitors or ARBs, and calcium channel blockers) should be used initially in patients with uncomplicated hypertension (**Table 4** lists common drugs by class). Recommended follow-up and

Table 3
Compelling indications

Indication	Recommended First-Line Drug Class(es)
Chronic kidney disease	*ACE inhibitor* (or ARB if intolerant)
Athrosclerotic cardiovascular disease	*β-Blocker* (preferred for patients with recent MI or angina), *ACE inhibitor* (or ARB if intolerant)
Diabetes	*ACE inhibitor* (or ARB if intolerant) indicated if complicated by diabetic nephropathy: otherwise *Thiazide Diuretic* or *CCB*
Recurrent stroke prevention	*Thiazide Diuretic, ACE inhibitor*
Heart failure	Guideline-based CHF treatment is recommended rather than isolated focus on hypertension; may include *Diuretic (Thiazide or Loop), β-Blocker, ACE inhibitor* (or ARB if intolerant), *aldosterone antagonist*

Abbreviations: CCB, calcium channel blocker; CHF, congestive heart failure; MI, myocardial infarction.

Table 4
Common drugs by class

Common Drugs by Class (Daily Dose Range, mg)	Advantages	Disadvantages/Side Effects	Line of Therapy
Thiazide diuretics HCTZ (12.5–50) *Chlorothalidone*[a] *(12.5–50)*	• Most effective in the elderly, those with isolated systolic hypertension, diabetics, African Americans, and those who are salt sensitive • *Inexpensive*	• May increase glucose, cholesterol, uric acid levels • Hypokalemia • Photosensitivity • Hyponatremia	1st line
ACE inhibitors Benazepril (10–80) Captopril (12.5–100) Enalapril (5–40) Lisinopirl (5–40) *Ramipril*[a] *(2.5–20)*	• Preferred for CKD, CHF, and diabetes • Works well with diuretics • *Generics usually inexpensive*	• Cough in 15% (switch to ARB) • Can increase SCr, acceptable up to 30% • Angioedema in 0.1%–0.7% • Hyperkalemia • Pregnancy category D	1st line
ARBs *Candesartan*[a] *(16–32)* Irbesartan (150–300) Losartan (25–100) Olmesartan (5–40) Valsartan (40–320)	• Works well with diuretics • Angioedema uncommon • Does not cause cough	• Dizziness • Hyperkalemia • Pregnancy category D	1st line
CCBs *Amlodipine*[a] *(2.5–10)* Diltiazem (120–360) Verapamil (120–480) Nifedipine (30–120)	• Well-tolerated and effective • Relatively inexpensive	• Diuretic-resistant edema (lesser problem if combined with ACE/ARB), headache, cardiac conduction defects • Constipation • Gingival hypertrophy	1st line
K+-sparing diuretics *Spironolactone*[a] *(25–100)* Triamterene (25–100)	• Most useful when a thiazide causes hypokalemia • Preferred in CHF if class II–IV with maximum medical therapy	• Hyperkalemia (rare with triamterene) • Gynecomastia • Weak antihypertensive	4th line
β-Blockers Atenolol (25–100) *Carvedilol*[a] *(6.25–50)* *Labetalol*[a] *(200–2400)* Metoprolol (25–400) Nadolol (40–320)	• Do not use β-blockers as initial therapy except in heart failure • Carvedilol is α- and β	• Masks hypoglycemia • Bronchospasm • Bradycardia • Worsens acute heart failure • Impairs peripheral circulation • Erectile dysfunction • Insomnia • Fatigue • Decreased exercise tolerance • Hypertriglyceridemia	5th line

(continued on next page)

Table 4 (continued)			
Common Drugs by Class (Daily Dose Range, mg)	**Advantages**	**Disadvantages/Side Effects**	**Line of Therapy**
Central β-agonists Methyldopa (500–3000) Clonidine (0.1–1.2)	Inexpensive	• Sedation • Dry mouth • Bradycardia • Rebound/withdrawal pertension • Constipation	5th line
Vasodilator Hydralazine (25–300)	Inexpensive	• Lupus reaction • Headache • Edema	5th line

Abbreviations: CCB, calcium channel blocker; CKD, chronic kidney disease; HCTZ, hydrochlorothiazide; SCr, serum creatinine.
 [a] Most effective agent in class.

monitoring by medication class are detailed in **Table 5**. In a patient with BP that is not well controlled with a particular agent, that medication should be titrated to its maximal effective dose before adding a second agent. When multiple antihypertensive medications are required, the use of combination therapy and once-daily dosing when possible can help improve adherence.

Resistant Hypertension

A patient whose BP is uncontrolled (>140/90 or >150/90 based on age and comorbidities) despite the use of 3 agents (one of which is a diuretic) at target doses is defined as having resistant hypertension.[40] The prevalence of resistant hypertension is increasing. NHANES data from 2005 to 2008 demonstrated approximately 13% of patients with hypertension are resistant.[54] Resistant hypertension is a complex, multifactorial disease, and many patients have significant underlying comorbidities. Initial assessment of these patients should include consideration of WCHT, salt consumption, and careful assessment of medication adherence with attention to side effects,

Table 5 Laboratory monitoring for medication side effects		
Drug Class	**Laboratory Tests**	**Frequency**
ACE inhibitors or ARBs	Potassium Serum creatinine[a]	• Before starting therapy (+) • 1–2 wk after starting or after dose increases (+)
Thiazide diuretics (+) Potassium sparing diuretics	Potassium[b] Serum creatinine[b] Sodium[c]	• Annually when on stable dose
β-blockers (+) Calcium channel blockers	No routine laboratory monitoring is required	

 [a] For patients started on ACE inhibitors or ARBs, increases in serum creatinine of up to 30% may generally be tolerated; consider specialty consultation when initiating ACE inhibitor or ARB in patients with significant renal impairment (stage IIIb chronic kidney disease or worse).
 [b] For patients started on diuretic therapy, fluid and electrolyte losses may result in potassium disturbances, oliguria, azotemia, and reversible increases in creatinine.
 [c] Particularly for elderly patients (>60 years), patients on multiple medications or with other comorbidities such as heart failure; diuretic therapy can lead to hypernatremia.

cost, or other issues. Secondary causes, particularly obstructive sleep apnea, are also appropriate to consider. These patients are appropriate referrals to an internal medicine or family physician, or to a hypertension specialist, if available.

SUMMARY AND DISCUSSION

Cardiovascular disease remains the leading cause of death for both women and men. The presence of hypertension confers a disproportionately higher risk for cardiovascular events compared with other traditional risk factors and is an effect more pronounced in women than men. Despite the significant cardiovascular risk, many hypertensive patients remain undiagnosed or uncontrolled, including a higher proportion of women than men after the age of 65.

Advancing age, race/ethnicity, diabetes, chronic kidney disease, and obesity are all independent risk factors for hypertension in women. Of these, obesity, which is present in more than 30% of women of reproductive age, is the most significant modifiable risk factor. The strongest nonmodifiable risk factor for hypertension in women is age. Although the incidence of hypertension increases after menopause, the role menopause plays on the incidence of hypertension remains controversial.

Hypertension developing as a result of COC therapy is common and reversible. Physicians must balance the risks and benefits of this therapy in women.

Besides hypertension and other traditional risk factors, PCOS (often associated with the metabolic syndrome) and a history of pre-eclampsia are important markers of increased cardiovascular risk in women. A history of these conditions should prompt the clinician to provide additional, ongoing guidance on improving these patients' modifiable risk factors to help mitigate excess cardiovascular risk.

Diagnosis and appropriate staging of hypertension require sequential high-quality BP measurements in the office setting corroborated, when possible, with home- or ambulatory-based readings. Initial evaluation should include careful assessment for signs of target organ damage and secondary causes, which significantly impact the timing and intensity of management.

Treatment of elevated BP or hypertension of any stage should include extensive and ongoing efforts to encourage lifestyle modifications. The choice of pharmacologic therapy, when initiated, should be individualized and should include medications with the best evidence for reducing cardiovascular morbidity and mortality.

REFERENCES

1. Mozaffarian D, Benjamin EJ, Go a S, et al. Heart disease and stroke statistics– 2015 update: a report from the American Heart Association. Circulation 2014; 131:e29–322.
2. Ehrenthal DB, Catov JM. Importance of engaging obstetrician/gynecologists in cardiovascular disease prevention. Curr Opin Cardiol 2013;28(5):547–53.
3. Edwards ST, Mafi JN, Landon BE. Trends and quality of care in outpatient visits to generalist and specialist physicians delivering primary care in the United States, 1997-2010. J Gen Intern Med 2014;29(6):947–55.
4. Bateman BT, Shaw KM, Kuklina EV, et al. Hypertension in women of reproductive age in the United States: NHANES 1999-2008. PLoS One 2012;7(4):e36171.
5. Egan BM, Zhao Y, Axon RN. US trends in prevalence, awareness, treatment, and control of hypertension, 1988-2008. JAMA 2010;303(20):2043–50.
6. Mosca L, Benjamin EJ, Berra K, et al. Effectiveness-based guidelines for the prevention of cardiovascular disease in women—2011 update: a guideline from the American Heart Association. Circulation 2011;123(11):1243–62.

7. Zahuranec DB, Lisabeth LD, Sánchez BN, et al. Intracerebral hemorrhage mortality is not changing despite declining incidence. Neurology 2014;82(24):2180–6.

8. Cheng S, Claggett B, Correia AW, et al. Temporal trends in the population attributable risk for cardiovascular disease: the atherosclerosis risk in communities study. Circulation 2014;130(10):820–8.

9. Wong ND, Thakral G, Franklin SS, et al. Preventing heart disease by controlling hypertension: impact of hypertensive subtype, stage, age, and sex. Am Heart J 2003;145(5):888–95.

10. Yancy CW, Jessup M, Bozkurt B, et al. 2013 ACCF/AHA guideline for the management of heart failure: a report of the American College of Cardiology Foundation/American Heart Association Task Force on practice guidelines. Circulation 2013;128(16):e240–327.

11. Hertz RP, Unger AN, Cornell JA, et al. Racial disparities in hypertension prevalence, awareness, and management. Arch Intern Med 2005;165(18):2098–104.

12. Ashaye MO, Giles WH. Hypertension in Blacks: a literature review. Ethn Dis 2003; 13(4):456–62. Available at: http://www.ncbi.nlm.nih.gov/pubmed/14632264. Accessed September 30, 2015.

13. Frieden TR. Forward: CDC health disparities and inequalities report—United States, 2011. MMWR Surveill Summ 2011;60(Suppl):1–2. Available at: http://www.ncbi.nlm.nih.gov/pubmed/21430612. Accessed September 30, 2015.

14. Turnbull F, Woodward M, Neal B, et al. Do men and women respond differently to blood pressure-lowering treatment? Results of prospectively designed overviews of randomized trials. Eur Heart J 2008;29(21):2669–80.

15. Law MR, Morris JK, Wald NJ. Use of blood pressure lowering drugs in the prevention of cardiovascular disease: meta-analysis of 147 randomised trials in the context of expectations from prospective epidemiological studies. BMJ 2009; 338:b1665.

16. Forman JP, Stampfer MJ, Curhan GC. Diet and lifestyle risk factors associated with incident hypertension in women. JAMA 2009;302(4):401–11.

17. Chasan-Taber L, Stampfer MJ. Epidemiology of oral contraceptives and cardiovascular disease. Ann Intern Med 1998;128(6):467–77. Available at: http://www.ncbi.nlm.nih.gov/pubmed/9499331. Accessed September 30, 2015.

18. Chasan-Taber L, Willett WC, Manson JE, et al. Prospective study of oral contraceptives and hypertension among women in the United States. Circulation 1996;94(3):483–9.

19. Woods JW. Oral contraceptives and hypertension. Hypertension 1988;11(3 Pt 2): II11–5. Available at: http://www.ncbi.nlm.nih.gov/pubmed/3280486. Accessed September 30, 2015.

20. Zhong G-C, Cheng J-H, Xu X-L, et al. Meta-analysis of oral contraceptive use and risks of all-cause and cause-specific death. Int J Gynaecol Obstet 2015;131(3): 228–33.

21. Pemu PI, Ofili E. Hypertension in women: part 1. J Clin Hypertens 2008;10(5): 406–10.

22. Centers for Disease Control and Prevention (CDC). U.S. medical eligibility criteria for contraceptive use, 2010. MMWR Recomm Rep 2010;59(RR-4):1–86. Available at: http://www.ncbi.nlm.nih.gov/pubmed/20559203. Accessed September 30, 2015.

23. Xu H, Eisenberg DL, Madden T, et al. Medical contraindications in women seeking combined hormonal contraception. Am J Obstet Gynecol 2014;210(3): 210.e1–5.

24. Roach REJ, Helmerhorst FM, Lijfering WM, et al. Combined oral contraceptives: the risk of myocardial infarction and ischemic stroke. Cochrane Database Syst Rev 2015;(8):CD011054.

25. Mortada R, Williams T. Metabolic syndrome: polycystic ovary syndrome. FP Essent 2015;435:30–42. Available at: http://www.ncbi.nlm.nih.gov/pubmed/26280343. Accessed September 30, 2015.

26. Ehrmann DA, Liljenquist DR, Kasza K, et al. Prevalence and predictors of the metabolic syndrome in women with polycystic ovary syndrome. J Clin Endocrinol Metab 2006;91(1):48–53.

27. Yildiz BO. Approach to the patient: contraception in women with polycystic ovary syndrome. J Clin Endocrinol Metab 2015;100(3):794–802.

28. Coylewright M, Reckelhoff JF, Ouyang P. Menopause and hypertension: an age-old debate. Hypertension 2008;51(4):952–9.

29. Reckelhoff JF, Fortepiani LA. Novel mechanisms responsible for postmenopausal hypertension. Hypertension 2004;43(5):918–23.

30. Hale GE, Shufelt CL. Hormone therapy in menopause: an update on cardiovascular disease considerations. Trends Cardiovasc Med 2015;25(6): 540–9.

31. Cobin RH, Futterweit W, Ginzburg SB, et al. American Association of Clinical Endocrinologists medical guidelines for clinical practice for the diagnosis and treatment of menopause. Endocr Pract 2006;12(3):315–37.

32. ACOG Practice Bulletin No. 141: management of menopausal symptoms. Obstet Gynecol 2014;123(1):202–16.

33. Benetos A, Labat C, Rossignol P, et al. Treatment with multiple blood pressure medications, achieved blood pressure, and mortality in older nursing home residents: the PARTAGE Study. JAMA Intern Med 2015;175(6):989–95.

34. Daskalopoulou SS, Rabi DM, Zarnke KB, et al. The 2015 Canadian Hypertension Education Program recommendations for blood pressure measurement, diagnosis, assessment of risk, prevention, and treatment of hypertension. Can J Cardiol 2015;31(5):549–68.

35. Mancia G, Bombelli M, Seravalle G, et al. Diagnosis and management of patients with white-coat and masked hypertension. Nat Rev Cardiol 2011;8(12): 686–93.

36. Sivén S, Niiranen T, Kantola I, et al. 1B.03: White-coat and masked hypertension as risk factors for progression to sustained hypertension: the Finn-home study. J Hypertens 2015;33(Suppl 1):e5–6.

37. Martin CA, McGrath BP. White-coat hypertension. Clin Exp Pharmacol Physiol 2014;41(1):22–9.

38. Screening for High Blood Pressure in Adults: U.S. Preventive Services Task Force Recommendation Statement. Ann Intern Med 2015;163(10):776–86.

39. Mancia G, Fagard R, Narkiewicz K, et al. 2013 ESH/ESC Guidelines for the management of arterial hypertension: the Task Force for the Management of Arterial Hypertension of the European Society of Hypertension (ESH) and of the European Society of Cardiology (ESC). J Hypertens 2013;31(7): 1281–357.

40. James PA, Oparil S, Carter BL, et al. 2014 Evidence-based guideline for the management of high blood pressure in adults. JAMA 2013;1097(5):1–14.

41. Chobanian AV, Bakris GL, Black HR, et al. The Seventh Report of the Joint National Committee on Prevention, Detection, Evaluation, and Treatment of High Blood Pressure: the JNC 7 report. JAMA 2003;289(19):2560–72.

42. National Coverage Determination (NCD) for Ambulatory Blood Pressure Monitoring (20.19). Available at: https://www.cms.gov/medicare-coverage-database/details/ncd-details.aspx?NCDId=254&ncdver=2&NCAId=6&ver=4&NcaName=Ambulatory+Blood+Pressure+Monitoring+(1st+Recon)&bc=AC AAAAAAIAAA. Accessed September 30, 2015.
43. Bushnell C, McCullough LD, Awad IA, et al. Guidelines for the prevention of stroke in women: a statement for healthcare professionals from the American Heart Association/American Stroke Association. Stroke 2014;45(5):1545–88.
44. Wilkins-Haug L, Celi A, Thomas A, et al. Recognition by women's health care providers of long-term cardiovascular disease risk after preeclampsia. Obstet Gynecol 2015;125(6):1287–92.
45. Snowden S, Nelson R. The effects of nonsteroidal anti-inflammatory drugs on blood pressure in hypertensive patients. Cardiol Rev 2011;19(4):184–91.
46. American College of Obstetricians and Gynecologists, Task Force on Hypertension in Pregnancy. Hypertension in pregnancy. Report of the American College of Obstetricians and Gynecologists' Task Force on Hypertension in Pregnancy. Obstet Gynecol 2013;122(5):1122–31.
47. Varon J, Marik PE. Clinical review: the management of hypertensive crises. Crit Care 2003;7(5):374–84.
48. Eckel RH, Jakicic JM, Ard JD, et al. 2013 AHA/ACC guideline on lifestyle management to reduce cardiovascular risk: a report of the American College of Cardiology/American Heart Association Task Force on Practice Guidelines. Circulation 2014;129(25 Suppl 2):S76–99.
49. Sacks FM, Svetkey LP, Vollmer WM, et al. Effects on blood pressure of reduced dietary sodium and the Dietary Approaches to Stop Hypertension (DASH) diet. DASH–Sodium Collaborative Research Group. N Engl J Med 2001;344(1):3–10.
50. Fildes A, Charlton J, Rudisill C, et al. Probability of an obese person attaining normal body weight: cohort study using electronic health records. Am J Public Health 2015;105:e1–6.
51. Wilhelm SM, Young J, Kale-Pradhan PB. Effect of bariatric surgery on hypertension: a meta-analysis. Ann Pharmacother 2014;48(6):674–82.
52. Cooper WO, Hernandez-Diaz S, Arbogast PG, et al. Major congenital malformations after first-trimester exposure to ACE inhibitors. N Engl J Med 2006;354(23): 2443–51.
53. Bullo M, Tschumi S, Bucher BS, et al. Pregnancy outcome following exposure to angiotensin-converting enzyme inhibitors or angiotensin receptor antagonists: a systematic review. Hypertension 2012;60(2):444–50.
54. Persell SD. Prevalence of resistant hypertension in the United States, 2003-2008. Hypertension 2011;57(6):1076–80.

Women's Health and Lung Development and Disease

Emily G. Kocurek, MD*, Anna R. Hemnes, MD

KEYWORDS

- Women • Interstitial lung disease • Pulmonary hypertension • Lung cancer
- Estrogen

KEY POINTS

- Lung structure and function in normal individuals is different in men and women.
- Many lung diseases have different prevalences, demographics, and courses in men and women, including chronic obstructive pulmonary disease, asthma, and interstitial lung diseases.
- Some diseases are limited to women whereas others are substantially more common in women.
- Recent epidemiologic and basic science work has begun to elucidate the sex-specific reasons for differences in lung disease in men and women.

INTRODUCTION

Although the lung is not traditionally thought of as an organ that is affected by sex-based differences, emerging literature elucidates major differences between men and women in development, physiology, and predilection to and outcomes in lung diseases. These differences are driven by differences in sex hormones, differential treatment effects, and differences in environmental exposures. However, in many cases the underlying etiology of these sex- and gender-based differences is unknown, and despite our emerging knowledge, diagnosis and treatment of lung disease is not yet sex specific. In this paper, we detail our existing knowledge regarding pulmonary disease in women and outline special considerations to keep in mind while caring for them in a primary care setting.

SEX-BASED DIFFERENCES IN PULMONARY PHYSIOLOGY

Divergence in the anatomy and molecular biology of the female and male respiratory systems commences in utero and continues throughout life, resulting in important

Conflicts of Interests: None.
Division of Allergy, Pulmonary and Critical Care Medicine, Vanderbilt University Medical Center, T1218 Medical Center North, 1161 21st Avenue South, Nashville, TN 37232, USA
* Corresponding author.
E-mail address: emily.g.kocurek@vanderbilt.edu

Obstet Gynecol Clin N Am 43 (2016) 307–323
http://dx.doi.org/10.1016/j.ogc.2016.01.003
0889-8545/16/$ – see front matter © 2016 Elsevier Inc. All rights reserved.

obgyn.theclinics.com

physiologic differences between the sexes. Sex hormones exert complex effects on lung maturation, which become functionally apparent at 16 weeks of gestation, and these effects persist throughout fetal development.[1] Androgens, for example, inhibit surfactant production and delay lung maturation in males, leading to an increased incidence of respiratory distress syndrome in male babies.[2] Androgens also promote increased airway branching, and researchers have observed that boy babies have larger lungs and more respiratory bronchioles at birth.[1] Sex differences endure into adulthood, and men are observed to have a larger airway diameter, number of alveoli, lung volume, and diffusion capacity compared with women.[3]

In addition to their anatomic differences, women are also exposed to a complex hormonal environment, and the effects of these hormones on the respiratory system are incompletely understood. Moreover, the hormonal environment is cyclical, and researchers have observed variations in respiratory physiology related to changing levels of estrogen in the menstrual cycle; for example, lung diffusion capacity nadirs in the follicular phase, and the lowest forced expiratory volume in 1 second (FEV_1) and forced vital capacity occur during the luteal phase.[4]

Although their cumulative effect on specific disease states remains to be elucidated, we know that estrogens influence almost every major part of the lung. Alveolar epithelial cells express estrogen/progesterone receptors, and in one study, mice that underwent ovariectomy experienced retarded alveolar development, which regenerated with the administration of estradiol.[5] Estrogen and progesterone influence alveolar fluid clearance, which could be of relevance in diseases such as cystic fibrosis and adult respiratory distress syndrmome.[6] Estrogen also has context-dependent effects on endothelial and smooth muscle proliferation, as well as on bronchial reactivity. In rats, chronic low-dose estrogen exposure yielded resistance to bronchoconstriction, but high doses of estrogen imparted sensitivity to a vasoconstrictive stimulus.[7] Finally, data suggest that sex hormones modulate immune and allergic responses; for instance, estradiol leads to degranulation in eosinophils and mast cells, and progesterone inhibits mast cells.[8]

OBSTRUCTIVE LUNG DISEASE

Women bear a significant and unrecognized amount of the burden of obstructive lung disease, and they experience increased susceptibility to disease and severity of illness when compared with men. To illuminate why this may be the case, we explore which risk factors are unique to women and how women are particularly affected by exposures.

Chronic Obstructive Pulmonary Disease

Chronic obstructive pulmonary disease (COPD), a chronic lung disease characterized by partially reversible airflow obstruction and inflammation, is the third leading cause of death in the United States, and the number of deaths from COPD exceeds those from lung and breast cancer combined.[9] The total number of deaths owing to COPD in women has exceeded men since 1999, and women made up about 57% of hospital discharges for COPD in 2010.[10,11] Unfortunately, women are more likely than men to have their COPD misdiagnosed or underdiagnosed. In one study observing primary care physicians, the likelihood that women were given a correct diagnosis of COPD was only 49.9%, compared with 64.6% of men. This discrepancy in diagnosis persisted even when physicians were given results of the patients' spirometry.[12] Symptoms suspicious for COPD that warrant performance of spirometry are shown in **Box 1**, and criteria for diagnosing and grading airflow limitation are shown in **Box 2**.[13]

Smoking is the major risk factor in both sexes for the development of COPD, and 250 million women still smoke worldwide.[14] Lung function seems to deteriorate more rapidly in women who continue to smoke, and women experience a greater decrease in lung function compared with men exposed to a similar amount of tobacco.[15] Secondhand smoke plays a role as well, and low-income women in particular are exposed to more environmental tobacco smoke.[16]

When examining the risks other than cigarette smoke for COPD, researchers have found that more nonsmoking women than men are diagnosed with COPD.[17] Research has shown that exposure to biologic dust increases the risk of COPD in women but not in men.[18] Additionally, more women than men are exposed to biomass fuel sources worldwide, which have been shown to increase the risk of COPD 2.4 times more than other fuel sources.[19]

Regarding disease severity, women describe more dyspnea when compared with men with similar lung function and tobacco use.[20] Women also experience more COPD exacerbations and a shorter interval of time before their first exacerbation, which may be explained by their increased incidence of diastolic dysfunction, which may worsen or imitate exacerbations.[21] Last, physicians should be aware that anxiety and depression are encountered more frequently in women than men with COPD and may complicate their disease.[22]

The cornerstones of COPD management include medications such as short- and long-acting anticholinergics and beta-agonists, inhaled corticosteroids, azithromycin, and roflumilast, as well as oxygen when needed, and pulmonary rehabilitation. Practitioners are urged to assess symptoms using questionnaires such as the COPD Assessment Test as well as the patient's risk for exacerbation and titrate medications accordingly. For details regarding therapy, we refer readers to goldcopd.org for a comprehensive treatment rubric. No sex differences in medication efficacy have been found. Both women and men report poor access to pulmonary rehabilitation, which has been shown to improve exercise capacity and health-related quality of life, as well as reduce hospitalizations.[23]

Primary care providers should be mindful of the possibility of COPD in their female patients. Spirometry is often warranted. Smoking is especially harmful in women, and women are also exposed to perhaps lesser recognized risk factors. Depression, anxiety, and diastolic dysfunction significantly impact women with COPD, and

---

Box 1
Consider chronic obstructive pulmonary disease and obtain spirometry if

Dyspnea
  Progressive
  Worse with exercise
  Persistent

Exposure to risk factors
  Tobacco smoke
  Home cooking and heating fuels
  Occupational dusts/chemicals

Chronic cough

Chronic sputum production

Family history of chronic obstructive pulmonary disease

Box 2
Severity of airflow limitation

Airflow limitation first confirmed by postbronchodilator FEV_1/FVC less than 0.70

Based on postbronchodilator FEV_1:

GOLD 1 (mild)
  FEV_1 ≥80% predicted

GOLD 2 (moderate)
  FEV_1 ≥50% but <80% predicted

GOLD 3 (severe)
  FEV_1 ≥30% but <50% predicted

GOLD 4 (very severe)
  FEV_1 <30% predicted

Abbreviations: FEV_1, forced expiratory volume in 1 second; FVC, forced vital capacity; GOLD, global initiative for chronic obstructive lung disease.
  Adapted from Global initiative for chronic obstructive lung disease pocket guide to COPD diagnosis, management, and prevention a guide for health care professionals. 2016. Available at: www.goldcopd.org.

---

physicians should identify and treat these conditions concomitantly. Pulmonary rehabilitation plays an integral role in therapy, and patients should be referred when at all possible.

Asthma

The prevalence and severity of asthma, which is a disease defined by reversible airflow limitation, inflammation, and airway hyperresponsiveness, seems to be related closely to levels of ovarian hormones in women, but this relationship is complex and incompletely understood. Keys to diagnosing asthma are listed in **Box 3**.[24] Girls who experience menarche younger than age 12 have a 2.08-times higher risk of having asthma compared with girls who reach menarche at age 12 or later.[25] After age 15, women are three times more likely than men to be hospitalized for an asthma-related event, independent of maintenance therapy or time to seeking medical help.[26] Pregnancy is not known to increase the risk of asthma.

Box 3
Consider asthma and obtain spirometry with features of recurrent airway obstruction

History of
  Cough
  Recurrent wheezing
  Recurrent dyspnea
  Recurrent chest tightness

Symptoms occur or worsen *at night* or with
  Exercise
  Viral infection
  Exposure to allergens and irritants
  Changes in weather
  Hard laughing or crying
  Stress
  Consider other causes of obstruction

In addition to the effects of menarche, monthly hormonal changes in women affect the airways. Both asthma symptoms and low peak flow rates appear when estrogen and progesterone concentrations are low.[27] To date, however, no studies have shown an increased rate of exacerbations during this time period, and more studies are needed to determine whether or not oral contraceptives might play a role in the modulation of asthma symptoms.

The prevalence of asthma does decrease at menopause, but women may have increased asthma symptoms during their transition to menopause.[28,29] Postmenopausal women who have not used hormone replacement therapy have a decreased risk of developing asthma compared with premenopausal women, but studies suggest an increased severity of symptoms when asthma is diagnosed during or after menopause.[29,30]

Primary care physicians should appreciate that female patients' phase of life may impact their risk for asthma as well as their asthma symptoms. There are, however, no current sex differences in recommendations of therapy for asthma. **Box 4** illustrates the recommended "stepwise approach" to the management of asthma in patients 12 years or older[24]; for additional information including alternative therapies we refer readers to the National Heart, Lung, and Blood Institute Asthma Guidelines.

Of note, many pregnant women have asthma, and the National Heart, Lung and Blood Institute as well as the Global Initiative for Asthma maintain that women should continue their current asthma regimen in pregnancy. Asthma medications are not associated with fetal abnormalities, and poorly managed asthma is associated with increased risk for preeclampsia, gestational diabetes, preterm birth, low birth weight, and perinatal mortality.[31]

Box 4
Stepwise approach to asthma management

Intermittent Asthma
Symptoms ≤ 2 d/wk
Nocturnal awakening $\leq 2\times$/mo
Short-acting beta$_2$-agonist for symptom control ≤ 2 d/wk
No interference with normal activity
  Step 1: Short-acting beta$_2$-agonist as needed

Persistent asthma: categorized as mild, moderate, or severe
Symptoms >2 d/wk up to throughout the day
Nighttime awakenings 3-4$\times$/month up to 7$\times$/wk
Short-acting beta$_2$-agonist >2 d/wk up to several times a day
  Step 2: Low-dose inhaled corticosteroid
  Step 3: Low-dose inhaled corticosteroid + long-acting beta$_2$ agonist *or* medium-dose inhaled corticosteroid
  Step 4: Medium-dose inhaled corticosteroid + long-acting beta$_2$ agonist
  Step 5: High-dose inhaled corticosteroid + long-acting beta$_2$ agonist and consider omalizumab if allergies
  Step 6: High-dose inhaled corticosteroid + long-acting beta$_2$ agonist + oral corticosteroid and consider omalizumab if allergies

Consider allergen immunotherapy at steps 2 to 3 if allergic asthma.

Consider consultation with asthma specialist beginning at step 3.

Data from Asthma care quick reference guidelines from the national asthma education and prevention program expert panel report 3. 2011. Available at: www.nhlbi.nih.gov/files/docs/guidelines/asthma_qrg.pdf. Accessed November 16, 2015.

INTERSTITIAL LUNG DISEASE

Interstitial lung disease (ILD) encompasses a broad category of disorders, so named because inflammation and fibrosis is proposed to occur in the interstitium of the lung, although in reality nearly all of the lung may be involved. Signs and symptoms that should make practitioners suspicious for ILD are listed in **Box 5**.[32]

There are more than 130 identified ILD's, caused by diverse insults as listed in **Box 6**, but this list is not exhaustive.[32] Inciting factors for some ILDs (such as sarcoidosis) are poorly understood and are beginning to be understood in others such as idiopathic pulmonary fibrosis. Sex disparities in ILD are also beginning to be elucidated. Sex disparities in ILD are most obvious for lymphangioleiomyomatosis (LAM), because this entity exclusively affects women, whereas connective tissue disease–ILD is more prevalent in women because connective tissue disease itself is more common in females, and idiopathic pulmonary fibrosis is more prevalent in elderly males.[33,34] A suggested workup for ILD is listed in **Box 7**.[32]

Primary care physicians should recognize ILD as a possibility in the differential diagnosis of patients with dyspnea. There are no currently recommended differences in therapy for ILD based on sex, and additional research is necessary to define and understand sex disparities in connective tissue disease–ILD and idiopathic pulmonary fibrosis.

Lymphangioleiomyomatosis

LAM is a rare pulmonary disease that uniquely affects women, with only four men ever reported with symptoms attributed to definite or probable LAM.[35] Untreated LAM results in a progressive decline in lung function that may culminate in death from respiratory failure at a relatively early age (median, 48 years).

Estrogen seems to be important to the pathogenesis of LAM, although the details are poorly understood. LAM cells are known to express estrogen and progesterone receptors, and LAM usually presents after puberty, may progress in pregnancy, and exhibits attenuated progression in menopause.[36–39]

Decline of lung function in patients with LAM is attributed to the influx of smooth musclelike cells of uncertain origin into the lung. These cells disrupt pulmonary lymphatics and produce cystic parenchymal damage. The underlying driver of disease

---

Box 5
Symptoms and signs suspicious for ILD

History of:
   Cough
   Dyspnea (especially insidious)
   Smoking
   Occupational or environmental exposures
   Connective tissue disease
   Certain medications
   Familial lung disease
   Recurrent pneumothorax

Physical exam:
   Exertional oxygen desaturation
   "Velcro" crackles
   Digital clubbing
   Extrapulmonary signs of systemic disease

Box 6
Classification of ILD

Known Cause

Connective tissue disease – ILD

Hypersensitivity pneumonitis
　Farmer's lung
　Hot tub lung
　Bird fancier's lung

Pneumoconioses
　Asbestosis
　Silicosis

Drug-induced ILD
　Chemotherapy
　Amiodarone
　Nitrofurantoin

Smoking-related ILD
　Langerhans cell histiocytosis
　Respiratory bronchiolitis-associated ILD
　Desquamative interstitial pneumonia

Radiation-induced ILD

Toxic inhalation-induced ILD
　Cocaine
　Ammonia

Unknown Cause or beginning to be understood

Idiopathic pulmonary fibrosis

Sarcoidosis

Other idiopathic interstitial pneumonias
　Cryptogenic organizing pneumonia
　Nonspecific interstitial pneumonia
　Lymphocytic interstitial pneumonia
　Acute interstitial pneumonia

Eosinophilic pneumonias

Lymphangioleiomyomatosis

Pulmonary alveolar proteinosis

Abbreviation: ILD, interstitial lung disease.
　Adapted from Ryu JH, Daniels CE, Hartman TE, et al. Diagnosis of interstitial lung diseases. Mayo Clin Proc 2007;82:977; with permission.

---

has been identified as constitutive activation of the mammalian target of rapamycin owing to loss of heterozygosity in tuberous sclerosis genes.[40] Given the high prevalence of LAM in patients with tuberous sclerosis, patients with this diagnosis are recommended to undergo regular screening for LAM; guidelines suggest either computed tomography (CT) scan of the chest at ages 18 and 30, or initial CT at age 18 and every 5 to 10 years thereafter if asymptomatic.[41,42]

LAM should be suspected in patients with the following features: spontaneous pneumothorax, chylous effusion, unexplained dyspnea, persistent or refractory asthma-type symptoms, or multicystic lung disease on chest imaging.[43] Eighty-two percent of patients experience their first pneumothorax before receiving a LAM diagnosis.[44] Delayed diagnosis is common.

Box 7
Workup of ILD and typical findings

Consider the following in addition to careful history and physical examination

Pulmonary function testing
   Reduced lung volumes
   Reduced DLCO

Chest radiograph
   Diffuse parenchymal infiltrates
   10% may be normal appearing

High-resolution computed tomography scan of the chest
   Consolidation
   Reticular pattern
   Nodular pattern
   Cystic airspaces
   Ground glass opacities
   Thickened interlobular septae
   Honeycombing

Laboratory testing
   Connective tissue disease serologies
   Hypersensitivity panel

Bronchoscopy in selected cases

Surgical lung biopsy in selected cases

Abbreviations: DLCO, diffusing capacity of the lung for carbon monoxide; ILD, interstitial lung disease.

Diagnosis is achieved with a combination of clinical symptoms, CT findings, vascular endothelial growth factor (VEGF)-D levels, and potentially tissue pathology. Typical pulmonary function testing in patients with LAM may be normal or show a decline in FEV_1, forced vital capacity, and diffusing capacity of the lung for carbon monoxide. Pulmonary function test patterns may be obstructive, nonspecific, or mixed.[43] Chest radiography may be normal, but CT will show thin-walled cysts of sub-centimeter to 3 cm in size.[45]

VEGF-D is produced by LAM cells and promotes lymphangiogenesis. VEGF-D is increased in 70% of patients with LAM, and levels greater than 800 pg/mL have a sensitivity of 73% and specificity of 100% for diagnosis.[46] If VEGF-D levels are normal, tissue diagnosis should be considered, especially if contemplating sirolimus.[43] Review by a pathologist with LAM expertise should be sought.

The Multicenter International Lymphangioleiomyomatosis Efficacy of Sirolimus (MILEs) trial demonstrated stabilization of FEV_1 and improvement in forced vital capacity with the administration of sirolimus, a mammalian target of rapamycin inhibitor, which was approved by the US Food and Drug Administration in May 2015 for the treatment of LAM; however, decline in lung function resumes with discontinuation of the drug.[47] Decline in FEV_1 and progressive dyspnea should prompt referral to a transplant center. Patients with LAM are perhaps best cared for in the LAM foundation's organized network of clinics.[43]

LUNG CANCER

Although lung cancer is the leading cause of death in both sexes, accumulating literature suggests that the disease is not homogenous in terms of risk factors for malignancy and tumor behavior between men and women. These distinctions have important clinical implications, not only for future prevention of disease and optimization of treatment strategies, but also potentially for the development of lung cancer screening methods specific to women.

Lung cancer kills more women than both breast and ovarian cancer combined, and its incidence has been increasing in women over the last 30 years, likely owing to the increased prevalence of female smokers in the United States during the 1960s and 1970s.[48] In fact, lung cancer deaths in women increased 16.8-fold between 1959 and 2010.[49] Women are diagnosed with lung cancer at an earlier age than men are diagnosed, with a significantly higher percentage of women diagnosed under age 50.[50]

Tobacco use is responsible for 80% of deaths due to lung cancer in women, and some studies suggest that women are more vulnerable to the effects of tobacco carcinogens than men.[51] Surprisingly, the majority (70%–80%) of lung cancer deaths in never smokers are women, and 15% of women compared with 2% of men with lung cancer have never smoked.[52] Additionally, tumor characteristics seem to be different between men and women, with women more likely to develop adenocarcinoma (41.1% of cancers), compared with men (34.1% of cancers).[50] Distinct molecular alterations are also more common in females with lung cancer, as described elsewhere in this paper.

Women seem to have improved lung cancer survival rates than men, independent of factors such as stage at diagnosis.[53] Some of their survival advantage has been attributed to an increased incidence of mutations such as epidermal growth factor receptor, which can be targeted with specific therapies.[54] ALK mutations can also be targeted specifically and may also be more common in women, particularly Asian women.[55] Studies have suggested that antiestrogen therapy in lung cancer may decrease mortality, but further investigation is needed.

Surgical resection of both small cell and non–small cell lung cancers affords women better survival rates than men, and women also show improved survival after radiation treatment.[56–58] In small cell lung cancer, chemotherapy seems to benefit women more than men, although certain chemotherapy drugs may have greater toxicity in women than men.[59] A basic algorithm for diagnosis and management of lung cancer is shown in **Box 8**[60]; however, treatment decisions are usually best made in a specialized multidisciplinary setting. For additional information we refer the reader to the third edition of *Diagnosis and Management of Lung Cancer* from the American College of Chest Physicians Evidence-Based Clinical Practice Guidelines, which can be found at www.chestnet.org.

Current screening guidelines for lung cancer indicate low-dose chest CT for individuals ages 55 to 74 with greater than or equal to a 30 pack-year smoking history, or if no longer smoking, cessation within the prior 15 years, or age greater than or equal to 50 years with a 20 pack-year history of smoking and one additional risk factor.[61] Because lung cancer seems to affect women at a younger age with less or no smoking history, and because women may exhibit a survival advantage when treated, further investigation into tailoring screening protocols specifically for women is warranted.

There are likely unique risk factors for lung cancer in women and different exposures than men that primary care physicians should keep in mind. These may alter the types and outcomes of lung cancer and its therapy. Further study is needed to determine whether there may be a benefit to antiestrogen therapy in lung cancer.

PULMONARY ARTERIAL HYPERTENSION

Pulmonary hypertension is characterized by increased pulmonary artery pressures that can result in right ventricular failure and death and is diagnosed via a mean

---

Box 8
Diagnosis and management of lung cancer

New, solid, indeterminate nodule on chest CT 8 to 30 mm

1. Assess surgical risk

2. If low to moderate surgical risk, assess clinical probability of malignancy. Consider use of quantitative model such as that from the Mayo Clinic.

3. If very low risk for malignancy, consider CT surveillance.
   Low to moderate risk for malignancy → PET to assess nodule.
   Depending on PET uptake and risk for malignancy, consider:
       CT surveillance
       Nonsurgical biopsy
       Surgical resection
   High risk for malignancy → PET to stage
   Metastasis → Biopsy most distant lesion → refer to medical/radiation oncology for chemotherapy or chemoradiation
   No metastasis → Biopsy confirms lung cancer → refer to thoracic surgery for resection. Note that patient may need lymph node staging via endobronchial ultrasound preoperatively.

4. If high surgical risk, consider nonsurgical biopsy or CT surveillance
   If nonsurgical biopsy, consider PET to stage
   Metastasis → Biopsy most distant lesion → refer to medical/radiation oncology for chemotherapy or chemoradiation
   No metastasis → Biopsy confirms lung cancer → refer to medical/radiation oncology and consider radiofrequency ablation or stereotactic body radiotherapy.

Abbreviation: CT, computed tomography.

---

pulmonary artery pressure of greater than 25 on right heart catheterization. Underlying disease pathogenesis is complex and is attributed to the intricate interplay of aberrant endothelial signaling (nitric oxide, endothelin), cell proliferation, thrombosis, and inflammation. The 2013 World Symposium of pulmonary hypertension assigned the following categories to pulmonary hypertension, according to the latest understanding of their underlying pathophysiology: group 1, pulmonary arterial hypertension (PAH); group 2, pulmonary venous hypertension owing to left heart disease; group 3, hypoxemic lung disease; group 4, chronic thromboembolic disease; and group 5, diverse diseases, including hematologic conditions and sarcoidosis.[62] Group 1 PAH includes both idiopathic and heritable PAH, and studies have shown a marked female prevalence, with a female to male ratio of 1.7 to 1.9:1 in mixed trials and 2:7:1 in heritable PAH, provoking interest in the role that sex plays in the development of PAH.[63] We focus our discussion on PAH, which is most highly influenced by gender, compared with the other groups of pulmonary hypertension.

Vascular remodeling in PAH consists of intimal hyperplasia and fibrosis, medial hypertrophy, and smooth muscle and endothelial dysfunction, with the most severe remodeling described as plexiform lesions. The most commonly mutated gene contributing to heritable PAH is the bone morphogenetic protein receptor type 2 (BMPR2) gene.[64] Although females seem clinically to be affected disproportionately, animal models have shown estrogen to be vasodilatory and beneficial to the pulmonary circulation.[65] Thus, attention has turned to estrogen metabolism as a potential explanation for this paradox.

Mutations in BMPR2 display variable penetrance, and the cytochrome P450 enzyme CYP1B1, which metabolizes estrogen to 2-hydroxyestradiol (2-OHE2) and

4-hydroxyestradiol, has been found to be ten times lower in affected compared with unaffected mutation carriers.[63] Lower CYP1B1 levels have been shown to lead to lower 2-OHE2 levels and higher 16-alpha-hydroxyestrogen levels.[66] Recently published data indicate that 16α-OHE in both heritable PAH patients and BMPR2 mutant mice promotes upregulation of the microRNA-29 family, a regulator of metabolism; furthermore, microRNA-29 antagonism improves the disease phenotype.[67]

The diagnosis of pulmonary hypertension should be entertained in patients with unexplained dyspnea or signs of right ventricular failure. The diagnosis is usually suggested by echocardiographic findings and should be confirmed with right heart catheterization. Evaluation focuses on elucidating potential causes as well as the degree of impairment and should include a complete history and physical as well as chest imaging, pulmonary function testing, and ventilation/perfusion scan to screen for chronic thromboembolic disease.[68] Treatment regimens are complex and include phosphodiesterase 5 inhibitors, endothelin receptor antagonists, and prostacyclin analogs, and these patients are generally best served at specialized centers.

Pregnancy in patients with pulmonary hypertension carries a prohibitive risk of maternal death owing to increased cardiac output and right ventricular demand.[69] Patients should be counseled to avoid pregnancy and to use two forms of birth control. Sterilization should be strongly considered. Estrogen-containing contraception generally should be avoided, with hysteroscopic sterilization and implantation of an intrauterine device being safer alternatives.[70] Pregnant patients with pulmonary hypertension should be referred to obstetricians specializing in high-risk pregnancies.

VENOUS THROMBOEMBOLISM

Although not exclusively a disease of women, venous thromboembolic disease occurs more frequently in women. This is owing to the presence of risk factors unique to women, such as pregnancy, oral contraceptive and pharmacologic estrogen exposure, and other risk factors more prevalent in women, such as antiphospholipid antibody syndrome. Estrogen exposure increases plasma fibrinogen and the activity of coagulation factors and promotes platelet aggregation. These coagulation changes are generally thought to be dose dependent as well.[71] A basic algorithm for diagnosis of pulmonary embolus is found in **Box 9** and a treatment algorithm is shown in **Box 10**.[72]

Box 9
Diagnosis of pulmonary embolism

Signs/symptoms of PE

Unstable → stabilize, consider massive PE

Stable →
  Estimate pretest probability via
    Modified Wells criteria
    Consider use of PERC

If pretest probability high, begin anticoagulation and perform CT angiogram

If pretest probability low/PERC positive, order D-dimer.
  D-Dimer negative → consider other diagnosis
  D-Dimer positive → perform CT angiogram
  CT angiogram positive → treat
  CT angiogram negative → consider D-dimer, reevaluate likelihood of diagnosis

Abbreviations: CT, computed tomography PE, pulmonary embolism; PERC, pulmonary embolism rule-out criteria.

Box 10
Treatment of VTE

Initiate anticoagulation
  LMWH
  Unfractionated heparin
  Fondaparinux
  Consider use of direct oral anticoagulant

Maintenance anticoagulation
  Warfarin
  Direct oral anticoagulant
  Low molecular weight heparin

General INR goal is 2 to 3

Consider LMWH if active malignancy

Heparin/fondaparinux must be continued for ≥ 5 days after initiation of warfarin and INR must be ≥ 2 for 2 consecutive days before discontinuation

LMWH may not be appropriate with underlying renal insufficiency

Abbreviations: INR, International Normalized Ratio; LMWH, low-molecular-weight heparin; VTE, venous thromboembolism.

Aside from the increased exposure to estrogens, pregnancy causes pelvic vascular congestion and compression by the enlarged uterus. Risks of venous thromboembolism (VTE) in pregnancy are estimated to 5- to 50-fold greater than the general population. Oral and transdermal contraceptive use in both young and older women increases the risk of VTE and in young women is the most important cause of VTE.[73,74] Additionally, hormone replacement therapy has been demonstrated to be associated with a 2-fold higher incidence of VTE.[75–77] Antiestrogens such as tamoxifen that are used in breast cancer therapy have also been associated with increased VTE risk.[78] Aside from recommending cessation of hormonal therapy when possible after VTE is identified, therapy recommendations and recurrence rates of VTE are not different in women. Moreover, in otherwise healthy young women without VTE risk factors, use of oral contraceptives is not contraindicated. The one exception to this is an anatomic variant found in women, May-Thurner syndrome. In this condition, an overlying right common iliac artery compresses the left common iliac vein into the vertebral body. This syndrome can be challenging to diagnose, but is predominantly in women and leads to left-sided deep venous thrombosis and chronic venous insufficiency. When identified, the vein may be stented to prevent recurrence, in addition to standard anticoagulation therapy.[79]

THORACIC COMPLICATIONS OF ENDOMETRIOSIS

Although endometriosis is generally thought to be a disease of the abdominal and pelvic organs, rarely the endometrial tissue can be also found in other organs, including the thorax. Within the thorax, endometriosis can affect the bronchus, pleura, parenchyma, and diaphragm.[80] The term definite thoracic endometriosis requires pathologic demonstration of endometrial tissue from thoracic cavity organs, whereas the thoracic endometriosis syndrome is used to describe clinical manifestations of thoracic endometriosis, such as pneumothorax, in association with menstruation or hemoptysis that occurs during menstruation only.[81,82] Within this spectrum of disease, pneumothorax is the most common. The term catamenial pneumothorax refers to the monthly occurrence of pneumothorax with menstruation, although in a small minority of patients the pneumothorax may occur at a time other than menses.[83] Often patients have a prior history of pelvic or uterine surgical procedures and the affected side is almost always the right.[84] Diagnosis can be confirmed by surgical exploration of the pleura when resection of endometrial tissue can occur as well, although immediate tube drainage of the pneumothorax is frequently required.[85] Even with surgical resection of the affected tissue, patients are usually treated with hormone suppression therapy postoperatively as well. Other, less common, presentations of thoracic endometriosis include hemothorax, hemoptysis, and pulmonary nodules.[82,86–89]

REFERENCES

1. Seaborn T, Simard M, Provost PR, et al. Sex hormone metabolism in lung development and maturation. Trends Endocrinol Metab 2010;21:729–38.
2. Torday JS, Nielsen HC. The sex difference in fetal lung surfactant production. Exp Lung Res 1987;12:1–19.
3. Hanna GM, Daniels CL, Berend N. The relationship between airway size and lung size. Br J Dis Chest 1985;79:183–8.
4. Farha S, Asosingh K, Laskowski D, et al. Effects of the menstrual cycle on lung function variables in women with asthma. Am J Respir Crit Care Med 2009;180:304–10.
5. Massaro D, Massaro GD. Estrogen regulates pulmonary alveolar formation, loss, and regeneration in mice. Am J Physiol Lung Cell Mol Physiol 2004;287:L1154–9.
6. Laube M, Küppers E, Thome UH. Modulation of sodium transport in alveolar epithelial cells by estradiol and progesterone. Pediatr Res 2011;69:200–5.
7. Degano B, Mourlanette P, Valmary S, et al. Differential effects of low and high-dose estradiol on airway reactivity in ovariectomized rats. Respir Physiol Neurobiol 2003;138:265–74.
8. Gilliver SC. Sex steroids as inflammatory regulators. J Steroid Biochem Mol Biol 2010;120:105–15.
9. World Health Organization (WHO). World health statistics. Geneva (Switzerland): World Health Organization; 2008.
10. Centers for Disease Control and Prevention (CDC). Deaths from chronic obstructive pulmonary disease – United States, 2000-2005. MMWR Morb Mortal Wkly Rep 2008;57:1229–32.
11. Centers for Disease Control and Prevention, National Center for Health Statistics. National hospital discharge survey. In: Education ALARaH, editor 2010.
12. Chapman KR, Tashkin DP, Pye DJ. Gender bias in the diagnosis of COPD. Chest 2001;119:1691–5.
13. Global initiative for chronic obstructive lung disease pocket guide to COPD diagnosis, management, and prevention a guide for health care professionals. 2016. Available at: www.goldcopd.org.
14. Fronczak A, Polańska K, Makowiec-Dabrowska T, et al. Smoking among women–strategies for fighting the tobacco epidemic. Przegl Lek 2012;69:1103–7 [in Polish].
15. Gan WQ, Man SF, Postma DS, et al. Female smokers beyond the perimenopausal period are at increased risk of chronic obstructive pulmonary disease: a systematic review and meta-analysis. Respir Res 2006;7:52.
16. Amos A, Greaves L, Nichter M, et al. Women and tobacco: a call for including gender in tobacco control research, policy and practice. Tob Control 2012;21:236–43.

17. Birring SS, Brightling CE, Bradding P, et al. Clinical, radiologic, and induced sputum features of chronic obstructive pulmonary disease in nonsmokers: a descriptive study. Am J Respir Crit Care Med 2002;166:1078–83.
18. Matheson MC, Benke G, Raven J, et al. Biological dust exposure in the workplace is a risk factor for chronic obstructive pulmonary disease. Thorax 2005;60: 645–51.
19. Po JY, FitzGerald JM, Carlsten C. Respiratory disease associated with solid biomass fuel exposure in rural women and children: systematic review and meta-analysis. Thorax 2011;66:232–9.
20. Watson L, Vestbo J, Postma DS, et al. Gender differences in the management and experience of Chronic Obstructive Pulmonary Disease. Respir Med 2004; 98:1207–13.
21. Almagro P, López García F, Cabrera F, et al. Comorbidity and gender-related differences in patients hospitalized for COPD. The ECCO study. Respir Med 2010;104:253–9.
22. Di Marco F, Verga M, Reggente M, et al. Anxiety and depression in COPD patients: The roles of gender and disease severity. Respir Med 2006;100: 1767–74.
23. Martinez CH, Raparla S, Plauschinat CA, et al. Gender differences in symptoms and care delivery for chronic obstructive pulmonary disease. J Womens Health (Larchmt) 2012;21:1267–74.
24. Asthma Care Quick Reference Guidelines from the National Asthma Education and Prevention Program Expert Panel Report 3. 2011. Available at: www.nhlbi. nih.gov/files/docs/guidelines/asthma_qrg.pdf. Accessed November 16, 2015.
25. Salam MT, Wenten M, Gilliland FD. Endogenous and exogenous sex steroid hormones and asthma and wheeze in young women. J Allergy Clin Immunol 2006; 117:1001–7.
26. Chen Y, Stewart P, Johansen H, et al. Sex difference in hospitalization due to asthma in relation to age. J Clin Epidemiol 2003;56:180–7.
27. Agarwal AK, Shah A. Menstrual-linked asthma. J Asthma 1997;34:539–45.
28. Real FG, Svanes C, Omenaas ER, et al. Lung function, respiratory symptoms, and the menopausal transition. J Allergy Clin Immunol 2008;121:72–80.e73.
29. Troisi RJ, Speizer FE, Willett WC, et al. Menopause, postmenopausal estrogen preparations, and the risk of adult-onset asthma. A prospective cohort study. Am J Respir Crit Care Med 1995;152:1183–8.
30. Balzano G, Fuschillo S, De Angelis E, et al. Persistent airway inflammation and high exacerbation rate in asthma that starts at menopause. Monaldi Arch Chest Dis 2007;67:135–41.
31. Lim A, Stewart K, König K, et al. Systematic review of the safety of regular preventive asthma medications during pregnancy. Ann Pharmacother 2011;45:931–45.
32. Ryu JH, Daniels CE, Hartman TE, et al. Diagnosis of interstitial lung diseases. Mayo Clin Proc 2007;82:976–86.
33. Fairweather D, Frisancho-Kiss S, Rose NR. Sex differences in autoimmune disease from a pathological perspective. Am J Pathol 2008;173:600–9.
34. American Thoracic Society. Idiopathic pulmonary fibrosis: diagnosis and treatment. International consensus statement. American Thoracic Society (ATS), and the European Respiratory Society (ERS). Am J Respir Crit Care Med 2000; 161:646–64.
35. Harknett EC, Chang WY, Byrnes S, et al. Use of variability in national and regional data to estimate the prevalence of lymphangioleiomyomatosis. QJM 2011;104: 971–9.

36. Gao L, Yue MM, Davis J, et al. In pulmonary lymphangioleiomyomatosis expression of progesterone receptor is frequently higher than that of estrogen receptor. Virchows Arch 2014;464:495–503.

37. Ryu JH, Moss J, Beck GJ, et al. The NHLBI lymphangioleiomyomatosis registry: characteristics of 230 patients at enrollment. Am J Respir Crit Care Med 2006; 173:105–11.

38. Johnson SR, Tattersfield AE. Decline in lung function in lymphangioleiomyomatosis: relation to menopause and progesterone treatment. Am J Respir Crit Care Med 1999;160:628–33.

39. Cohen MM, Freyer AM, Johnson SR. Pregnancy experiences among women with lymphangioleiomyomatosis. Respir Med 2009;103:766–72.

40. Henske EP, McCormack FX. Lymphangioleiomyomatosis - a wolf in sheep's clothing. J Clin Invest 2012;122:3807–16.

41. Johnson SR, Cordier JF, Lazor R, et al. European Respiratory Society guidelines for the diagnosis and management of lymphangioleiomyomatosis. Eur Respir J 2010;35:14–26.

42. Krueger DA, Northrup H. Tuberous sclerosis complex surveillance and management: recommendations of the 2012 International Tuberous Sclerosis Complex Consensus Conference. Pediatr Neurol 2013;49:255–65.

43. Berg JZ, Young L. Lymphangioleiomyomatosis. In: Hemnes A, editor. Gender, sex hormones, and respiratory disease: a comprehensive guide. 1st edition. New York: Springer; 2015. p. 173–88.

44. Almoosa KF, Ryu JH, Mendez J, et al. Management of pneumothorax in lymphangioleiomyomatosis: effects on recurrence and lung transplantation complications. Chest 2006;129:1274–81.

45. Abbott GF, Rosado-de-Christenson ML, Frazier AA, et al. From the archives of the AFIP: lymphangioleiomyomatosis: radiologic-pathologic correlation. Radiographics 2005;25:803–28.

46. Young LR, Vandyke R, Gulleman PM, et al. Serum vascular endothelial growth factor-D prospectively distinguishes lymphangioleiomyomatosis from other diseases. Chest 2010;138:674–81.

47. McCormack FX, Inoue Y, Moss J, et al. Efficacy and safety of sirolimus in lymphangioleiomyomatosis. N Engl J Med 2011;364:1595–606.

48. Giovino GA. Epidemiology of tobacco use in the United States. Oncogene 2002; 21:7326–40.

49. Thun MJ, Carter BD, Feskanich D, et al. 50-year trends in smoking-related mortality in the United States. N Engl J Med 2013;368:351–64.

50. Radzikowska E, Głaz P, Roszkowski K. Lung cancer in women: age, smoking, histology, performance status, stage, initial treatment and survival. Population-based study of 20 561 cases. Ann Oncol 2002;13:1087–93.

51. Risch HA, Howe GR, Jain M, et al. Are female smokers at higher risk for lung cancer than male smokers? A case-control analysis by histologic type. Am J Epidemiol 1993;138:281–93.

52. Sun S, Schiller JH, Gazdar AF. Lung cancer in never smokers–a different disease. Nat Rev Cancer 2007;7:778–90.

53. Thomas L, Doyle LA, Edelman MJ. Lung cancer in women: emerging differences in epidemiology, biology, and therapy. Chest 2005;128:370–81.

54. Yang SH, Mechanic LE, Yang P, et al. Mutations in the tyrosine kinase domain of the epidermal growth factor receptor in non-small cell lung cancer. Clin Cancer Res 2005;11:2106–10.

55. Fan L, Feng Y, Wan H, et al. Clinicopathological and demographical characteristics of non-small cell lung cancer patients with ALK rearrangements: a systematic review and meta-analysis. PLoS One 2014;9:e100866.
56. de Perrot M, Licker M, Bouchardy C, et al. Sex differences in presentation, management, and prognosis of patients with non-small cell lung carcinoma. J Thorac Cardiovasc Surg 2000;119:21–6.
57. Siddiqui F, Bae K, Langer CJ, et al. The influence of gender, race, and marital status on survival in lung cancer patients: analysis of Radiation Therapy Oncology Group trials. J Thorac Oncol 2010;5:631–9.
58. Spiegelman D, Maurer LH, Ware JH, et al. Prognostic factors in small-cell carcinoma of the lung: an analysis of 1,521 patients. J Clin Oncol 1989;7:344–54.
59. Singh S, Parulekar W, Murray N, et al. Influence of sex on toxicity and treatment outcome in small-cell lung cancer. J Clin Oncol 2005;23:850–6.
60. Gould MK, Donington J, Lynch WR, et al. Evaluation of individuals with pulmonary nodules: when is it lung cancer? Diagnosis and management of lung cancer, 3rd ed: American College of Chest Physicians evidence-based clinical practice guidelines. Chest 2013;143:e93S–120S.
61. Wood DE. National Comprehensive Cancer Network (NCCN) clinical practice guidelines for lung cancer screening. Thorac Surg Clin 2015;25:185–97.
62. Simonneau G, Gatzoulis MA, Adatia I, et al. Updated clinical classification of pulmonary hypertension. J Am Coll Cardiol 2013;62:D34–41.
63. Loyd JE, Butler MG, Foroud TM, et al. Genetic anticipation and abnormal gender ratio at birth in familial primary pulmonary hypertension. Am J Respir Crit Care Med 1995;152:93–7.
64. Aldred MA, Vijayakrishnan J, James V, et al. BMPR2 gene rearrangements account for a significant proportion of mutations in familial and idiopathic pulmonary arterial hypertension. Hum Mutat 2006;27:212–3.
65. Lahm T, Crisostomo PR, Markel TA, et al. Selective estrogen receptor-alpha and estrogen receptor-beta agonists rapidly decrease pulmonary artery vasoconstriction by a nitric oxide-dependent mechanism. Am J Physiol Regul Integr Comp Physiol 2008;295:R1486–93.
66. Austin ED, Cogan JD, West JD, et al. Alterations in oestrogen metabolism: implications for higher penetrance of familial pulmonary arterial hypertension in females. Eur Respir J 2009;34:1093–9.
67. Chen X, Talati M, Fessel JP, et al. The estrogen metabolite 16alphaOHE exacerbates BMPR2-associated PAH through miR-29-mediated modulation of cellular metabolism. Circulation 2015;133(1):82–97.
68. Badesch DB, Champion HC, Sanchez MA, et al. Diagnosis and assessment of pulmonary arterial hypertension. J Am Coll Cardiol 2009;54:S55–66.
69. Hemnes AR, Kiely DG, Cockrill BA, et al. Statement on pregnancy in pulmonary hypertension from the pulmonary vascular research institute. Pulm Circ 2015;5:435–65.
70. Hemnes AR, Robbins IM. Hysteroscopic sterilization in women with pulmonary vascular disease. Mayo Clin Proc 2008;83:1188–9 [author reply: 1189].
71. Bonnar J. Coagulation effects of oral contraception. Am J Obstet Gynecol 1987;157:1042–8.
72. Dupras D, Bluhm J, Felty C, et al. Institute for clinical systems improvement. Venous thromboembolism diagnosis and treatment. 2013. Available at: http://bit/ly/VTE0113.

73. Hulley S, Furberg C, Barrett-Connor E, et al. Noncardiovascular disease outcomes during 6.8 years of hormone therapy: Heart and Estrogen/progestin Replacement Study follow-up (HERS II). JAMA 2002;288:58–66.
74. Peragallo Urrutia R, Coeytaux RR, McBroom AJ, et al. Risk of acute thromboembolic events with oral contraceptive use: a systematic review and meta-analysis. Obstet Gynecol 2013;122:380–9.
75. Miller J, Chan BK, Nelson HD. Postmenopausal estrogen replacement and risk for venous thromboembolism: a systematic review and meta-analysis for the U.S. Preventive Services Task Force. Ann Intern Med 2002;136:680–90.
76. Perez Gutthann S, García Rodríguez LA, Castellsague J, et al. Hormone replacement therapy and risk of venous thromboembolism: population based case-control study. BMJ 1997;314:796–800.
77. Grodstein F, Stampfer MJ, Goldhaber SZ, et al. Prospective study of exogenous hormones and risk of pulmonary embolism in women. Lancet 1996;348:983–7.
78. Fisher B, Costantino JP, Wickerham DL, et al. Tamoxifen for prevention of breast cancer: report of the National Surgical Adjuvant Breast and Bowel Project P-1 Study. J Natl Cancer Inst 1998;90:1371–88.
79. Patel NH, Stookey KR, Ketcham DB, et al. Endovascular management of acute extensive iliofemoral deep venous thrombosis caused by May-Thurner syndrome. J Vasc Interv Radiol 2000;11:1297–302.
80. Jubanyik KJ, Comite F. Extrapelvic endometriosis. Obstet Gynecol Clin North Am 1997;24:411–40.
81. Alifano M, Jablonski C, Kadiri H, et al. Catamenial and noncatamenial, endometriosis-related or nonendometriosis-related pneumothorax referred for surgery. Am J Respir Crit Care Med 2007;176:1048–53.
82. Channabasavaiah AD, Joseph JV. Thoracic endometriosis: revisiting the association between clinical presentation and thoracic pathology based on thoracoscopic findings in 110 patients. Medicine (Baltimore) 2010;89:183–8.
83. Legras A, Rousset-Jablonski C, Bobbio A, et al. Pneumothorax in women of childbearing age: an update classification based on clinical and pathologic findings. Chest 2014;145:354–60.
84. Rousset-Jablonski C, Alifano M, Plu-Bureau G, et al. Catamenial pneumothorax and endometriosis-related pneumothorax: clinical features and risk factors. Hum Reprod 2011;26:2322–9.
85. Korom S, Canyurt H, Missbach A, et al. Catamenial pneumothorax revisited: clinical approach and systematic review of the literature. J Thorac Cardiovasc Surg 2004;128:502–8.
86. Alifano M, Roth T, Broët SC, et al. Catamenial pneumothorax: a prospective study. Chest 2003;124:1004–8.
87. Joseph J, Sahn SA. Thoracic endometriosis syndrome: new observations from an analysis of 110 cases. Am J Med 1996;100:164–70.
88. Puma F, Carloni A, Casucci G, et al. Successful endoscopic Nd-YAG laser treatment of endobronchial endometriosis. Chest 2003;124:1168–70.
89. Slabbynck H, Laureys M, Impens N, et al. Recurring catamenial pneumothorax treated with a Gn-RH analogue. Chest 1991;100:851.

Primary Care Endocrinology in the Adult Woman

Celeste C. Thomas, MD, MS*, Meltem Zeytinoglu, MD, MBA

KEYWORDS

- Diabetes in women • Thyroid disease in women • Osteoporosis
- Bone mineral density

KEY POINTS

- The gynecologist has a critical role in identifying women at risk for diabetes mellitus, encouraging healthful lifestyle choices, managing the disease, and providing access to resources for education and support.
- Identifying an appropriate treatment goal (eg, hemoglobin A1c) for each individual patient will decrease the number of people with uncontrolled diabetes.
- Women with thyroid disease often present first to their gynecologist reporting menstrual irregularities or infertility. Identifying and treating thyroid disease is essential in the pregnant patient.
- Osteoporosis and low bone mineral density affect a substantial proportion of older women.
- Lifestyle interventions and therapeutic options are available and the gynecologist plays an important role in optimizing risk factor assessment, screening, and providing treatment when appropriate.

DIABETES MELLITUS
Background

An estimated 29 million Americans have diabetes mellitus and it is predicted that as many as 1 in 3 American adults will have the disease by 2050.[1,2] Diabetes mellitus is a group of metabolic diseases characterized by hyperglycemia resulting from defects in insulin action, insulin secretion, or both. The chronic hyperglycemia of diabetes results in disturbances of carbohydrate, fat, and protein metabolism and is associated with long-term damage, dysfunction, and failure of various organs, especially the eyes, kidneys, nerves, heart, and blood vessels.[3] Diabetes is a leading cause

No financial disclosures.

Section of Adult and Pediatric Endocrinology, Diabetes, and Metabolism, Department of Medicine, University of Chicago, Chicago, IL, USA

* Corresponding author. 5841 South Maryland Avenue, MC 1027, Chicago, IL 60637.

E-mail address: cthomas5@medicine.bsd.uchicago.edu

Obstet Gynecol Clin N Am 43 (2016) 325–346

http://dx.doi.org/10.1016/j.ogc.2016.01.005

obgyn.theclinics.com

of blindness, end-stage renal disease, and nontraumatic lower limb amputations in the United States. It is also a major cause of cardiovascular disease and stroke.[4] The increasing incidence is particularly challenging in women because the disease affects both mothers and their unborn children. Gestational diabetes serves as a harbinger of type 2 diabetes and provides an opportunity to delay or prevent the onset of the disease. Gynecologists are in a unique position to identify women at risk for diabetes and intervene to reduce the disease burden.

Pathophysiology and Classification

The pathophysiology of diabetes mellitus remains under study and varies for each subtype of the group of diseases. Type 1 diabetes mellitus (T1DM) is an autoimmune disease associated with selective destruction of insulin-producing pancreatic β-cells and accounts for 5% to 10% of prevalent diabetes.[5] The destructive process usually results in absolute insulin deficiency. Latent autoimmune diabetes of adults presents with a slower progression of β-cell destruction.[6] Ketosis-prone diabetes presents with a transient secretory defect of β-cells at the time of onset with remarkable recovery of β-cell activity during the period(s) of remission.[7,8] The most common type of diabetes, type 2 diabetes mellitus (T2DM), is characterized by tissue resistance to the glucose-lowering effects of insulin as well as β-cell failure.[9] Normally, pancreatic β-cells respond to insulin resistance, which occurs with obesity and transiently at times of disrupted sleep and stress, by increasing their output of insulin to meet the needs of tissues. T2DM develops when there is a failure of the β-cell to adequately compensate for this insulin resistance. Gestational diabetes mellitus (GDM) is important to distinguish from preexisting T2DM or even T1DM or latent autoimmune diabetes of adults that was undiagnosed before pregnancy. Metabolic changes that develop during pregnancy are significant and occur over time with increasing insulin resistance with growth of the conceptus.[10] GDM occurs when insulin secretion fails to compensate for physiologic insulin resistance.

Maturity-onset diabetes of the young (MODY) describes a group of disorders caused by multiple gene mutations (ie, monogenic diabetes). MODY should be suspected if a type 2 diabetes–like condition occurs in 2 or more generations and the pattern of inheritance is consistent with autosomal-dominant inheritance.[11] MODY may first be identified as GDM and in a small study, 5% (2/40) of women with GDM were found to have a MODY mutation.[12] There are also a number of secondary causes of diabetes mellitus, including cystic fibrosis, chronic pancreatitis, hemochromatosis, pancreatic neoplasia, other endocrinopathies such as Cushing's syndrome or acromegaly, and drug-induced diabetes mellitus.

Prevention

The Diabetes Prevention Program (DPP) reported that, in subjects with impaired glucose tolerance, an intensive lifestyle intervention and metformin reduced the rate of developing diabetes by 58% and 31%, respectively, compared with placebo.[13] In a follow-up study, diabetes incidence in the 10 years after DPP randomization was decreased by 34% in the lifestyle group and 18% in the metformin group compared with placebo.[14]

Type 1 Diabetes TrialNet is an international group of researchers studying ways to prevent and delay the progression of T1DM.[15] Studies are conducted in individuals at risk for T1DM in an effort to delay the development of the clinical disease.

Assessment of Overall Risk and Screening Recommendations

T2DM often goes undiagnosed until complications appear. Among the estimated 29 million Americans in 2012 with diabetes mellitus, more than 25% were undiagnosed.[16]

Risk factors for T2DM are listed in **Box 1**. The US Preventive Services Task Force revised its recommendations in October 2015 to advise screening for abnormal blood glucose as part of a cardiovascular risk assessment in adults aged 40 to 70 years who are overweight or obese.[17] The American Diabetes Association recommends universal screening for T2DM of adults older than 45 years. Adults of any age who are overweight (body mass index $\geq$25 or 23 kg/m^2 in Asian Americans) and who have 1 or more additional risk factors for diabetes should also be screened, and if tests are normal, repeat screening should occur at 3-year intervals. Considering risk factors other than age when screening for diabetes mellitus is important because young adults with T2DM are suffering significant microvascular and macrovascular complications.

Options for screening include hemoglobin A1c, fasting plasma glucose, and oral glucose tolerance tests. Criteria for diagnosis are listed in **Table 1**.

Clinical Presentation

The traditional paradigms of T2DM occurring only in adults and T1DM occurring only in children are no longer accurate, because both diseases present in both cohorts. Assigning a type of diabetes to an individual often depends on the circumstances present at the time of diagnosis, with many individuals not necessarily fitting clearly into a single category. Children with T1DM typically present with the hallmark symptoms of polyuria, polydipsia, polyphagia and occasionally with diabetic ketoacidosis. The onset of T1DM may be variable in adults and may not present with the classic symptoms seen in children. Autoimmune and monogenic diabetes often masquerade as T2DM in youth and adults. Occasionally, patients with T2DM may present with diabetic ketoacidosis. The initial evaluation includes appropriate laboratory studies, including autoimmune markers and consideration of testing for monogenic diabetes, to evaluate the disease. Clinical presentation and disease progression vary considerably in all types of diabetes.

Management

Patients with T1DM require exogenous insulin. Optimal insulin dosing incorporates the carbohydrate content of the meal, body weight and lean muscle mass, exercise, illness, stress, and the effects of a patient's menstrual cycle and other medications.

Box 1
Risk factors for development of T2DM

Advancing age

Overweight/obesity

Family history of T2DM

High-risk race/ethnicity including Native American, African American, Latino, Asian American, Pacific Islander

Physical inactivity and decreased muscle mass

History of gestational diabetes mellitus or prediabetes

Certain medications (eg, glucocorticoids, thiazide diuretics, atypical antipsychotics)

Other conditions associated with insulin resistance (eg, hypertension, dyslipidemia, polycystic ovarian syndrome, disrupted sleep, obstructive sleep apnea, cardiovascular disease, or other endocrinopathies)

Abbreviation: T2DM, type 2 diabetes mellitus.

Table 1
Criteria for diagnosis of prediabetes and diabetes

	Prediabetes	Diabetes
Hemoglobin A1c (%)	5.7–6.4	≥6.5
Fasting plasma glucose (mg/dL)	100–125	≥126
2-h oral glucose tolerance test (mg/dL; after 75 g glucose load)	140–199	≥200
Random plasma glucose (mg/dL)	—	≥200[a]

[a] Only diagnostic in a patient with classic symptoms of hyperglycemia (polyuria, polydipsia, polyphagia).

Most people with T1DM should be treated with multiple-dose insulin injections also known as basal/bolus insulin (3–4 injections per day of basal and prandial insulin) or continuous subcutaneous insulin infusion therapy. Patients must be educated in how to match carbohydrate intake with prandial insulin dose and preprandial blood glucose level. Anticipated physical activity should also be considered. Insulin analogues are often used to reduce the risk of hypoglycemia. For many patients, especially those with hypoglycemia unawareness or frequent nocturnal hypoglycemia, continuous glucose monitoring should be considered.

Management of prediabetes and overt T2DM can be achieved with a focus on supporting intensive lifestyle modifications that incorporate patient preferences. Adequate support for behavior change is essential including offering high-quality diabetes self-management education, diabetes self-management support, and medical nutrition therapy designed to encourage healthful eating patterns. Depression is a common comorbid condition and psychosocial assessment and screening should be considered. After or in addition to lifestyle interventions, metformin is the preferred initial pharmacologic agent for T2DM, if not contraindicated, and should be offered with the largest meal of the day initially at a low dose (eg, 500 mg once daily) to improve tolerance and then titrated to the maximum dose tolerated. Recommended second agents if glycemic targets are not achieved on metformin include glucagonlike peptide 1 receptor agonists (administered via subcutaneous injection), dipeptidyl peptidase 4 inhibitors, thiazolidinediones, and sodium/glucose cotransporter 2 inhibitors. Glucagonlike peptide-1 receptor agonists and sodium/glucose cotransporter 2 inhibitors offer the additional benefit of weight loss. Costs must be considered. Sulfonylureas are less favored given associated weight gain and risk of hypoglycemia. Pharmacologic therapies are summarized in **Table 2**. Combination tablets including metformin and dipeptidyl peptidase 4 inhibitors or sodium/glucose cotransporter 2 inhibitors are available. In some patients with newly diagnosed T2DM, insulin therapy is initiated early. Owing to the progressive nature of T2DM, insulin therapy is eventually indicated for many patients with T2DM.

Lowering hemoglobin A1c values to less than 7% has been shown to reduce microvascular complications. Achieving this goal early in the disease course is associated with long-term reductions in macrovascular disease. For many patients, targeting A1c less than 6.5% is appropriate if it can be achieved without significant hypoglycemia. For other patients, especially those with comorbid conditions and a greater likelihood for severe hypoglycemia, less stringent A1c goals (eg, <8%) may be more appropriate.

As for the general population, all individuals with diabetes should receive routine vaccinations including pneumococcal and annual influenza vaccinations. Referrals should be considered and are listed in **Box 2**.

The American Diabetes Association recommends that all women with risk factors be tested for undiagnosed diabetes at the first prenatal visit.[18] Women of childbearing age with diabetes should be counseled regarding the importance of strict glycemic control before conception as well as the teratogenic effects of some antihypertensive and lipid-lowering agents. Observational studies show an increased risk of diabetic embryopathy, especially congenital heart disease, anencephaly, and microcephaly that increases in a direct relationship with hemoglobin A1c. It is recommended that the preconception A1c be less than 7% if that level can be achieved without hypoglycemia.[18] Before conception, women with pregestational diabetes should be evaluated for hypothyroidism and should undergo evaluation for preexisting renal disease and be referred for an ophthalmologic examination. Management of diabetes in pregnancy is beyond the scope of this text.

Summary

Diabetes is manageable and its complications can be prevented. The first step is to be aware of its presence by screening those at risk. If diabetes is diagnosed, the physician must then identify glycemic targets (eg, hemoglobin A1c) for the individual patient and intervene as necessary with lifestyle and pharmacologic therapies to achieve the target. Approximately 15% of people with diabetes receive their care from an endocrinologist[19] and there are not enough endocrinologists to care for the increasing number of people with diabetes. The obstetrician–gynecologist has an important role in caring for women with diabetes and reducing the disease burden by working to motivate those with GDM to continue lifestyle interventions postpartum.

THE THYROID GLAND
Background

The American Thyroid Association estimates that 20 million Americans have some form of thyroid disease. Women are 5 to 8 times more likely than men to have thyroid disorders and approximately 1 woman in 8 will develop a thyroid disorder during her lifetime. Undiagnosed thyroid disease puts women at increased risk for infertility, cardiovascular diseases, and osteoporosis. Pregnant women with undiagnosed or inadequately treated hypothyroidism have an increased risk of miscarriage, preterm delivery, and severe developmental problems in their offspring. The obstetrician–gynecologist has a critical role in identifying symptoms and providing treatment or referral for management of thyroid disease.

Thyroid hormone synthesis and action

Thyroid-stimulating hormone (TSH, also called thyrotropin) is one of several hormones produced by the anterior pituitary gland. TSH is stored in granules and released into the circulation in a highly regulated manner in response to stimulation by hypothalamic thyrotropin-releasing hormone.[20] TSH acts on the thyroid gland by binding to its receptor, where it activates synthesis of thyroid hormone. Thyroid hormone directly blocks pituitary secretion of TSH and decreases thyrotropin-releasing hormone stimulation of TSH release.[20] Thyroid hormones are critical for fetal development and the activity of thyroid hormone influences multiple aspects of metabolism.

There are 2 biologically active thyroid hormones: thyroxine (T4) and 3,5,3'-triiodothyronine (T3). T4 is the primary secretory product of the thyroid gland. It is converted to T3 in the peripheral tissues.

Table 2
Common pharmacologic agents to treat DM

Class	Medications	Primary Action(s)	Approximate Reduction in Glycosylated Hemoglobin (%)	Advantages	Disadvantages
Biguanides	Metformin (immediate release) Metformin extended release	Decreases hepatic glucose production	1–1.5	First agent if no contraindications Low risk of hypoglycemia Low cost Weight neutral	Lactic acidosis risk (rare) Contraindications including chronic kidney disease, hypoxia, iodinated contrast
GLP-1 receptor agonists	Exenatide Exenatide extended release Liraglutide Albiglutide Dulaglutide	Glucose-dependent increase in insulin secretion Glucose-dependent decrease in glucagon secretion Slows gastric emptying Induces satiety	1–1.5	Low risk of hypoglycemia when used alone Weight loss Decreases postprandial glucose excursions	Gastrointestinal side effects (nausea, vomiting, diarrhea) Acute pancreatitis C-cell hyperplasia, medullary thyroid tumors in animals Injection, requires training for use High cost of medication
DPP-4 inhibitors	Sitagliptin Saxagliptin Linagliptin Alogliptin	Glucose-dependent increase in insulin secretion Glucose-dependent decrease in glucagon secretion — —	0.5–1	No hypoglycemia Generally well-tolerated Weight neutral	Angioedema, urticaria Acute pancreatitis Arthralgias Increased heart failure hospitalizations with saxagliptin High cost of medication
SGLT2 inhibitors	Canagliflozin Dapagliflozin Empagliflozin	Inhibits glucose reabsorption by the kidney resulting in glucosuria	0.5–1	No hypoglycemia Weight loss Decreases blood pressure Durable	Genitourinary infections Polyuria Volume depletion, hypotension, dizziness Euglycemic ketoacidosis High cost of medication

Sulfonylureas	Glipizide (immediate release) Glipizide extended release Glyburide Glimepiride	Increases insulin secretion unrelated to meals	1–1.5	Extensive experience Low cost of medication	High risk of hypoglycemia, often significant and prolonged in older patients Weight gain Low durability High risk in advanced age
TZDs	Pioglitazone Rosiglitazone	Increases insulin sensitivity	1–1.5	No hypoglycemia Durable	Weight gain Edema Contraindicated in CHF Bone fractures Bladder cancer
Bile acid sequestrants	Colesevelam	Increases Incretin levels	0.5–1	No hypoglycemia Decrease LDL-C	Increases triglyceride levels May affect absorption of other medications

Insulins	• Rapid-acting insulin analogs
	  ○ Lispro
	  ○ Aspart
	  ○ Glulisine
	• Short-acting
	  ○ Human regular
	• Intermediate-acting
	  ○ Human NPH
	• Basal insulin analogs
	  ○ Glargine
	  ○ Detemir
	  ○ Degludec
		Increases peripheral glucose uptake and disposal
		Decreases hepatic glucose production
			—	Unlimited efficacy in diabetes mellitus	Hypoglycemia
					Weight gain
					Mitogenic effects
					Injection, requires training for use

Not all Food and Drug Administration–approved agents are listed here.

Abbreviations: CHF, congestive heart failure; DPP-4, dipeptidyl peptidase 4; GLP, glucagonlike peptide, LDL-C, low-density lipoprotein cholesterol; NPH, neutral protamine Hagedorn; SGLT2, sodium/glucose cotransporter 2.

Box 2
Recommended referrals for patients with diabetes mellitus

Ophthalmologist for annual dilated eye examination

Dentist for comprehensive oral examinations

Registered dietician for medical nutrition therapy

Certified diabetes educator for diabetes self-management education and support

Mental health professional, if needed, for diabetes-related distress or comorbid depression

Podiatrist

Perturbations of Thyroid Function and Structure

Hypothyroidism

In iodine-sufficient areas of the world like the United States, hypothyroidism is most often caused by chronic lymphocytic thyroiditis, the result of an autoimmune process leading to diffuse lymphocytic infiltration of the gland.[21] Autoimmune thyroid diseases have been estimated to be nearly 10 times more common in women than in men[22] and are heritable.[23] Autoimmune hypothyroidism is often called Hashimoto's thyroiditis.[24] In the early stages, patients most often have normal thyroid hormone levels (ie, euthyroid) and the only evidence of autoimmune thyroiditis is the presence of antithyroid antibodies in a patient's serum. As the disease progresses, thyroid function is variable ranging from euthyroidism to thyrotoxicosis. Further progression over time often results in atrophic thyroiditis and hypothyroidism. The percentages of women with thyroid antibodies increases with age from approximately 10% during reproductive years to nearly 20% in older women.[21]

Primary hypothyroidism may also occur as a result of treatment of hyperthyroidism, thyroid cancer, or benign nodular thyroid disease with radioactive iodine or surgery. External beam radiation for non–thyroid-related head and neck malignancies also increases the risk of hypothyroidism. Some drugs, especially tyrosine kinase inhibitors, check point inhibitors, and amiodarone, may also induce hypothyroidism via various mechanisms including alterations in T4 and T3 metabolism.[25]

Hypothyroidism may be either subclinical or overt. Subclinical hypothyroidism is characterized by a serum TSH above the upper reference limit in combination with a normal free T4. This designation is only applicable when the hypothalamic–pituitary–thyroid axis is normal, and there is no recent or ongoing illness. Subclinical thyroid dysfunction is a common finding in older adults, occurring in 10% to 15% among those age 65 and older, and may contribute to multiple common problems of older age, including mood disorders, cognitive dysfunction, muscular discomfort, and cardiovascular disease.[26] Based on the currently available evidence, recommendations advise treatment of subclinical hypothyroidism at TSH values greater than 10 mIU/L.[27] An elevated TSH, in combination with a subnormal free T4, is consistent with a diagnosis of overt hypothyroidism.

Notably, subclinical hypothyroidism in pregnancy is a special case and may be associated with adverse outcomes for both the mother and offspring. Current guidelines recommend levothyroxine replacement in pregnant women with subclinical hypothyroidism who have circulating antithyroid antibodies.[28] In addition, treatment with levothyroxine before conception has been shown to reduce the miscarriage rate and to increase live birth rate in women with subclinical hypothyroidism undergoing assisted reproduction.[29]

Central hypothyroidism occurs when there is insufficient production of TSH owing to pituitary or hypothalamic tumors (eg, craniopharyngiomas, meningiomas), inflammatory or infiltrative diseases, hemorrhagic or ischemic necrosis of the pituitary gland (eg, Sheehan's syndrome, a unique case in women), or surgical and radiation treatment for pituitary or hypothalamic disease. In central hypothyroidism, serum TSH may be mildly elevated or normal with subnormal serum free T4. Resistance to thyroid hormone is a syndrome of reduced end-organ responsiveness to thyroid hormone. Diagnosis is based on persistent elevations of thyroid hormone levels in the absence of TSH suppression (levels are usually normal or slightly increased).

Clinical manifestations and diagnosis of hypothyroidism Early in the disease course, most patients with autoimmune thyroiditis are euthyroid or have subclinical hypothyroidism with elevated TSH and normal thyroid hormone levels. As time passes, hypothyroidism develops. The signs and symptoms of hypothyroidism (**Table 3**) are nonspecific and tend to be more subtle than those of thyrotoxicosis (**Table 4**). Other clinical and metabolic endpoints that may be affected by hypothyroidism include resting heart rate, serum cholesterol, serum creatine kinase levels, anxiety level, sleep pattern, and menstrual cycle abnormalities.

In a patient who has not recently experienced acute illness, subnormal serum free T4 levels establishes the diagnosis of hypothyroidism whether primary, in which serum TSH is increased, or central, in which serum TSH is normal or low.

Management in nonpregnant women Hypothyroidism is usually managed with supplemental thyroid hormone in the form of T4 as levothyroxine. Some patients are also treated with T3 as liothyronine (usually in combination with T4), whereas others may be treated with desiccated thyroid hormone. The goal of treatment is to provide resolution of the patients' symptoms and signs of hypothyroidism and to achieve normalization of serum TSH with improvement in thyroid hormone concentrations while avoiding overtreatment, especially in the elderly. An American Thyroid Association task force found no consistently strong evidence for the superiority of alternative preparations (eg, levothyroxine–liothyronine combination therapy, or thyroid extract therapy) over monotherapy with levothyroxine, in improving health outcomes. It concluded that levothyroxine should remain the standard of care for treating hypothyroidism.[30] Because coadministration of food and levothyroxine is likely to impair levothyroxine absorption, it is recommended that levothyroxine be taken either 60 minutes before breakfast or at bedtime ($\geq$3 hours after the evening meal) for optimal and consistent absorption. Ideally, levothyroxine will not be taken within 4 hours of other medications and

Table 3 Symptoms of hypothyroidism	
Common	Amenorrhea/other menstrual irregularities
	Infertility
	Dry skin
	Cold sensitivity
	Fatigue
	Muscle cramps
	Voice changes
	Constipation
Less Common	Carpal tunnel syndrome
	Sleep apnea

Table 4 Symptoms of thyrotoxicosis	
Common	Fatigue Weight loss Heat intolerance Palpitations Tremulousness Nervousness, anxiety, irritability Diaphoresis Increased appetite Menstrual irregularities/infertility
Less common	Hyperdefecation Neck fullness Eye symptoms Dyspnea Velvety skin Onycholysis Proximal muscle weakness

Data from Graf H. Werner and Ingbar's the thyroid: a fundamental and clinical text. Philadelphia: Lippincott Williams & Wilkins; 2012.

supplements, especially those containing calcium, iron, or soy. Women of advanced age should be started on a low dose (eg, 25 μg), and this dose should be titrated slowly. Normal serum TSH ranges are higher in older populations. Based on the current evidence the American Thyroid Association states it is reasonable to raise the target serum TSH to 4 to 6 mIU/L in persons greater than age 70 to 80 years.[30]

Management in pregnant women In pregnancy, thyroid hormone requirements are increased. Untreated hypothyroidism during pregnancy may adversely affect maternal and fetal outcomes. Adverse outcomes include increased incidence of spontaneous miscarriage, preterm delivery, preeclampsia, maternal hypertension, and postpartum hemorrhage. Other potential outcomes include low birth weight, impaired intellectual and psychomotor development of the offspring, and stillbirth.[28] The specifics of the management recommendations in pregnancy are beyond the scope of this document. For women with pre-existing hypothyroidism who are already on thyroid hormone replacement, patients should be advised to increase their dose of thyroid hormone by 25–30% as soon as pregnancy is suspected. Obstetricians should target a TSH concentration of <2.5 mIU/L for women in the first trimester of pregnancy.[31]

Thyrotoxicosis
Thyrotoxicosis is a clinical state that results from inappropriately high thyroid hormone action in tissues. Thyrotoxicosis has multiple etiologies, including excess thyroid hormone produced by the thyroid gland (hyperthyroidism) and excess thyroid hormone from ectopic locations or ingestion. In the United States, the prevalence of hyperthyroidism is approximately 1.2% (0.5% overt and 0.7% subclinical); the most common causes include Graves' disease, toxic multinodular goiter, and toxic adenoma[21] (**Table 5**).

Graves' disease is an autoimmune disorder in which thyrotropin receptor antibodies stimulate the TSH receptor, increasing thyroid hormone production.[32] It is the most common cause of hyperthyroidism in the United States.

In toxic multinodular goiter and toxic adenomas, autonomous hormone production can be caused by activating mutations of genes regulating thyroid hormone

Table 5
Causes of thyrotoxicosis

Autoimmune	Graves' disease
Nodular thyroid disease	Toxic adenoma, toxic multinodular goiter
Destructive process	Painless thyroiditis, subacute thyroiditis, acute thyroiditis
Drug induced	Amiodarone, iodinated contrast
Unusual	TSH-producing pituitary adenomas Trophoblastic disease Factitious ingestion of thyroid hormone Struma ovarii Metastases from follicular thyroid cancer

Abbreviation: TSH, thyroid-stimulating hormone.

synthesis.[33] Hormone production may progress from subclinical to overt hyperthyroidism, and the administration of iodinated contrast to such patients may result in iodine-induced hyperthyroidism.[34] Although toxic nodular goiter is less common than Graves' disease, its prevalence increases with age and in the presence of iodine deficiency. Stuma ovarii is a less common cause of hyperthyroidism in women. It is a rare teratoma that contains mostly thyroid tissue and may present as a solid or complex mass.

The mechanism of hyperthyroidism in subacute and painless thyroiditis is inflammation of thyroid tissue with release of preformed hormone into the circulation. Painless thyroiditis is the etiology of hyperthyroidism in about 10% of patients and includes that occurring in the postpartum period (postpartum thyroiditis) and in 5% to 10% of amiodarone-treated patients.[35] Subacute thyroiditis is thought to be caused by viral infection and is characterized by fever and thyroid pain.

When hyperthyroidism is suspected, diagnostic accuracy improves when both a serum TSH and free T4 are assessed. In overt hyperthyroidism, usually both serum free T4 and T3 estimates are increased, and serum TSH is below the threshold needed for detection. As is the case with T4, protein-binding impacts total T3 measurements. Assays for estimating free T3 are less widely validated than those for free T4, and measurement of total T3 is preferred in clinical practice. Subclinical hyperthyroidism is defined as a normal serum-free T4 estimate and normal total T3 with subnormal serum TSH concentration.

The diagnosis of hyperthyroidism in pregnancy should be made using serum TSH values, and total T4 and T3 with reference range adjusted to 1.5 times the nonpregnant range or trimester-specific normal reference ranges. Graves' disease is also the most common cause of hyperthyroidism during pregnancy. Hyperthyroidism caused by a choriocarcinoma or human chorionic gonadotropin–producing molar pregnancy presents with a diffuse hyperactive thyroid gland similar to Graves' disease, but in these patients the serum human chorionic gonadotropin is higher than expected and thyroid receptor antibodies are not present.

Patients with overt Graves' hyperthyroidism should be treated with 1 of 3 therapies: antithyroid medication, radioactive iodine, or thyroidectomy.[35] Patients are often referred to endocrinologists to discuss their options. Patients with a high likelihood of remission, including women with small glands and negative or low antibody titers, often select antithyroid drugs, as do older adults with comorbidities and increased surgical risk. Women who are planning a pregnancy in the future (>6 months after therapy) often select radioactive iodine to avoid antithyroid drugs during pregnancy. Surgery is often the intervention of choice when there is symptomatic compression, very large goiters, or when thyroid malignancy is suspected. Surgery is also the choice for women planning a pregnancy in less than 4 to 6 months and in patients with severe disease and moderate to severe Graves' orbitopathy. When surgery is considered, referral to a center with extensive experience is advised.

Contraindications to radioactive iodine therapy include pregnancy, lactation, thyroid cancer, and women planning a pregnancy within 4 to 6 months.

Thyroid nodules and thyroid cancer

Thyroid nodules are common and most often benign. The prevalence of nodules depends on the population studied and the method(s) used to detect the nodules. Studies suggest a prevalence of 2% to 6% with palpation, 19% to 35% with ultrasound, and 8% to 65% in autopsy data.[36] Thyroid nodules are more common in women and with advancing age.[37] Referral to an endocrinologist is recommended after identification of a thyroid nodule to exclude thyroid cancer, which occurs in 5% to 15% depending on age, sex, radiation exposure history, family history, and other factors.[38]

Summary

Thyroid disease is common among the patients seen in an obstetrics and gynecology clinic, including pregnant patients. The gynecologists' role in evaluation, management, and referral, when appropriate, will prevent these patients from experiencing sequelae of untreated disease and improve their quality of life.

OSTEOPOROSIS
Background

The estimated prevalence of osteoporosis and low bone mass in the US population, older than 50 years is 53.6 million individuals, or more than one-half of the population in this demographic. Approximately two-thirds of these individuals are women, many of whom seek primary medical care in the gynecologist's clinic.[39] The major clinical outcome of osteoporosis and osteopenia or low bone mineral density (BMD) is fractures, and it is estimated that 1 out of every 2 women will sustain an osteoporotic fracture in their lifetime.[40] The gynecologist has a key role in identifying risk factors, screening, and providing treatment or referral for management of these conditions.

Bone metabolism involves a tightly coordinated balance between bone formation and resorption. Genetics, physical activity, nutrition, and risk factors for secondary osteoporosis play a large role in perturbing or maintaining this balance. Additionally, throughout the woman's life, various events including reproduction, lactation, and most notably, menopause shift this balance. Awareness of how these phases affect bone health can enable the physician to optimize care for this population.

Assessment of Overall Risk

Several lifestyle factors such as vitamin D insufficiency, low calcium intake, a high-sodium diet, reduced physical activity, recurrent falls, immobilization, alcohol abuse, smoking, underweight, and weight loss contribute to an increased risk of low BMD, osteoporosis, and fracture. Additionally, there is an extensive list of physiologic states, systemic disorders, and medications that may result in increased risk for low BMD and osteoporosis (**Table 6**).[40,41] Clinicians should be aware of these conditions and regularly assess patients for these risk factors. Appropriate diagnostic studies to evaluate for secondary causes should be tailored to the index of suspicion for individual conditions.

Table 6
Secondary causes of osteoporosis in premenopausal and postmenopausal women

Genetic	Parental history of hip fracture
	Cystic fibrosis
	Hypophosphatasia
	Osteogenesis imperfecta
	Homocystinuria
	Marfan syndrome
	Menkes Steely hair syndrome
	Ehlers-Danlos syndrome
	Glycogen storage diseases
	Riley-Day syndrome
	Gaucher's disease
	Hemochromatosis
	Porphyria
Endocrine	Hypogonadal states (primary or secondary)
	Central obesity
	Hyperparathyroidism
	Hypercalciuria
	Hyperthyroidism
	Diabetes mellitus
	Acromegaly
	Adrenal insufficiency
	Cushing's syndrome
Rheumatologic	Rheumatoid arthritis
	Systemic lupus erythematosus
	Ankylosing spondylitis
	Sarcoidosis
	Other inflammatory and autoimmune conditions
Gastrointestinal/ nutritional	Calcium, vitamin D, and nutrient deficiencies
	Celiac disease and other malabsorptive states (eg, after bariatric surgery, cystic fibrosis, inflammatory bowel disease)
	Liver and biliary disease
Hematologic	Leukemias and lymphomas
	Hemophilia
	Sickle cell disease
	Multiple myeloma
	Thalassemia
	Monoclonal gammopathy
Neurologic	Epilepsy
	Multiple sclerosis
	Stroke
	Spinal cord injury
	Parkinson's disease
Musculoskeletal	Connective tissue disorders
	Marfan syndrome
	Muscular dystrophy
Other	Excessive alcohol intake
	Smoking
	Depression
	Human immunodeficiency virus/AIDS infection
	Mastocytosis
	Chronic obstructive pulmonary disease
	Idiopathic scoliosis
	Weight loss
	End-stage renal disease
	Posttransplantation
	Amyloidosis

(continued on next page)

Table 6 (continued)	
Medications	Glucocorticoids
	Immunosuppressants (cyclosporine and tacrolimus)
	Gonadotropin-releasing hormone agonists
	Depo Provera contraception
	Aromatase inhibitors
	Tamoxifen (in premenopausal women)
	Chemotherapeutic agents (cyclophosphamide, methotrexate)
	Serotonin reuptake inhibitors
	Barbiturates
	Antiepileptic drugs (phenytoin, carbamezapime)
	Antitretroviral therapies (tenofavir)
	Proton pump inhibitors
	Aluminum antacids
	Thiazoledinediones
	Excessive vitamin A
	Heparin

Data from Cosman F, De Beur SJ, LeBoff MS, et al. Clinician's guide to prevention and treatment of osteoporosis. Osteoporos Int 2014;25(10):2359–81; and Cohen A, Shane E. Evaluation and management of the premenopausal woman with low BMD. Curr Osteoporos Rep 2013;11(4):276–85.

Screening for Osteoporosis

Indications for BMD evaluation in women are listed in **Table 7**.[40,42] Sites tested include the lumbar spine, femoral neck, and total hip. In cases of primary hyperparathyroidism, very obese patients, or where hip and/or spine BMD is not measurable, clinicians should also measure forearm BMD.

Table 7
Indications for bone mineral density evaluation and vertebral imaging in women

Bone Mineral Density Testing	Add Vertebral Imaging
All women >65 y	Women ≥70 y with BMD ≤-1.0 at lumbar spine, femoral neck, or total hip
Postmenopausal women <65 y if risk factors such as low body weight, previous fracture, high risk medication use (see **Table 6**), or a disease or condition associated with bone loss is present	Women between 65–69 y with BMD ≤-1.5 at lumbar spine, femoral neck, or total hip
Perimenopausal women with clinical risk factors for fracture	Postmenopausal women ≥50 y with: 1. History of fragility fracture in adulthood 2. Historical height loss of ≥1.5 inches (≥4 cm) 3. Prospective height loss of ≥0.8 inches (≥2 cm) from prior measurement 4. Recent or long-term glucocorticoid treatment.
History of fragility fracture in adulthood	—
Women with risk factors for secondary osteoporosis	—

Abbreviation: BMD, bone mineral density.
Data from Cosman F, De Beur SJ, LeBoff MS, et al. Clinician's guide to prevention and treatment of osteoporosis. Osteoporos Int 2014;25(10):2359–81; and Schousboe JT, Shepherd JA, Bilezikian JP, et al. Executive summary of the 2013 international society for clinical densitometry position development conference on bone densitometry. J Clin Densitom 2013;16(4):455–66.

Although vertebral fractures can result in kyphosis, back pain, and restrictive lung disease, the majority are clinically silent.[43] Nevertheless, vertebral fractures are a major predictor of future fracture risk at multiple sites.[44] Thus, for a comprehensive assessment of fracture risk, there are also criteria for the addition of vertebral imaging.

Although routine BMD screening is not recommended for premenopausal women, indications for evaluation in the premenopausal woman include a history of fragility fracture, secondary conditions associated with low bone mass or accelerated bone loss, and when considering or monitoring pharmacologic therapy for osteoporosis. When assessing for early or accelerated bone loss in the premenopausal patient, it is critical to first address the patient's reproductive history to determine whether low bone mass is occurring in the context of pregnancy or lactation.

Diagnosis of Osteoporosis and Low Bone Mineral Density

The diagnostic criteria for osteoporosis and low bone mass are based on the World Health Organization (WHO) classification system. In postmenopausal women, osteoporosis is defined by BMD at the lumbar spine, femoral neck, or total hip, that is, 2.5 or more standard deviations below the mean BMD (T-score $\leq$ -2.5) of the young adult reference population. Severe osteoporosis is present when women have both a

---

Box 3
Recommendations for historical and lifestyle mediators of bone health

Estrogen exposure history
  Age at menarche
  Parity/fertility history
  Age at menopause
  Prior or current use of oral contraceptives, hormone replacement therapies

Height or weight loss

Family history of osteoporosis; parental history of hip fractures

Personal or family history of nephrolithiasis, hypercalciuria, or other metabolic bone disorders

Exercise, both weight bearing and muscle strengthening

Barriers to exercise

When applicable, provide a prescription for physical therapy for strengthening exercises, balance, and posture, and fall prevention

Nutrition – estimate daily calcium intake[a] and add calcium supplements

Goal, for most women older than 50 years, is 1200 mg/day (recommend lower intake in women with nephrolithiasis, primary hyperparathyroidism, hypercalcuria)
  Milk (8 oz serving) 300 mg
  Yogurt (6 oz serving) 300 mg
  Cheese (1 oz or 1 cubic in) 200 mg

Sun exposure

Vitamin D intake by supplements

Recommend therapeutic supplementation, or maintenance dose of 800 to 1000 IU daily for most women older than 50

Alcohol and tobacco use

Provide support for avoidance of excess alcohol and tobacco cessation when appropriate

  [a] Data from The National Osteoporosis Foundation Clinician's Guide to Prevention and Treatment of Osteoporosis.

Table 8
Pharmacologic prevention and management of osteoporosis and low bone mineral density

Drug	Other Indications	Risk Reduction	Potential Adverse Effects	Contraindications
Prevention of postmenopausal osteoporosis				
Estrogen	Relief of vasomotor symptoms Postmenopausal vulvovaginal atrophy	Vertebral and hip fractures	Increased risk of venous thromboembolism, breast cancer, stroke, and increased risk of cardiovascular disease (if used after the first 10 y of menopause). Should be used in combination with progestin in women with intact uterus.	History of breast or endometrial cancer Undiagnosed abnormal genital bleeding History of venous thromboembolism or known thrombophilic disorder Liver disease History of coronary or cerebrovascular disease Gallbladder disease Hypertriglyceridemia Migraine Pregnancy
Bazedoxifene/conjugated Estrogen 0.45 mg/20 mg/d	Treatment of moderate-to-severe vasomotor symptoms	Vertebral fractures	Same as estrogen, plus muscle spasms, nausea, diarrhea, dyspepsia, abdominal pain, dizziness, neck pain. Should only be used in postmenopausal women with intact uterus.	Same as estrogen alone

Prevention and treatment of postmenopausal osteoporosis

Bisphosphonates

Drug / Dose	Indication	Fractures	Side effects	Contraindication
Alendronate				
35 mg/wk or 5 mg/d for prevention 70 mg/wk or 10 mg/d for treatment	Treatment of glucocorticoid-induced osteoporosis	Vertebral and hip fractures	Gastrointestinal intolerance, flulike symptoms, musculoskeletal pain (rare), hypocalcemia, ocular inflammation, osteonecrosis of jaw (rare), atypical femoral fractures (rare)	Kidney disease (GFR < 35 mL/min)
Risedronate				
35 mg/wk or 5 mg/d for prevention and treatment	—	Vertebral and nonvertebral fractures	Same as above	Kidney disease (GFR <35 mL/min)
Ibandronate				
2.5 mg/d or 150 mg once monthly 3 mg every 3 mo (intravenous)	—	Vertebral fractures	Gastrointestinal intolerance, gastro-esophogeal inflammation, flu-like symptoms, hypocalcemia, ocular inflammation, osteonecrosis of jaw (rare), atypical femoral fractures (rare)	Kidney disease (GFR < 35 mL/min)
Zoledronate				
5 mg every 2 y (intravenous over 15 min) for prevention and every year for treatment	Prevention and treatment of osteoporosis in women expected to be on glucocorticoid treatment for ≥12 mo Prevention of new fractures in women with a recent low-trauma osteoporotic fracture	Vertebral fractures, hip fractures, and nonvertebral fractures	Flulike symptoms, hypocalcemia, ocular inflammation, osteonecrosis of jaw (rare), atypical femoral fractures (rare)	Kidney disease (GFR < 35 mL/min)

(continued on next page)

Table 8
(continued)

Drug	Other Indications	Risk Reduction	Potential Adverse Effects	Contraindications
Raloxifene				
60 mg/d	Reduction of risk of invasive breast cancer in postmenopausal women with osteoporosis	Vertebral fractures	Increased risk of venous thromboembolism, increase in hot flashes, leg cramps	History of venous thromboembolism
Treatment of postmenopausal osteoporosis				
Denosumab				
60 mg every 6 mo (subcutaneous injection)	—	Vertebral, nonvertebral, and hip fractures	Serious skin infections (cellulitis) osteonecrosis of jaw (rare), atypical femoral fractures (rare)	Hypocalcemia and vitamin D deficiency must be corrected before starting denosumab Use with caution in cases of renal impairment
Teriparatide				
20 μg/d (subcutaneous injection)	Treatment of glucocorticoid-induced osteoporosis	Vertebral fractures and nonvertebral fractures.	Osteosarcoma (in rats, has not been confirmed in humans).	Hyperparathyroidism Other bone diseases (Paget's, osteomalacia, rickets) History of radiation therapy History of bone cancer or metastatic bone cancer

Use FRAX tool and clinical judgment to determine if treatment may be beneficial in patients with low bone mineral density.
Vitamin D and calcium levels should be replete before initiating therapy.
Abbreviation: GFR, glomerular filtration rate.

T-score of -2.5 or less and a fracture. Additionally, the clinical diagnosis of osteoporosis can be made when there is a low-trauma hip fracture (independent of T-score), or the presence of a low-trauma spine, distal forearm, humerus, or pelvis fracture in an individual with low BMD. Postmenopausal women with T-scores between -1.0 and -2.5 at the lumbar spine, femoral neck, or total hip are considered to have low bone mass, or osteopenia, and women whose T-scores are greater than -1.0 are considered to have a normal BMD.

Whereas in perimenopausal and postmenopausal women the diagnosis of osteoporosis can be made using WHO diagnostic T-score criteria alone, in premenopausal women, the relationship between fracture risk and BMD is less well-defined, and T-scores cannot be used. In this case, the recommendation of the International Society for Clinical Densitometry is to use an age-, sex-, and ethnicity-matched reference population (Z-score) in lieu of T-scores. Here, a Z-score of -2.0 or lower is used to define "low BMD for chronologic age" or "below the expected range for age." Those above -2.0 are considered "within the expected range for age.[42]"

Management

All women, regardless of BMD and clinical risk for osteoporosis, need to be counseled on the importance of lifestyle factors in reducing the risk of osteoporosis and fractures. In addition to assessing for clinical risk factors for osteoporosis, we recommend that the provider obtain a comprehensive history as detailed in **Box 3**.

In women with vertebral or hip fractures, or osteoporosis based on T-score, the need for pharmacologic therapy is obvious. In women with low BMD, however, the benefits of treatment, weighed against the potential risks, is not always clear. The WHO FRAX tool (available at: www.shef.ac.uk/FRAX/)[45] for estimation of 10-year absolute fracture risk can be used to estimate fracture risk in postmenopausal women. Individuals with low BMD and a 10-year probability of hip fracture 3% or greater, or of major osteoporosis-related fracture 20% or greater should be considered for treatment.

Several pharmacologic therapies are available for prevention and treatment (**Table 8**). Before initiating therapy, low calcium intake and vitamin D deficiency must be corrected. The choice of agent is individualized to the patient based on efficacy, severity of fracture risk, side effect profile, patient preference, and cost. Oral bisphosphonates, especially alendronate, are used as first-line therapy because of their demonstrated efficacy, tolerability, and low cost. In patients with very low BMD, more potent antiresorptive therapies (zoledronate, denosumab), or anabolic therapy may be indicated. Individuals who do not tolerate oral bisphosphonates owing to gastrointestinal side effects may be treated with zoledronate or denosumab. In individuals with markedly low BMD or in whom other therapies have failed, anabolic therapy with teriparatide may be considered. In these instances, the primary care provider may wish to refer to an endocrinologist or bone specialist for further therapy. Women's health providers may also consider referral in any case where there is uncertainty about the potential benefits and risk of specific therapies; where there is uncertainty about the need for a drug holiday or use of sequential therapies; or where there is concern for treatment failure.

For women who have been on oral bisphosphonates for 5 years, or intravenous bisphosphoantes for 3 years, reassessment of fracture risk is recommended. For those women who remain at high risk, continuation of treatment for up to 10 years with oral, or 6 years with intravenous bisphosphonates may be considered. For those women who are not at high fracture risk after 3–5 years of bisphosphonate therapy, a drug holiday of 2–3 years may be considered. In both instances of continuing therapy and drug holidays, ongoing re-evaluation of risk should be considered.[46]

In general, a repeat BMD is indicated 1 year after a therapy has been started or changed, and then every 2 years thereafter. For women with normal BMD, intervals may be extended.

Summary

Osteoporosis and low BMD affect a substantial proportion of older women and some younger women with risk factors for secondary osteoporosis. The morbidity and mortality of osteoporotic fractures is substantial. Nevertheless, there are many lifestyle interventions and therapeutic options available for these conditions, and the gynecologist can play a key role in optimizing risk factor assessment, screening, and providing treatment when appropriate.

REFERENCES

1. Centers for Disease Control and Prevention (CDC). National diabetes statistics report, 2014. Atlanta (GA): CDC; 2014. p. 2014.
2. Boyle JP, Thompson TJ, Gregg EW, et al. Projection of the year 2050 burden of diabetes in the US adult population: dynamic modeling of incidence, mortality, and prediabetes prevalence. Popul Health Metr 2010;8:29.
3. World Health Organization (WHO). Definition and diagnosis of diabetes mellitus and intermediate hyperglycemia: report of a WHO/IDF Consultation. Vol (WHO, IDF, eds). Geneva (Switzerland): WHO; 2006.
4. Centers for Disease Control and Prevention (CDC). National diabetes Statistics report: estimates of diabetes and its Burden in the United States, 2014. Atlanta (GA): CDC; 2014.
5. Hober D, Sauter P. Pathogenesis of type 1 diabetes mellitus: interplay between enterovirus and host. Nat Rev Endocrinol 2010;6(5):279–89.
6. Fourlanos S, Dotta F, Greenbaum CJ, et al. Latent autoimmune diabetes in adults (LADA) should be less latent. Diabetologia 2005;48(11):2206–12.
7. Mauvais-Jarvis F, Sobngwi E, Porcher R, et al. Ketosis-prone type 2 diabetes in patients of sub-Saharan African origin clinical pathophysiology and natural history of β-cell dysfunction and insulin resistance. Diabetes 2004;53(3):645–53.
8. Umpierrez GE, Smiley D, Kitabchi AE. Narrative review: ketosis-prone type 2 diabetes mellitus. Ann Intern Med 2006;144(5):350–7.
9. Halban PA, Polonsky KS, Bowden DW, et al. β-Cell failure in type 2 diabetes: postulated mechanisms and prospects for prevention and treatment. Diabetes Care 2014;37(6):1751–8.
10. Barbour LA, McCurdy CE, Hernandez TL, et al. Cellular mechanisms for insulin resistance in normal pregnancy and gestational diabetes. Diabetes Care 2007; 30(Suppl 2):S112–9.
11. Naylor RN, Greeley S, Bell GI. Genetics and pathophysiology of neonatal diabetes mellitus. J Diabetes Investig 2011;2(3):158–69.
12. Stoffel M, Bell KL, Blackburn CL, et al. Identification of glucokinase mutations in subjects with gestational diabetes mellitus. Diabetes 1993;42(6):937–40.
13. Knowler WC, Barrett-Connor E, Fowler SE, et al. Reduction in the incidence of type 2 diabetes with lifestyle intervention or metformin. N Engl J Med 2002; 346(6):393–403.
14. Diabetes Prevention Program Research Group, Knowler WC, Fowler SE, et al. 10-year follow-up of diabetes incidence and weight loss in the Diabetes Prevention Program Outcomes Study. Lancet 2009;374(9702):1677–86.

15. Skyler JS. Update on worldwide efforts to prevent type 1 diabetes. Ann N Y Acad Sci 2008;1150(1):190–6.
16. Centers for Disease Control and Prevention (CDC). National diabetes statistics report: estimates of diabetes and its burden in the United States, 2014. Atlanta (GA): CDC; 2014.
17. Selph S, Dana T, Blazina I, et al. Screening for type 2 diabetes mellitus: a systematic review for the U.S. Preventive Services Task Force. Ann Intern Med 2015; 162(11):765–76.
18. American Diabetes Association. 12. Management of diabetes in pregnancy. Diabetes Care 2015;38(Suppl 1):S77–9.
19. Vigersky RA, Fish L, Hogan P, et al. The clinical endocrinology workforce: current status and future projections of supply and demand. J Clin Endocrinol Metab 2014;99(9):3112–21.
20. Fauci A, Braunwald E, Kasper D, et al. Harrison's principles of internal medicine. 17th edition. New York: McGraw-Hill Prof Med/Tech; 2008.
21. DeGroot LJ, Jameson JL. Endocrinology. Philadelphia: W B Saunders Co; 2006.
22. Kumar V, Abbas AK, Fausto N, et al. Robbins and Cotran pathologic basis of disease, professional edition. New York: Elsevier Health Sciences; 2014.
23. Brix TH, Hegedüs L. Twin studies as a model for exploring the aetiology of autoimmune thyroid disease. Clin Endocrinol 2012;76(4):457–64.
24. Mackay IR, Rose NR. The autoimmune diseases. Cambridge (MA): Academic Press; 2013.
25. Kappers MHW, van Esch JHM, Smedts FMM, et al. Sunitinib-induced hypothyroidism is due to induction of type 3 deiodinase activity and thyroidal capillary regression. J Clin Endocrinol Metab 2011;96(10):3087–94.
26. Biondi B, Cooper DS. The clinical significance of subclinical thyroid dysfunction. Endocr Rev 2013;29(1):76–131.
27. Surks MI, Ortiz E, Daniels GH, et al. Subclinical thyroid disease: scientific review and guidelines for diagnosis and management. JAMA 2004;291(2):228–38.
28. De Groot L, Abalovich M, Alexander EK, et al. Management of thyroid dysfunction during pregnancy and postpartum: an endocrine society clinical practice guideline. J Clin Endocrinol Metab 2013;97(8):2543–65.
29. Velkeniers B, Van Meerhaeghe A, Poppe K, et al. Levothyroxine treatment and pregnancy outcome in women with subclinical hypothyroidism undergoing assisted reproduction technologies: systematic review and meta-analysis of RCTs. Hum Reprod Update 2013;19(3):251–8.
30. JonklaasJacqueline CB, Bianco AC, Bauer AJ, et al. Guidelines for the treatment of hypothyroidism: prepared by the American Thyroid Association task force on thyroid hormone replacement. Thyroid 2014;24(12):1670–751.
31. Stagnaro-Green A, Abalovich M, Alexander E, et al. The American Thyroid Association Taskforce on Thyroid Disease During Pregnancy and Postpartum. Thyroid 2011;21(10):1081–125.
32. Weetman AP. Graves' disease. N Engl J Med 2000;343(17):1236–48.
33. Tonacchera M, Agretti P, Chiovato L, et al. Activating thyrotropin receptor mutations are present in nonadenomatous hyperfunctioning nodules of toxic or autonomous multinodular goiter. J Clin Endocrinol Metab 2013;85(6):2270–4.
34. Krohn K, Führer D, Bayer Y, et al. Molecular pathogenesis of euthyroid and toxic multinodular goiter. Endocr Rev 2013;26(4):504–24.
35. Bahn Chair RS, Burch HB, Cooper DS, et al, American Thyroid Association, American Association of Clinical Endocrinologists. Hyperthyroidism and other causes of thyrotoxicosis: management guidelines of the American Thyroid

Association and American association of clinical endocrinologists. Thyroid 2011; 21(6):593–646.

36. Dean DS, Gharib H. Epidemiology of thyroid nodules. Best Pract Res Clin Endocrinol Metab 2008;22(6):901–11.

37. Tan GH, Gharib H. Thyroid incidentalomas: management approaches to nonpalpable nodules discovered incidentally on thyroid imaging. Ann Intern Med 1997; 126(3):226–31.

38. Cooper DS, Doherty GM, Haugen BR, et al. Revised American Thyroid Association management guidelines for patients with thyroid nodules and differentiated thyroid cancer. Thyroid 2009;19(11):1167–214.

39. Wright NC, Looker AC, Saag KG, et al. The recent prevalence of osteoporosis and low bone mass in the United States based on bone mineral density at the femoral neck or lumbar spine. J Bone Miner Res 2014;29(11):2520–6.

40. Cosman F, De Beur SJ, LeBoff MS, et al. Clinician's guide to prevention and treatment of osteoporosis. Osteoporos Int 2014;25(10):2359–81.

41. Cohen A, Shane E. Evaluation and management of the premenopausal woman with low BMD. Curr Osteoporos Rep 2013;11(4):276–85.

42. Schousboe JT, Shepherd JA, Bilezikian JP, et al. Executive summary of the 2013 international society for clinical densitometry position development conference on bone densitometry. J Clin Densitom 2013;16(4):455–66.

43. Nevitt MC, Ettinger B, Black DM, et al. The association of radiographically detected vertebral fractures with back pain and function: a prospective study. Ann Intern Med 1998;128(10):793–800.

44. Klotzbuecher CM, Ross PD, Landsman PB, et al. Patients with prior fractures have an increased risk of future fractures: a summary of the literature and statistical synthesis. J Bone Miner Res 2000;15(4):721–39.

45. Kanis JA, McCloskey E, Johansson H, et al. FRAX® with and without bone mineral density. Calcif Tissue Int 2012;90(1):1–13.

46. Adler RA, El-Hajj Fuleihan G, Bauer DC, et al. Managing Osteoporosis in Patients on Long-Term Bisphosphonate Treatment: Report of a Task Force of the American Society for Bone and Mineral Research. J Bone Miner Res 2016;31(1):16–35.

Primary Care Evaluation and Management of Gastroenterologic Issues in Women

Vijaya L. Rao, MD*, Dejan Micic, MD, Karen E. Kim, MD

KEYWORDS

- Colorectal cancer • Irritable bowel syndrome • Peptic ulcer disease
- Gallbladder disorders • Inflammatory bowel disease • Gastroesophageal reflux
- Barrett's esophagus

KEY POINTS

- Colorectal cancer is the third most common malignancy among women and colonoscopy is the screening test of choice.
- Irritable bowel syndrome is a diagnosis of exclusion, for which dietary and lifestyle modifications are first-line therapies.
- *Helicobacter pylori* infection and nonsteroidal anti-inflammatory drugs *are* the primary risk factors for peptic ulcer disease; eradication of *H pylori* and proton pump inhibitors are the cornerstones of therapy.
- Inflammatory bowel diseases, classified as Crohn's disease or ulcerative colitis, are increasing in incidence with increased sophistication of medical therapy.
- Gastroesophageal reflux typically responds to antisecretory therapies; further testing is required when disease complications are suspected, patients fail therapy, or the diagnosis must be confirmed.

INTRODUCTION

Gastrointestinal disorders commonly present to the primary care setting where initial preventive, diagnostic, and treatment strategies are implemented. Both gastrointestinal and liver diseases result in heavy economic and social costs in the United States.[1] Therefore, focusing on the initial presentations and appropriate management of common gastrointestinal disorders has the ability to curtail unnecessary costs in diagnosis

The authors have nothing to disclose.
Section of Gastroenterology, Hepatology and Nutrition, The University of Chicago Medical Center, 5841 South Maryland Avenue, Chicago, IL 60637, USA
* Corresponding author. MC 4076, Room M421, 5841 South Maryland Avenue, Chicago, IL 60637.
E-mail address: VIJAYA.RAO@UCHOSPITALS.EDU

Obstet Gynecol Clin N Am 43 (2016) 347–366
http://dx.doi.org/10.1016/j.ogc.2016.01.006
0889-8545/16/$ – see front matter © 2016 Elsevier Inc. All rights reserved.

obgyn.theclinics.com

and treatment strategies. In this review, we describe the presentation, diagnosis, and management of common gastrointestinal disorders with a focus on the evaluation and management of gastrointestinal disorders in women.

COLORECTAL CANCER

Colorectal cancer (CRC) is the third most common cancer as well as the third leading cause of cancer-related deaths among women and men. The estimated lifetime risk of developing CRC is 4.7%, although the incidence has been decreasing at a rate of approximately 3% per year from 2002 to 2011, likely as a result of greater adherence to screening recommendations. In the United States, the median age of diagnosis is 68 with a precipitous increase in cases after age 50.[2]

Clinical evaluation of patients in a primary care setting should include a risk assessment for CRC based on a detailed history and physical examination. Family history is integral because patients with first-degree relatives with CRC or advanced adenomas should be screened at an earlier age and potentially at more frequent intervals, depending on the relative's age of diagnosis. Signs and symptoms that should warrant diagnostic endoscopic evaluation include the development of iron deficiency anemia, hematochezia or rectal bleeding, and weight loss or changes in bowel habits, although primary prevention with screening is the key to reducing morbidity and mortality from CRC.

Current Screening Modalities and Guidelines

The evolving landscape of CRC screening tools over the last 2 decades can make the decision of how and when to screen patients daunting for providers. Available screening modalities are stratified into either "cancer detection" or "cancer prevention" tests.[3] Cancer detection tests include stool-based testing such as high sensitivity guaiac-based fecal occult blood test, fecal immunochemical test (FIT), and multitarget fecal DNA testing. These tests have a low sensitivity for polyps and an even lower sensitivity for malignancy as compared with cancer prevention tests, which are able to detect both premalignant as well as malignant lesions, with the preferred modality being colonoscopy. Alternative cancer detection tests include flexible sigmoidoscopy, colonoscopy, computed tomography, colonography, and double contrast barium enema. Physicians should discuss the risks, benefits, and limitations of each test with patients, taking into account their individual clinical picture including age and comorbidities. Screening recommendations are summarized in **Table 1**.

The United States Preventive Services Task Force recommends initiation of CRC screening at age 50 in patients who are average risk for CRC. Recent studies have sought to compare the efficacy of cancer prevention to cancer detection tests in detecting CRC. When the stool-based FIT was compared with colonoscopy, it was found that more advanced adenomas were detected via colonoscopy than with FIT (1.9% vs 0.9%). The difference in the rate of detection of nonadvanced adenomas was more pronounced, at 4.2% via colonoscopy versus 0.4% via FIT testing, whereas the rate of CRC at 10 years was similar in both groups at 0.1%.[4] However, the higher detection rate and diagnostic yield of colonoscopy with respect to premalignant lesions is important to note because advanced adenomas are often considered a surrogate marker for CRC. Therefore, colonoscopy is preferred because it may not only reduce the rate of death from CRC, but also the incidence of disease.

Table 1
Screening examination options for adults at average risk for colorectal cancer

Test Option	Testing Interval if Negative Result
Cancer detection	
High sensitivity guaiac-based fecal occult blood testing [Hemoccult Sensa]	Every year
Fecal immunochemical test	Every year
Fecal DNA testing	Every 3 y
Cancer Prevention	
Endoscopic examinations	
Colonoscopy	Every 10 y
Flexible sigmoidoscopy	Every 5 y
Radiologic Examinations	
Computed tomographic colonography	Every 5 y

Adapted from Kim KE. Early Detection and Prevention of Colorectal Cancer. Thorofare (NJ): SLACK incorporated; 2009. p. 109–23.

High-Risk Populations

In patients who have a family history of 2 or more first-degree relatives with CRC at any age or one first-degree relative with CRC or an advanced adenoma (adenoma ≥1 cm in size, or with high-grade dysplasia or villous elements) diagnosed at age younger than 60 years, colonoscopy is recommended every 5 years starting at age 40 or 10 years younger than the age at diagnosis of the youngest affected relative. A family history of small tubular adenomas (<1 cm) in first-degree relatives does not influence the screening recommendations for CRC.[3]

Although the majority of diagnosed CRC is believed to be sporadic, hereditary cancer syndromes conferring a high lifetime risk of CRC have been identified in up to 5% to 6% of cases.[5] Hereditary syndromes that affect CRC screening guidelines include familial adenomatous polyposis, MUTYH-associated polyposis, and hereditary nonpolyposis CRC. The presence of inflammatory bowel disease (IBD) such as Crohn's disease (CD) or ulcerative colitis (UC) also affects interval of screening for CRC, with general recommendations to begin screening 8 years after disease diagnosis[6,7] (**Fig. 1**).

Several risk factors for CRC have been identified such as diabetes mellitus, alcohol use, tobacco use, and obesity.[8–11] Although these factors may predispose to the development of CRC, they do not currently affect CRC screening recommendations.

Colorectal Cancer in Women

Although the current screening guidelines for CRC do not distinguish between men and women, significant gender differences do exist, which may ultimately lead to the development of customized guidelines in the future.

The Colorectal Neoplasia Screening With Colonoscopy in Asymptomatic Women at Regional Navy/Army Medical Centers (CONCeRN) study, published in 2005, found that in a population of age-matched men and women adjusted for family history and fecal occult blood test results, men were found to be nearly twice as likely to have advanced neoplasia at colonoscopy as women (8.6% vs 3.5%).[12] Several other studies have also confirmed a sex-based disparity in the prevalence of adenomas and advanced neoplasia between men and women.[13,14]

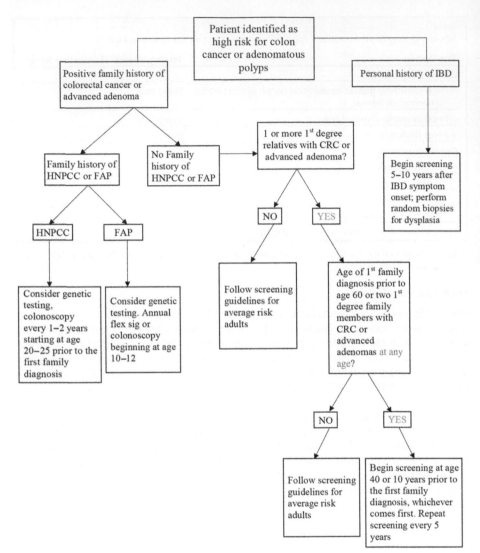

Fig. 1. Algorithm for initiation of colorectal cancer screening in a high-risk population. CRC, colorectal cancer; FAP, familial adenomatous polyposis; HNPCC, hereditary non polyposis colorectal cancer; IBD, inflammatory bowel disease. (*Adapted from* Kim KE. Early Detection and Prevention of Colorectal Cancer. Thorofare (NJ): SLACK incorporated; 2009. p. 109–23.)

Data have also suggested that the location of neoplasm in women is predominantly right sided, indicating that the usefulness and diagnostic yield of flexible sigmoidoscopy, which only evaluates the left colon, is significantly lower in women.[12]

Overall, it is estimated that only 52% of adults aged 50 to 75 adhere to recommended CRC guidelines. Healthy People 2020 is a public health initiative that sets 10-year national objectives with a goal to reach 70.5% adherence to CRC screening guidelines by 2020. Patients of white, non-Hispanic descent, higher education levels, and those who have access to private insurance had rates of adherence 14% to 42% higher than minority patients, patients with lower income, and patients with lower education levels.

Acknowledging such disparities in CRC screening is important in the primary care setting to ultimately decrease barriers to CRC screening.[15]

IRRITABLE BOWEL SYNDROME

Irritable bowel syndrome (IBS) is one of the most commonly diagnosed gastroenterologic conditions, accounting for a large number of physician visits in both gastroenterology and primary care practices.[16] In North America, the prevalence is estimated to be 11.8%.[17] This is a particularly important topic among women, because there is a 2:1 female predominance in patients diagnosed with IBS in the United States.[18] Interestingly, the gender difference seems to wane with age; there are 4 times more female patients with IBS under the age of 30.[19]

Diagnosis

Patients with IBS most commonly suffer from irregular bowel habits in conjunction with abdominal pain or discomfort. The Rome III diagnostic criteria for IBS require the presence of recurrent abdominal pain and/or discomfort for at least 3 days per month during the last 3 months with onset of greater than 6 months prior.[20] These symptoms must also be associated with 2 or more of the following: improvement with defecation, change in stool frequency, or change in stool appearance or form. IBS is typically considered a diagnosis of exclusion, requiring initial evaluation for organic or structural causes, especially in the setting of symptom onset after age 50, unexplained iron deficiency anemia, rectal bleeding, weight loss, and nocturnal abdominal pain.[21] All patients with suspected IBS should undergo age appropriate CRC screening and a complete blood count. In patients with diarrhea, testing for celiac disease as well colonoscopy with random biopsies should be considered. Obtaining serum or stool inflammatory markers such as C-reactive protein or fecal calprotectin can aid in the initial evaluation.[22]

The Rome III criteria further stratify IBS into subtypes based on the predominant feature of the bowel complaint: IBS with constipation (IBS-C), IBS with diarrhea (IBS-D), mixed-type, and unclassified. IBS-C tends to have the greatest predilection toward females; there is no sex difference found for IBS-D.[23]

Pathophysiology

The pathophysiology behind the development of IBS has not been clearly elucidated. Although there is some speculation it may be related to underlying colonic dysmotility, no predominant pattern of dysmotility has emerged. However, patients with IBS do experience visceral hypersensitivity, or an increased sensation in response to stimuli. Several studies have shown that IBS patients have increased pain caused by balloon distention in the intestine compared with controls, suggestive of such visceral hypersensitivity.[24,25] Altered gut immune activation, intestinal permeability, and intestinal and colonic microbiome have also been implicated as potential etiologies.[26,27]

Many patients with IBS associate symptoms with food allergies, despite the low prevalence of true food allergies in Western countries (1%–3%).[28] Some patients may be intolerant of certain foods, but IBS is not a true food allergy. Often, patients cannot accurately identify a correlation between symptoms and a particular food therefore recommending patients to keep a food and symptom diary may be helpful.

Psychosocial distress likely plays a significant role in the development of IBS. Research has showed that female patients with IBS are more likely to have experienced physical, verbal, or sexual abuse and also have higher rates of depression and anxiety.[29–31]

Management

A strong clinician–patient relationship with continuity of care is paramount in the management of IBS. Because IBS is a symptom-based disorder, tailoring the treatment plan to the patient's predominant complaint may be most beneficial. First-line therapies often include over-the-counter medications such as probiotics, a bowel slowing agent for patients with IBS-D, and laxatives or fiber supplementation for IBS-C patients. These medications often have a favorable cost and adverse effect profile.

In recent years, successful therapeutic strategies have relied heavily on lifestyle and dietary modifications. An increase in physical activity has been shown to improve gastrointestinal symptoms related to IBS.[32] Several restrictive diets have been studied in the treatment of IBS, but currently, evidence supports diets that are low in fermentable oligosaccharides, disaccharides, monosaccharides, and polyols (FODMAPs). FODMAPs consist of poorly absorbed, highly fermentable, short-chain carbohydrates and are found in wheat, select fruits and vegetables, onions, sorbitol, and some dairy products. FODMAPs can lead to increased intestinal water secretion and fermentation, which causes increased production of short-chain fatty acids and gas, which in turn is hypothesized to adversely affect individuals with gastrointestinal visceral hypersensitivity.[32,33]

Questions regarding the use of probiotics and antibiotics commonly arise in clinical settings. Probiotics may improve symptoms of IBS, but current data are not strong enough to recommend routine use. With regard to antibiotics, rifaximin has been studied and also may provide relief in some patients but should be used with caution because symptoms may recur after completion of a 14-day course.[34]

In patients who do not respond to over-the-counter symptom-based treatments or diet and lifestyle modifications, prescription pharmacologic agents may be considered. Antispasmodics have anticholinergic properties that may improve IBS symptoms by relaxing smooth muscle in the intestine. Dicyclomine or hyoscyamine are commonly used and may provide short-term symptomatic relief for IBS patients with cramping abdominal pain.[20]

Management of Irritable Bowel Syndrome with Constipation

Two prosecretory agents have been approved for patients with IBS-C. Lubiprostone activates chloride channels, stimulating intestinal fluid secretion, and can improve bowel and abdominal symptoms.[35] Linactolide is guanylate cyclase agonist with similar effects on intestinal fluid secretion and transit. There is strong evidence in its efficacy for patients with persistent constipation despite treatment with laxatives such as polyethylene glycol.[36,37] Prokinetic effects of selective serotonin-reuptake inhibitors may be also be effective in IBS-C patients.

Management of Irritable Bowel Syndrome with Diarrhea

A recent metaanalysis showed that the use of antidepressants showed significant improvement in abdominal pain in IBS patients.[38] Tricyclic antidepressants can also slow transit time given their anticholinergic effects, providing relief in patients with IBS-D. Serotonin modulators, such as 5HT-3 receptor antagonists, may help to alleviate visceral hypersensitivity in IBS.

In summary, the management of IBS should focus on symptom-based therapies as well as avoidance of triggers for patients' symptoms. First-line therapies for the treatment of IBS should include diet and lifestyle modifications and the trial of over-the-counter medications. For patients with refractory symptoms, several prescription pharmacologic options are available but should be used judiciously by providers.

PEPTIC ULCER DISEASE

A peptic ulcer is defined as a disruption of the mucosal integrity in the stomach or duodenum which penetrates the muscularis mucosa and deeper layers of the luminal wall (**Fig. 2**). The prevalence of peptic ulcer disease (PUD) is 5% to 10%, approximately 2% of which are symptomatic.[39]

Clinical Presentation

In PUD patients who develop symptoms, they most commonly present with dyspepsia, defined by epigastric pain or burning, postprandial fullness, and early satiety. Symptoms may vary depending on ulcer location, with the pain of duodenal ulcerations occurring 2 to 3 hours postprandially or nocturnally in the setting of low pH. Classically, gastric ulcer symptoms typically worsen after food intake, which may result in anorexia or weight loss. However, these symptoms are not necessarily specific for PUD.

In many individuals, PUD may be asymptomatic and the first presentation may be a complication such as gastrointestinal bleeding, perforation, penetration, or obstruction. Bleeding is the most common complication and occurs in an estimated 15% to 20% of patients, manifesting as melena, coffee-ground emesis, or in cases of a brisk bleed, hematochezia. In cases of chronic gastrointestinal bleeding, ulcers can present as unexplained iron deficiency anemia.

Risk Factors

The 2 major risk factors in the development of PUD include use of nonsteroidal anti-inflammatory drugs (NSAIDs) or *Helicobacter pylori* infection, which account for 90% of all ulcers.

An estimated 25% of patients who use NSAIDs chronically develop PUD. Patients who are over the age of 65, have a history of ulcer or GI bleeding in the past, are on a high dose of NSAIDs, or are concomitantly using corticosteroids or other anticoagulants are at greatest risk for development of PUD.[40] Proton pump inhibitors (PPIs) are currently the antisecretory drug of choice in the prevention and treatment of NSAID-induced ulcers, although cessation of NSAID use is recommended as well if an ulcer is identified.

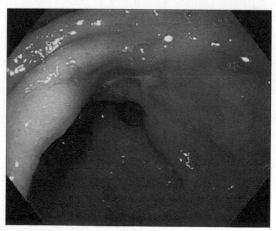

Fig. 2. Endoscopic appearance of a nonbleeding, clean-based peptic ulceration with surrounding erythema at the prepyloric region of the stomach.

Helicobacter pylori infection is more common in developing countries, but in the United States the prevalence is estimated to be approximately 30% to 40%.[41] *H pylori* infection induces an inflammatory response resulting in varying degrees of chronic active gastritis, which can lead to PUD. In addition to PUD, the presence of *H pylori* also predisposes to gastric adenocarcinoma and mucosa-associated lymphoid tissue lymphoma. Nonendoscopic testing for *H pylori* includes serum antibody testing, urea breath test, and fecal antigen test. Options for endoscopic testing of gastric tissues includes histology, rapid urease testing, culture or polymerase chain reaction. Caution must be used with urease testing because the use of PPIs, antibiotics, and bismuth compounds decreases test sensitivity.[42]

In immunocompromised hosts, viral etiologies for PUD such as herpes simplex type I or cytomegalovirus should also be suspected. Other less common conditions that may lead to the development of PUD include sarcoidosis, systemic mastocytosis, mesenteric ischemia, and Zollinger–Ellison syndrome.

Endoscopic Evaluation and Management

Endoscopic evaluation should be performed in patients who have symptoms of dyspepsia and are greater than age 55. Alarm symptoms such as gastrointestinal bleeding, anemia, early satiety, unexplained weight loss, dysphagia, odynophagia, recurrent vomiting, or significant family history of gastrointestinal malignancy should also warrant endoscopic evaluation.[43]

If endoscopy confirms PUD, all patients should receive PPI therapy but specific recommendations vary based on ulcer characteristics, presence of complications, and presumed etiology of the ulcer. Patients who have high-risk endoscopic stigmata of ulcer hemorrhage, such as active bleeding, a nonbleeding visible vessel, or adherent clot should receive intravenous PPI therapy after endoscopic intervention.[43] All patients with evidence of PUD on endoscopy should be tested for *H pylori*.

In patients with NSAID-induced ulcerations, PPI therapy should be maintained for a minimum of 8 weeks with discontinuation of NSAID use. If there is a need for continued use of NSAIDs or anticoagulation, patients should remain on concomitant PPI therapy.

There are several regimens available for the treatment of *H pylori* infections, the most common being triple therapy with a PPI in combination with clarithromycin and either amoxicillin or metronidazole for 10 to 14 days. Alternative regimens include a PPI with bismuth, metronidazole, and tetracycline. Testing to confirm eradication is recommended 4 or more weeks after completion of therapy, with the urease breath test being the most reliable nonendoscopic test to do so.[44] If there is failure to eradicate after initial treatment, a second-line course of therapy may be used, but should not include repeating metronidazole or clarithromycin given high rates of resistance to these antibiotics.

For patients with uncomplicated *H pylori* associated duodenal ulcers, 10 to 14 days of PPI therapy in conjunction with antibiotics should be sufficient for healing. For gastric or complicated duodenal *H pylori* positive ulcers, 8 to 12 weeks and 4 to 8 weeks of PPI use is recommended, respectively (**Table 2**).

Given the low risk of malignancy in patients with duodenal ulcers, a repeat upper endoscopy is not recommended routinely unless symptoms persist or recur. In patients with gastric ulcerations, the decision for endoscopic surveillance should be individualized. However, repeat endoscopy after 12 weeks of PPI therapy should be considered strongly if the ulcer has any of the following characteristics: unclear etiology, greater than 2 cm, an appearance suspicious for malignancy, if the ulcer was not

Table 2
Guidelines for proton pump inhibitor therapy in the treatment of peptic ulcer disease

Type of Ulcer	Length of Proton Pump Inhibitor Therapy
Idiopathic	Indefinite
NSAID related	8 wk or as long as NSAIDs are continued
Uncomplicated duodenal *Helicobacter pylori*-related ulcer	10–14 d
Complicated duodenal *H pylori*-related ulcer	4–8 wk
Gastric *H pylori*-related ulcer	8–12 wk

Abbreviation: NSAID, nonsteroidal antiinflammatory drug.

biopsied on the initial endoscopy, or if the initial endoscopy was performed for bleeding.[45]

GALLBLADDER DISORDERS
Biliary Colic

Biliary colic classically presents as epigastric or right upper quadrant pain that is episodic in nature and triggered by eating, with progressive worsening 3 to 4 hours postprandially. This pain is presumably caused by spasm of the cystic duct when transiently obstructed by a gallstone. Pain lasting longer than 6 hours may be concerning for acute cholecystitis, secondary to inflammation of the gallbladder wall.

True biliary colic can be difficult to differentiate from nonspecific dyspepsia, but is an important distinction for clinicians to make; symptoms of gas and bloating are not characteristic features. A detailed history and physical examination should be completed as well as laboratory work including liver and pancreatic function tests. Abdominal ultrasound should be ordered as a first-line imaging study given its low risk and high sensitivity and specificity (95%) for the detection of gallstones.[46]

Cholelithiasis and Cholecystitis

Women are affected by cholelithiasis approximately twice as often as men with up to a 4:1 female predominance in the reproductive years.[47,48] Advanced age, family history, obesity, ileal CD, hypertriglyceridemia, and total parenteral nutrition are also risk factors for the development of cholelithiasis.

Approximately one-third of patients with cholelithiasis are symptomatic. As mentioned, abdominal ultrasonography should be completed, but if negative and clinical suspicion remains high, endoscopic ultrasonography can be performed to evaluate for missed stones or sludge. Magnetic resonance cholangiopancreatography is a noninvasive imaging study that can provide high-quality images of the biliary and pancreatic ducts and is particularly sensitive in the detection of choledocholithiasis.

Acute cholecystitis is typically caused by prolonged obstruction of the cystic duct by a gallstone; acalculous cholecystitis accounts for 5% to 10% of cases.[49] Patients may have persistent severe biliary-type pain localized to the right upper quadrant in conjunction with findings of fever and leukocytosis. Jaundice may also occur, even in the absence of choledocholithiasis. Findings on ultrasonography in acute cholecystitis includes intramural gas, thickening of the gallbladder wall and pericholecystic fluid collection. If a hepatobiliary iminodiacetic acid scan is performed, the gallbladder may not be visualized secondary to occlusion of the cystic duct.[50,51]

Cholecystectomy is the treatment of choice for both symptomatic cholelithiasis and acute cholecystitis. Nonoperative therapies, such as shock wave lithotripsy or bile dissolution therapy, have largely fallen out of favor given the high rate of gallstone recurrence. For pain control during acute bouts of biliary colic, NSAIDs are the drug of choice; a recent metaanalysis showed comparable efficacy to opioids and significant reduction in the proportion of patients with severe complications.[52]

Gallbladder Disease and Pregnancy

Gallstones are common during pregnancy as a result of decreased gallbladder motility and emptying with subsequent bile stasis, which predisposes to stone formation. Higher circulating levels of reproductive hormones such as estrogen and progesterone increase cholesterol circulation.[53,54] The major risk factor for the development of gallstones is obesity before pregnancy. If suspected, ultrasound remains the first-line diagnostic imaging study of choice given its safety and reliability. Pregnant patients should first be treated conservatively with supportive care such as analgesics and intravenous fluids. For recurrent, refractory biliary colic or acute cholecystitis, cholecystectomy can still be performed safely, but may be more technically difficulty later in the pregnancy.

INFLAMMATORY BOWEL DISEASE

The IBDs can be classified into 2 main entities, CD and UC. Although the pathogenesis of IBD is not well-understood, the current premise is that defects in the immune system allow for aberrant immune responses to intraluminal antigens, which ultimately lead to bowel damage.[55] In UC, acute and chronic inflammation confined exclusively to the mucosa of the colorectum is the hallmark of the disease. The inflammation is characteristically superficial in nature, and seems to begin in the rectum with variable extension to more proximal portions of the colon (**Fig. 3**). The majority of the symptoms of UC are derived from an inflamed rectum and correspond to a loss of compliance and loss of discriminant sensation: tenesmus, incomplete evacuation, urgency, and hematochezia. Persistent inflammation and mucosal ulceration can subsequently lead to the recognized acute complications of UC including toxic megacolon, perforation, and bleeding; prolonged inflammation can result in the development of dysplasia and CRC.[49]

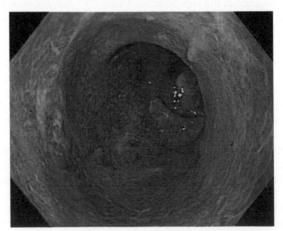

Fig. 3. Endoscopic appearance of ulcerative colitis demonstrating a granular mucosa with loss of normal vascular pattern in a circumferential and continuous pattern.

In CD, acute and chronic transmural inflammation results in a progressive disease course with complications including the development of perianal abscesses or fistulas, luminal stricturing, and intraabdominal or enterocutaneous fistulas. The endoscopic appearance of CD can affect any portion of the gastrointestinal track with a characteristic patchy inflammation ranging from superficial aphthous ulcerations to deep serpiginous ulcerations (**Fig. 4**). A variety of clinical courses ranging from mild to severe disease are evident and based on the disease location, extent, and phenotype.[56] In a population-based study, at presentation, 56.2% of individuals were between the ages of 17 and 40 with an extent characterized by ileal disease in 45.1%, ileocolonic in 18.6% and 32.0% with colonic disease.[57] The rate of complication (defined by the development of stricturing or penetrating disease behavior) occurred in 33.7% within 5 years and 50.8% at 20 years with a corresponding surgical rate of 81.6% within 6 months of disease behavior change.[57] Prognostic factors associated with the development of a progressive disease include disease location and presence of perianal disease in addition to a diagnosis before age 40, an initial requirement in the use of corticosteroids for disease control and the presence of severe endoscopic lesions (defined by extensive and deep ulcerations covering >10% of the mucosal area).[58–62]

Given the progressive disease course in IBD, medical therapies are designed to alter dysregulated inflammatory responses. The current use of immunosuppressant and biologic therapies has been demonstrated to decrease the risk of surgery in both CD and UC over the past 6 decades in a systematic review of population-based studies.[63,64] With the ability to alter the natural history of a progressive gastrointestinal condition, the goals of treatment now include the induction and maintenance of mucosal (and histologic) healing.[65]

Inflammatory Bowel Disease Therapy

Historically, a step-up approach to medical care has included the use of aminosalicylate derivatives, corticosteroids, methotrexate, thiopurines and biologic agents (anti–tumor necrosis factor and antiintegrin inhibitors) with separate goals of an induction of clinical remission and maintenance of disease control. More recent evidence has advocated for an earlier use of biologic therapies, combination therapies and surgery in appropriate severe presentations of disease while minimizing the risks of

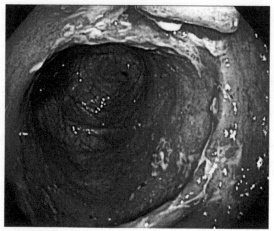

Fig. 4. Endoscopic appearance of Crohn's disease demonstrating patchy linear ulcerations with normal intervening mucosa with a preserved vascular pattern.

overtreatment. Although a uniform prognostication or therapeutic algorithm is not in current use, more aggressive disease monitoring with objective assessments are in wider clinical use to assess responses to therapeutic changes and target more defined goals of mucosal healing and durable remission. Given the recent advances in the therapies and objective endpoints in disease monitoring, early referral to an expert IBD center is appropriate.

Inflammatory Bowel Disease and Pregnancy

Given the common young age at diagnosis, females with IBD commonly require management of IBD in pregnancy. The growing current experience suggests that most women will have a good outcome.[66] Proper disease management requires collaboration between the patient, gastroenterologist, and obstetrician, all of whom are comfortable and experienced with the common IBD medications. Overall rates of fertility among patients with stable IBD are similar to age-matched controls, with the one exception among females who have previously undergone an ileal pouch anal anastomosis, which has been associated with a 3-fold decreased rate of fertility.[67,68] Although concerns exist as to the effect of IBD medications on the fetus, the primary concern in pregnancy should be the risk of disease flare if medications are stopped. Disease activity at conception has been associated with higher rates of preterm delivery, preeclampsia, preterm premature rupture of membranes, and low birth weight.[69,70] During the course of a pregnancy, women are not at an increased risk of disease flare; therefore, the goal should be induction of remission before a pregnancy with maintenance of therapy throughout the pregnancy.[71] Most medications used in IBD are compatible with pregnancy and breastfeeding (**Table 3**) with the primary exceptions of methotrexate and

Table 3
FDA classification of therapies in IBD

Medication	Brand(s)	Route of Administration	FDA Classification
Sulfasalazine	Azulfidine	PO	B
Mesalamine	Asacol	PO	C
	Pentasa	PO	B
	Lialda	PO	B
	Apriso	PO	B
Balsalazide	Colazol	PO	B
Olsalazine	Dipentum	PO	B
Mesalamine	Canasa	Rectal	B
	Rowasa	Rectal	B
Azathioprine	Imuran	PO	D
6-mercaptopurine	Purinethol	PO	D
Methotrexate	Trexall	PO	X
Thalidomide	Thalomid	PO	X
Infliximab	Remicade	IV	B
Adalimumab	Humira	SQ	B
Certolizumab pegol	Cimzia	SQ	B
Golimumab	Simponi	SQ	B
Natalizumab	Tysabri	IV	C
Vedolizumab	Entyvio	IV	B

Abbreviations: FDA, Food and Drug Administration; IBD, inflammatory bowel disease; IV, intravenous; PO, per os; SQ, subcutaneous.

thalidomide (Food and Drug Administration category X), which should be stopped a minimum of 3 months and ideally 6 months before a pregnancy.[66] The biologic therapies are Food and Drug Administration category B and to date are not associated with a consistent pattern of adverse pregnancy outcome.[66] Current evidence suggests that the risks of birth defects, infectious complications, or impairment in developmental milestones are not increased among children exposed to biologic therapies.[66,72,73] Ultimately, an interdisciplinary approach with active engagement of the patient and appropriate communication through providers is needed to provide the expected favorable outcomes in pregnancy.

GASTROESOPHAGEAL REFLUX DISEASE

Gastroesophageal reflux disease (GERD) is one of the most common disorders of the gastrointestinal tract and is defined as troublesome symptoms or mucosal damage secondary to the abnormal reflux of gastric contents into the esophagus.[74] Although the reflux of gastric contents into the esophagus is a physiologic event, given the definition requiring mucosal damage or abnormal symptoms, the diagnosis of GERD can be made using a combination of presenting symptoms and/or objective testing.[75] When defined by using patient-centered symptoms, prevalence rates of GERD in North America range from 18.1% to 27.8%.[76]

GERD occurs when the normal antireflux barrier between the stomach and the esophagus is impaired, either transiently or permanently. Defects in the esophagogastric barrier, such as lower esophageal sphincter incompetence, transient lower esophageal sphincter relaxations, and hiatal hernia, are the primary factors involved in the development of GERD.[77] Symptoms develop when the offensive factors in the gastroduodenal contents, such as acid, pepsin, bile acids, and trypsin, overcome several lines of esophageal defense, including esophageal acid clearance and mucosal resistance. Primary risk factors for the predictors of erosive GERD include overweight status, alcohol use, and smoking status.[78]

It is neither practical nor necessary to initiate diagnostic testing on every patient with symptoms of GERD and therefore clinical symptom-based and empiric medical therapies remain as the frontline evaluation in patients suspected to have GERD. Further testing is only required when disease complications are suspected, patients fail therapy, or the diagnosis must be confirmed owing to atypical symptoms or before a change in treatment strategy is initiated.[79]

Endoscopy is the test of choice to evaluate the mucosa in patients with symptoms of GERD. Endoscopy is indicated in those who do not respond to initial therapy, when there are alarm symptoms suggesting complicated disease (dysphagia, odynophagia, bleeding, weight loss, or anemia) and when sufficient duration of disease places an individual at risk for Barrett's esophagus.[74] Cross-sectional studies of patients undergoing endoscopy have suggested that approximately 20% of patients with upper gastrointestinal symptoms have esophagitis, 20% have endoscopy-negative reflux disease, 10% have PUD, 2% have Barrett's esophagus, and 1% may have malignancy.[80] Findings related to a diagnosis of GERD include the presence of erosive esophagitis, peptic strictures, and a columnar-lined esophagus (Barrett's esophagus).[75]

Ambulatory esophageal pH monitoring is an important tool in the diagnosis and management of GERD. Esophageal pH monitoring can detect and quantify gastroesophageal reflux and correlate symptoms temporally with reflux. The primary indications for ambulatory 24-hour esophageal pH monitoring are[81] to document excessive acid reflux in patients with suspected GERD but without endoscopic esophagitis, to assess reflux frequency, and to assess symptom association.[81] Standard ambulatory 24-hour esophageal pH monitoring measures distal esophageal acid exposure by using a single pH electrode catheter that is, passed through the nose and positioned 5 cm above the superior margin of the manometrically determined lower esophageal sphincter. Typical ambulatory esophageal pH monitoring units have an event marker that can be activated by the patient during the study to indicate the timing of symptoms, meals, and recumbent positioning. At the end of the study, data are downloaded to a computer, which generates a pH tracing and a data summary. Given limitations in patient tolerance to ambulatory catheter-based esophageal pH monitoring systems and difficulties with prolonged measurement periods, an ambulatory wireless capsule-based pH monitoring system has been developed. Upon endoscopic placement, recording data are then transmitted to a device worn on the patient's waist. The wireless system has the advantage of recording 48 to 96 hours of pH data. The capsule pH probe falls off after several days and is passed in the stool. The wireless capsule-based pH monitoring system may be better tolerated, causing less interference with daily activities, and has a higher overall satisfaction rate for patients with GERD.

Gastroesophageal Reflux Disease Therapy

Lifestyle interventions remain an important part of therapy in GERD and include counseling on weight loss, tobacco and alcohol cessation, avoidance of late-night meals, and foods that can aggravate reflux (caffeine, chocolate, spicy foods, and highly acidic foods).[75] Medical options include antacids, histamine-receptor antagonists and PPI therapy. A metaanalysis including 43 studies assessing rates of healing of erosive esophagitis demonstrated higher rates of healing with PPI therapy (83.6% ± 11.4%) compared with histamine receptor antagonists (51.9% ± 17.1%), sucralfate (39.2% ± 22.4%), and placebo (28.2% ± 15.6%). Furthermore, patients exposed to PPI therapy had faster rates of heartburn symptom relief and more complete heartburn relief.[82] After a standard 8-week treatment course of PPI therapy for erosive esophagitis or GERD-related symptoms, PPI therapy should be limited to the lowest effective dose to decrease the risk of complications of medical therapy including low but defined risks of enteric infections including *Clostridium difficile* infection and community-acquired pneumonia.[83,84] Although debate has surrounded the use of PPI therapy and bone fractures, a population-based Canadian study was unable to find an association between PPI use and accelerated bone mineral density loss.[85] Multiple studies have been unable to determine an association between PPI use and cardiovascular outcomes, initially hypothesized owing to similarities in PPI metabolism and activation of the antiplatelet therapy clopidogrel.[86,87]

Gastroesophageal Reflux Disease and Pregnancy

Symptoms of GERD have been reported to effect 30% to 80% of females during the course of a pregnancy.[88] Factors related to the development of GERD in pregnancy include a decrease in the lower esophageal sphincter pressure mediated by smooth muscle relaxation effects of progesterone in combination with estrogen.[89,90] Furthermore, a gravid uterus and alterations in gastrointestinal motility are hypothesized to promote GERD through an increase in intra-abdominal pressure and delayed gastric emptying, respectively.[89] Invasive diagnostic procedures are commonly reserved during the course of pregnancy for those with severe or refractory symptoms to medical management. Although lifestyle changes are typically used first in the management of GERD in pregnancy, antacids, histamine receptor antagonists, and PPI therapy can be used effectively. A Swedish cohort including 553 children born to 547 mothers did not demonstrate an increased risk of congenital malformations among children born to mothers using histamine receptor antagonists or omeprazole therapy.[91] A subsequent metaanalysis including 7 studies and 1530 exposed females to PPI therapy in pregnancy found no association with major congenital malformation, spontaneous abortion, or preterm delivery.[92] Given the commonly short duration of reflux symptoms in pregnancy, most cases can be managed symptomatically with a combination of lifestyle and medical therapies.

Barrett's Esophagus

Complications associated with GERD include the development of erosive esophagitis, peptic strictures and Barrett's esophagus. Barrett's esophagus can be found in 5% to 15% of patients who have endoscopy for symptoms of GERD. Although screening for Barrett's esophagus in the general population remains controversial, a number of studies highlight risk factors associated with the presence of Barrett's esophagus. These include male sex, older age (>40 years) and prolonged duration of symptoms (>13 years).[93–95] Barrett's esophagus is suspected endoscopically when the pale pink squamous mucosa of the distal esophagus is replaced to varying extent with salmon pink columnar mucosa (**Fig. 5**). In Barrett's esophagus, the squamocolumnar junction is displaced proximal to the gastroesophageal junction, and the diagnosis is confirmed with a biopsy finding of intestinal metaplasia, characterized by mucin-containing goblet cells. Barrett's esophagus may be divided into short segment and long segment types according to whether the metaplasia is longer or shorter than 3 cm. It is more common to find dysplasia and cancer in a patient with long segment Barrett's esophagus, but patients with short segment Barrett's esophagus are also at increased risk. Therefore, surveillance endoscopy is commonly practiced in the United States. Four quadrant biopsies every 2 cm of the Barrett's mucosa allows for sampling and detection of dysplasia, with repeat surveillance intervals determined based on the pathologic findings.[95,96] Although the absolute annual risk of development of adenocarcinoma among individuals with Barrett's esophagus remains low (0.12%), the demonstration of dysplasia is associated with increased risks of the development of esophageal

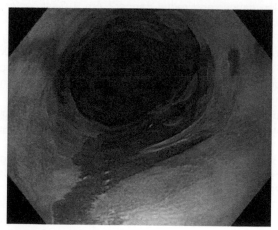

Fig. 5. Endoscopic appearance of Barrett's esophagus with the replacement of the pale pink squamous mucosa of the distal esophagus by salmon pink columnar mucosa.

adenocarcinoma.[97] Fortunately, most patients with high-grade dysplasia can be treated with various endoscopic eradication therapies as opposed to the requirement of esophagectomy.[96] PPI therapy remains an essential medical therapy in patients with Barrett's esophagus and GERD symptoms, although its role in the sole reduction of development of dysplasia among patients with Barrett's esophagus remains controversial.[96]

REFERENCES

1. Sandler RS, Everhart JE, Donowitz M, et al. The burden of selected digestive diseases in the United States. Gastroenterology 2002;122(5):1500–11.
2. SEER Stat fact sheets: colon and rectum cancer. Available at: http://seer.cancer.gov/statfacts/html/colorect.html. Accessed September 29, 2015.
3. Rex DK, Johnson DA, Anderson JC, et al. American College of Gastroenterology guidelines for colorectal cancer screening 2009 [corrected]. Am J Gastroenterol 2009;104(3):739–50.
4. Quintero E, Castells A, Bujanda L, et al. Colonoscopy versus fecal immunochemical testing in colorectal-cancer screening. N Engl J Med 2012;366(8):697–706.
5. Stoffel EM, Kastrinos F. Familial colorectal cancer, beyond Lynch syndrome. Clin Gastroenterol Hepatol 2014;12(7):1059–68.
6. Farraye FA, Odze RD, Eaden J, et al. AGA technical review on the diagnosis and management of colorectal neoplasia in inflammatory bowel disease. Gastroenterology 2010;138(2):746–74, 774.e1–4; [quiz: e12–3].
7. Leighton JA, Shen B, Baron TH, et al. ASGE guideline: endoscopy in the diagnosis and treatment of inflammatory bowel disease. Gastrointest Endosc 2006; 63(4):558–65.
8. Botteri E, Iodice S, Bagnardi V, et al. Smoking and colorectal cancer: a meta-analysis. JAMA 2008;300(23):2765–78.
9. Cho E, Smith-Warner SA, Ritz J, et al. Alcohol intake and colorectal cancer: a pooled analysis of 8 cohort studies. Ann Intern Med 2004;140(8):603–13.
10. Karahalios A, English DR, Simpson JA. Weight change and risk of colorectal cancer: a systematic review and meta-analysis. Am J Epidemiol 2015;181(11):832–45.
11. Yuhara H, Steinmaus C, Cohen SE, et al. Is diabetes mellitus an independent risk factor for colon cancer and rectal cancer? Am J Gastroenterol 2011;106(11): 1911–21 [quiz: 22].
12. Schoenfeld P, Cash B, Flood A, et al. Colonoscopic screening of average-risk women for colorectal neoplasia. N Engl J Med 2005;352(20):2061–8.
13. Ferlitsch M, Reinhart K, Pramhas S, et al. Sex-specific prevalence of adenomas, advanced adenomas, and colorectal cancer in individuals undergoing screening colonoscopy. JAMA 2011;306(12):1352–8.
14. Regula J, Rupinski M, Kraszewska E, et al. Colonoscopy in colorectal-cancer screening for detection of advanced neoplasia. N Engl J Med 2006;355(18): 1863–72.
15. Healthy people 2020. 2014. Available at: www.healthypeople.gov/2020/leading-health-indicators/2020-lhi-topics/Clinical-Preventive-Services/data. Accessed September 29, 2015.
16. Everhart JE, Ruhl CE. Burden of digestive diseases in the United States part I: overall and upper gastrointestinal diseases. Gastroenterology 2009;136(2):376–86.
17. Lovell RM, Ford AC. Global prevalence of and risk factors for irritable bowel syndrome: a meta-analysis. Clin Gastroenterol Hepatol 2012;10(7):712–21.e4.

18. Brandt LJ, Chey WD, Foxx-Orenstein AE, et al. An evidence-based position statement on the management of irritable bowel syndrome. Am J Gastroenterol 2009; 104(Suppl 1):S1–35.
19. Garcia Rodriguez LA, Ruigomez A, Wallander MA, et al. Detection of colorectal tumor and inflammatory bowel disease during follow-up of patients with initial diagnosis of irritable bowel syndrome. Scand J Gastroenterol 2000;35(3):306–11.
20. Ford AC, Moayyedi P, Lacy BE, et al. American College of Gastroenterology monograph on the management of irritable bowel syndrome and chronic idiopathic constipation. Am J Gastroenterol 2014;109(Suppl 1):S2–26 [quiz: S7].
21. Chey WD, Kurlander J, Eswaran S. Irritable bowel syndrome: a clinical review. JAMA 2015;313(9):949–58.
22. Menees SB, Powell C, Kurlander J, et al. A meta-analysis of the utility of C-reactive protein, erythrocyte sedimentation rate, fecal calprotectin, and fecal lactoferrin to exclude inflammatory bowel disease in adults with IBS. Am J Gastroenterol 2015; 110(3):444–54.
23. Shiotani A, Miyanishi T, Takahashi T. Sex differences in irritable bowel syndrome in Japanese university students. J Gastroenterol 2006;41(6):562–8.
24. Nozu T, Kudaira M, Kitamori S, et al. Repetitive rectal painful distention induces rectal hypersensitivity in patients with irritable bowel syndrome. J Gastroenterol 2006;41(3):217–22.
25. Zuo XL, Li YQ, Shi L, et al. Visceral hypersensitivity following cold water intake in subjects with irritable bowel syndrome. J Gastroenterol 2006;41(4):311–7.
26. Dupont HL. Review article: evidence for the role of gut microbiota in irritable bowel syndrome and its potential influence on therapeutic targets. Aliment Pharmacol Ther 2014;39(10):1033–42.
27. Simren M, Barbara G, Flint HJ, et al. Intestinal microbiota in functional bowel disorders: a Rome foundation report. Gut 2013;62(1):159–76.
28. Rona RJ, Keil T, Summers C, et al. The prevalence of food allergy: a meta-analysis. J Allergy Clin Immunol 2007;120(3):638–46.
29. Blanchard EB, Scharff L. Psychosocial aspects of assessment and treatment of irritable bowel syndrome in adults and recurrent abdominal pain in children. J Consult Clin Psychol 2002;70(3):725–38.
30. Drossman DA. Abuse, trauma, and GI illness: is there a link? Am J Gastroenterol 2011;106(1):14–25.
31. Tang YR, Yang WW, Wang YL, et al. Sex differences in the symptoms and psychological factors that influence quality of life in patients with irritable bowel syndrome. Eur J Gastroenterol Hepatol 2012;24(6):702–7.
32. Murray K, Wilkinson-Smith V, Hoad C, et al. Differential effects of FODMAPs (fermentable oligo-, di-, mono-saccharides and polyols) on small and large intestinal contents in healthy subjects shown by MRI. Am J Gastroenterol 2014;109(1):110–9.
33. Halmos EP, Power VA, Shepherd SJ, et al. A diet low in FODMAPs reduces symptoms of irritable bowel syndrome. Gastroenterology 2014;146(1):67–75.e5.
34. Menees SB, Maneerattannaporn M, Kim HM, et al. The efficacy and safety of rifaximin for the irritable bowel syndrome: a systematic review and meta-analysis. Am J Gastroenterol 2012;107(1):28–35 [quiz: 6].
35. Drossman DA, Chey WD, Johanson JF, et al. Clinical trial: lubiprostone in patients with constipation-associated irritable bowel syndrome–results of two randomized, placebo-controlled studies. Aliment Pharmacol Ther 2009;29(3):329–41.
36. Chey WD, Lembo AJ, Lavins BJ, et al. Linaclotide for irritable bowel syndrome with constipation: a 26-week, randomized, double-blind, placebo-controlled trial to evaluate efficacy and safety. Am J Gastroenterol 2012;107(11):1702–12.

37. Videlock EJ, Cheng V, Cremonini F. Effects of linaclotide in patients with irritable bowel syndrome with constipation or chronic constipation: a meta-analysis. Clin Gastroenterol Hepatol 2013;11(9):1084–92.e3 [quiz: e68].
38. Ruepert L, Quartero AO, de Wit NJ, et al. Bulking agents, antispasmodics and antidepressants for the treatment of irritable bowel syndrome. Cochrane Database Syst Rev 2011;(8):CD003460.
39. Aro P, Storskrubb T, Ronkainen J, et al. Peptic ulcer disease in a general adult population: the Kalixanda study: a random population-based study. Am J Epidemiol 2006;163(11):1025–34.
40. Lanza FL, Chan FK, Quigley EM. Guidelines for prevention of NSAID-related ulcer complications. Am J Gastroenterol 2009;104(3):728–38.
41. Peterson WL, Fendrick AM, Cave DR, et al. Helicobacter pylori-related disease: guidelines for testing and treatment. Arch Intern Med 2000;160(9):1285–91.
42. Midolo P, Marshall BJ. Accurate diagnosis of Helicobacter pylori. Urease tests. Gastroenterol Clin North Am 2000;29(4):871–8.
43. Laine L, Jensen DM. Management of patients with ulcer bleeding. Am J Gastroenterol 2012;107(3):345–60 [quiz: 61].
44. Howden CW, Chey WD, Vakil NB. Clinical rationale for confirmation testing after treatment of helicobacter pylori infection: implications of rising antibiotic resistance. Gastroenterol Hepatol (N Y) 2014;10(7 Suppl 3):1–19.
45. Banerjee S, Cash BD, Dominitz JA, et al. The role of endoscopy in the management of patients with peptic ulcer disease. Gastrointest Endosc 2010;71(4):663–8.
46. Ahmed A, Cheung RC, Keeffe EB. Management of gallstones and their complications. Am Fam Physician 2000;61(6):1673–80, 1687–8.
47. Diehl AK. Epidemiology and natural history of gallstone disease. Gastroenterol Clin North Am 1991;20(1):1–19.
48. Schirmer BD, Winters KL, Edlich RF. Cholelithiasis and cholecystitis. J Long Term Eff Med Implants 2005;15(3):329–38.
49. Beaugerie L, Svrcek M, Seksik P, et al. Risk of colorectal high-grade dysplasia and cancer in a prospective observational cohort of patients with inflammatory bowel disease. Gastroenterology 2013;145(1):166–75.e8.
50. Bellows CF, Berger DH, Crass RA. Management of gallstones. Am Fam Physician 2005;72(4):637–42.
51. Dayer E, Yoshida H, Izui S, et al. Quantitation of retroviral gp70 antigen, autoantibodies, and immune complexes in extravascular space in arthritic MRL-lpr/lpr mice. Use of a subcutaneously implanted tissue cage model. Arthritis Rheum 1987;30(11):1274–82.
52. Colli A, Conte D, Valle SD, et al. Meta-analysis: nonsteroidal anti-inflammatory drugs in biliary colic. Aliment Pharmacol Ther 2012;35(12):1370–8.
53. Everson GT. Gastrointestinal motility in pregnancy. Gastroenterol Clin North Am 1992;21(4):751–76.
54. Everson GT. Pregnancy and gallstones. Hepatology 1993;17(1):159–61.
55. Rutgeerts P, Vermeire S, Van Assche G. Biological therapies for inflammatory bowel diseases. Gastroenterology 2009;136(4):1182–97.
56. Cheifetz AS. Management of active Crohn disease. JAMA 2013;309(20):2150–8.
57. Thia KT, Sandborn WJ, Harmsen WS, et al. Risk factors associated with progression to intestinal complications of Crohn's disease in a population-based cohort. Gastroenterology 2010;139(4):1147–55.
58. Allez M, Lemann M, Bonnet J, et al. Long term outcome of patients with active Crohn's disease exhibiting extensive and deep ulcerations at colonoscopy. Am J Gastroenterol 2002;97(4):947–53.

59. Beaugerie L, Seksik P, Nion-Larmurier I, et al. Predictors of Crohn's disease. Gastroenterology 2006;130(3):650–6.

60. Loly C, Belaiche J, Louis E. Predictors of severe Crohn's disease. Scand J Gastroenterol 2008;43(8):948–54.

61. Vermeire S, Ferrante M, Rutgeerts P. Recent advances: personalised use of current Crohn's disease therapeutic options. Gut 2013;62(10):1511–5.

62. Solberg IC, Vatn MH, Hoie O, et al. Clinical course in Crohn's disease: results of a Norwegian population-based ten-year follow-up study. Clin Gastroenterol Hepatol 2007;5(12):1430–8.

63. Cosnes J, Nion-Larmurier I, Beaugerie L, et al. Impact of the increasing use of immunosuppressants in Crohn's disease on the need for intestinal surgery. Gut 2005;54(2):237–41.

64. Frolkis AD, Dykeman J, Negron ME, et al. Risk of surgery for inflammatory bowel diseases has decreased over time: a systematic review and meta-analysis of population-based studies. Gastroenterology 2013;145(5):996–1006.

65. Lichtenstein GR, Hanauer SB, Sandborn WJ. Management of Crohn's disease in adults. Am J Gastroenterol 2009;104(2):465–83 [quiz: 4, 84].

66. Ng SW, Mahadevan U. My treatment approach to management of the pregnant patient with inflammatory bowel disease. Mayo Clin Proc 2014;89(3):355–60.

67. Hudson M, Flett G, Sinclair TS, et al. Fertility and pregnancy in inflammatory bowel disease. Int J Gynaecol Obstet 1997;58(2):229–37.

68. Waljee A, Waljee J, Morris AM, et al. Threefold increased risk of infertility: a meta-analysis of infertility after ileal pouch anal anastomosis in ulcerative colitis. Gut 2006;55(11):1575–80.

69. Boyd HA, Basit S, Harpsoe MC, et al. Inflammatory bowel disease and risk of adverse pregnancy outcomes. PLoS One 2015;10(6):e0129567.

70. Mahadevan U, Sandborn WJ, Li DK, et al. Pregnancy outcomes in women with inflammatory bowel disease: a large community-based study from Northern California. Gastroenterology 2007;133(4):1106–12.

71. Nielsen OH, Andreasson B, Bondesen S, et al. Pregnancy in ulcerative colitis. Scand J Gastroenterol 1983;18(6):735–42.

72. Casanova MJ, Chaparro M, Domenech E, et al. Safety of thiopurines and anti-TNF-alpha drugs during pregnancy in patients with inflammatory bowel disease. Am J Gastroenterol 2013;108(3):433–40.

73. Mahadevan U, Cucchiara S, Hyams JS, et al. The London Position Statement of the World Congress of Gastroenterology on Biological Therapy for IBD with the European Crohn's and Colitis Organisation: pregnancy and pediatrics. Am J Gastroenterol 2011;106(2):214–23 [quiz: 24].

74. DeVault KR, Castell DO. Updated guidelines for the diagnosis and treatment of gastroesophageal reflux disease. Am J Gastroenterol 2005;100(1):190–200.

75. Katz PO, Gerson LB, Vela MF. Guidelines for the diagnosis and management of gastroesophageal reflux disease. Am J Gastroenterol 2013;108(3):308–28 [quiz: 29].

76. El-Serag HB, Sweet S, Winchester CC, et al. Update on the epidemiology of gastro-oesophageal reflux disease: a systematic review. Gut 2014;63(6):871–80.

77. Orlando RC. Pathogenesis of gastroesophageal reflux disease. Gastroenterol Clin North Am 2002;31(4 Suppl):S35–44.

78. Labenz J, Jaspersen D, Kulig M, et al. Risk factors for erosive esophagitis: a multivariate analysis based on the ProGERD study initiative. Am J Gastroenterol 2004;99(9):1652–6.

79. Pandolfino JE, Vela MF. Esophageal-reflux monitoring. Gastrointest Endosc 2009; 69(4):917–30, 930.e1.
80. Moayyedi P, Talley NJ, Fennerty MB, et al. Can the clinical history distinguish between organic and functional dyspepsia? JAMA 2006;295(13):1566–76.
81. McGarvey LP, Heaney LG, Lawson JT, et al. Evaluation and outcome of patients with chronic non-productive cough using a comprehensive diagnostic protocol. Thorax 1998;53:738–43.
82. Chiba N, De Gara CJ, Wilkinson JM, et al. Speed of healing and symptom relief in grade II to IV gastroesophageal reflux disease: a meta-analysis. Gastroenterology 1997;112(6):1798–810.
83. Bavishi C, Dupont HL. Systematic review: the use of proton pump inhibitors and increased susceptibility to enteric infection. Aliment Pharmacol Ther 2011; 34(11–12):1269–81.
84. Johnstone J, Nerenberg K, Loeb M. Meta-analysis: proton pump inhibitor use and the risk of community-acquired pneumonia. Aliment Pharmacol Ther 2010;31(11): 1165–77.
85. Targownik LE, Leslie WD, Davison KS, et al. The relationship between proton pump inhibitor use and longitudinal change in bone mineral density: a population-based study [corrected] from the Canadian Multicentre Osteoporosis Study (CaMos). Am J Gastroenterol 2012;107(9):1361–9.
86. Gerson LB, McMahon D, Olkin I, et al. Lack of significant interactions between clopidogrel and proton pump inhibitor therapy: meta-analysis of existing literature. Dig Dis Sci 2012;57(5):1304–13.
87. Kwok CS, Jeevanantham V, Dawn B, et al. No consistent evidence of differential cardiovascular risk amongst proton-pump inhibitors when used with clopidogrel: meta-analysis. Int J Cardiol 2013;167(3):965–74.
88. van der Woude CJ, Metselaar HJ, Danese S. Management of gastrointestinal and liver diseases during pregnancy. Gut 2014;63(6):1014–23.
89. Ali RA, Egan LJ. Gastroesophageal reflux disease in pregnancy. Best Pract Res Clin Gastroenterol 2007;21(5):793–806.
90. Richter JE. Gastroesophageal reflux disease during pregnancy. Gastroenterol Clin North Am 2003;32(1):235–61.
91. Kallen B. Delivery outcome after the use of acid-suppressing drugs in early pregnancy with special reference to omeprazole. Br J Obstet Gynaecol 1998;105(8): 877–81.
92. Gill SK, O'Brien L, Einarson TR, et al. The safety of proton pump inhibitors (PPIs) in pregnancy: a meta-analysis. Am J Gastroenterol 2009;104(6):1541–5 [quiz: 1540, 1546].
93. Conio M, Filiberti R, Blanchi S, et al. Risk factors for Barrett's esophagus: a case-control study. Int J Cancer 2002;97(2):225–9.
94. Eloubeidi MA, Provenzale D. Clinical and demographic predictors of Barrett's esophagus among patients with gastroesophageal reflux disease: a multivariable analysis in veterans. J Clin Gastroenterol 2001;33(4):306–9.
95. Wang KK, Sampliner RE. Updated guidelines 2008 for the diagnosis, surveillance and therapy of Barrett's esophagus. Am J Gastroenterol 2008;103(3):788–97.
96. Spechler SJ, Sharma P, Souza RF, et al. American Gastroenterological Association medical position statement on the management of Barrett's esophagus. Gastroenterology 2011;140(3):1084–91.
97. Hvid-Jensen F, Pedersen L, Drewes AM, et al. Incidence of adenocarcinoma among patients with Barrett's esophagus. N Engl J Med 2011;365(15):1375–83.

Primary Care for the Older Adult Patient

Common Geriatric Issues and Syndromes

Katherine Thompson, MD[a],*, Sandra Shi, MD[b],
Carmela Kiraly, MD[b]

KEYWORDS

- Geriatric syndromes • Dementia • Polypharmacy • Falls • Advance directives
- Women's health

KEY POINTS

- Dementia is a common contributor to morbidity and mortality in older adults and should be assessed for and managed in the primary care setting.
- Falls are the leading cause of injury in older adults. Exercise and minimizing medications are two evidence-based interventions to lower fall risk.
- Polypharmacy is common and poses significant risks to older adults. Evidence-based tools exist to help minimize polypharmacy in older adults.
- Advance care planning, including completion of a living will and durable power of attorney for health care, should be considered with all older adult patients.

INTRODUCTION

Older adults are the fastest growing segment of the US population[1] and represent a growing proportion of most primary care practices. Women account for 56% of adults older than the age of 65 and 67% of adults older than the age of 85 in the United States.[1] The older adult population is heterogeneous. Many older adults are healthier and more active than their younger counterparts, whereas a large number of older adults have multiple advanced illnesses and complex health care needs. In addition, functional and cognitive decline is common in this population. The ability to recognize and treat geriatric syndromes and facilitate care planning in complex older adult patients can help mitigate functional decline and loss of independence.

---

[a] Department of Medicine, University of Chicago, 5841 South Maryland Avenue, MC 6098, Chicago, IL 60637, USA; [b] Department of Medicine, University of Chicago, 5841 South Maryland Avenue, MC 7082, Chicago, IL 60637, USA
* Corresponding author.
E-mail address: Katherine.thompson@uchospitals.edu

Obstet Gynecol Clin N Am 43 (2016) 367–379
http://dx.doi.org/10.1016/j.ogc.2016.01.010
0889-8545/16/$ – see front matter © 2016 Elsevier Inc. All rights reserved.

COGNITIVE IMPAIRMENT AND DEMENTIA
Epidemiology

Dementia, defined as neurocognitive decline marked by impairment in cognitive functions, such as memory, speech, and reasoning, is a significant contributor to the morbidity and mortality of older adults in the United States and worldwide. It is estimated that about 14% of US adults older than age 70 have dementia.[2] This includes more than 5 million people older than the age of 65 in the United States who have Alzheimer disease, the most common form of dementia. Of these, nearly two-thirds are women.[3,4] This number is expected to grow annually with the growth of the older adult population. The projected estimated incidence of Alzheimer disease will double in the next 50 years from 2000 to 2050.

Alzheimer disease is currently the sixth leading cause of death in the United States,[5] placing it ahead of common pathologies, such as diabetes, liver, and kidney diseases as a cause of mortality. It is a comorbidity to other health problems. A recent study evaluating the contribution of individual diseases to death in older adults with multiple diseases found that dementia was the second most common contributor to death after heart failure.[6] Care for older adults with dementia is costly. The annual cost of care for persons with dementia in the United States is estimated to be about $226 billion.[3] Caregivers for those with dementia are often unpaid, with high emotional and physical burdens of caregiving. Many patients with dementia eventually require nursing home care and about two-thirds of individuals with dementia die in nursing homes.[7]

Diagnosis

Dementia is a syndrome rather than a specific illness. A diagnosis of dementia is made through a combination of history provided by the patient; history from a knowledgeable informant, such as a close friend or family member; and bedside mental status examination. The hallmark of dementia includes impairment in multiple cognitive domains. Functional decline is also characteristic of the syndrome and differentiates dementia from mild cognitive impairment, where there is some objective memory deficit but no functional deficit.[8]

Alzheimer disease is the most common cause of dementia, representing about 60% to 80% of cases.[2] Other common dementia syndromes include vascular dementia, Lewy body dementia, Parkinson disease with dementia, and frontotemporal dementia, each marked by characteristic features, but frequently with overlapping signs and symptoms (**Table 1**). Some illnesses, such as delirium and depression, can mimic symptoms of dementia and should be excluded. Other illnesses can lead to reversible or treatable cognitive dysfunction, such as thyroid disorders, vitamin B_{12} deficiency, neurosyphilis, human immunodeficiency virus, and alcohol abuse. One meta-analysis found that 9% of people with dementia-like symptoms had other potentially reversible conditions; therefore, evaluation should include an assessment for possible treatable causes.[9]

Risk Factors and Screening

Many risk factors for dementia have been identified. The most significant risk factor is advancing age, followed by family history.[2] Several genetic risk factors have been identified, including presence of the apolipoprotein E-e4 gene and the presence of Down syndrome. Other environmental and health-related risk factors include history of head injury, fewer years of formal education, physical frailty, alcohol abuse, diagnosis of mild cognitive impairment, and cardiovascular disease risk factors (hypertension, hyperlipidemia, obesity, insulin resistance, tobacco abuse).

Table 1
Common dementia syndromes

Syndrome	Characteristic Features
Alzheimer disease	Memory impairment is early/presenting feature Insidious onset, progressive course Most common cause of dementia
Vascular dementia	Vascular disease on neuroimaging Diverse symptoms based on affected area of brain Impaired judgment and executive dysfunction is common
Lewy body dementia	Parkinson-like movement disorder (preceded by or concurrent with cognitive symptoms) Visual hallucinations Fluctuations in cognition
Parkinson disease with dementia	Movement disorder precedes dementia Earlier executive and visuospatial dysfunction Memory and language impairments less prominent
Frontotemporal dementia	Frontotemporal atrophy on neuroimaging Earlier onset (sixth decade most common) Marked behavioral or language changes

The US Preventative Services Task Force has recommended against screening for dementia in older adults[10] because of insufficient evidence to assess the benefits and harms. In its statement, however, the Task Force does note that early identification of cognitive decline may enable patients to make diagnostic and treatment decisions and enable clinicians to anticipate problems that patients may have in understanding or adhering to recommended therapies. Additionally, early identification of dementia may enable patients or caregivers to anticipate and plan for future problems that may develop as a result of disease progression.[10]

Evaluation

Dementia is a clinical diagnosis. The diagnostic evaluation should involve assessment for subjective cognitive complaints, evidence of decline in functioning, objective assessment of cognition, and selected testing to rule out reversible causes of cognitive decline or diagnoses mimicking dementia. Initial history should be obtained from the patient, and also from a reliable informant or caregiver, because dementia can impair the patient's ability to provide accurate historical details. History should focus on early signs and symptoms of dementia, such as memory loss that disrupts daily routines; misplacing items; repeating stories or questions; word-finding issues; missed appointments; or changes in personality, mood, or judgment. Often, symptoms first become apparent around times of life change, such as death of a household member, move to a new home, or travel. Risk factors should be assessed. Medications should be reviewed to identify any that can impair cognition including anticholinergics, sedative-hypnotics, and psychotropic drugs. A thorough functional history should be obtained to assess for decline from a previous level of functioning. Patients with dementia often have impairments first noted in such activities as financial management, medication management, or driving. Objective memory testing should be performed by using one of several validated tools, such as the Mini-Mental State examination,[11] Mini-Cog,[12] or Montreal Cognitive Assessment.[13] Neuropsychologic testing may be obtained in instances where the diagnosis is unclear or more information about specific cognitive deficits is required.

A thorough neurologic examination should be part of the initial physical examination. This examination should evaluate for any focal neurologic deficits consistent with prior stroke, language problems, parkinsonian signs, or gait abnormalities. Patients with more advanced dementia may exhibit hyperreflexia, frontal release signs, or dysphagia. Depression should be screened for, and delirium, particularly if an acute confused state is noted. Basic laboratory tests include thyroid-stimulating hormone and vitamin B_{12} levels.[14] Routine testing for syphilis and human immunodeficiency virus is not recommended, but may be appropriate for patients with specific risk factors. Neuroimaging with nonenhanced computed tomography or MRI is recommended.[14] Currently, the National Institute of Aging-Alzheimer's Association Workgroups do not advocate the use of Alzheimer disease biomarkers or genetic testing for routine diagnostic purposes.[15]

Management

Principles of management for dementia include consideration of pharmacotherapy (**Table 2**), management of comorbid disease processes, assessment of safety issues, management of behavioral symptoms, caregiver support, and planning for disease progression. Although the clinical course of dementia is highly variable, the average time from diagnosis to death is about 4.5 years,[16] with a slow progressive decline in cognitive functioning during that time. In the mild stage of dementia, patients may still be able to drive and live independently with some increase in assistance and supervision. In the moderate stage, patients generally need assistance with instrumental activities of daily living and can no longer live alone. In the severe stage, patients progressively lose the ability to perform activities of daily living, eventually becoming nonverbal, incontinent, and bedbound.

In earlier stages of dementia, aggressive management of comorbid disease processes, particularly those that carry an association with cerebrovascular disease, may help slow further decline and maximize patient quality of life. As dementia progresses to later stages, clinicians should consider eliminating therapies without short-term benefit. Pharmacotherapy (see **Table 2**) may be considered at all stages; however, effects are modest at best, and possible treatment benefit should be carefully weighed against potential harms including side effects and contribution to polypharmacy in a patient already at risk for nonadherence. Safety issues should be

Table 2
Pharmacologic agents for Alzheimer disease treatment

Class	Agents	Benefit	Side Effects	Notes
Acetylcholinesterase inhibitor	Donepezil Galantamine Rivastigmine	Delay or slower decline in symptom progression Approved for mild, moderate, severe disease	Nausea Diarrhea Anorexia Syncope	Uptitrate slowly to maximal dose Rivastigmine available in transdermal patch
N-methyl-D-aspartate receptor antagonist	Memantine	Delay or slower decline in symptom progression Approved for moderate and severe disease	Dizziness Confusion Headache Constipation	Uptitrate slowly to maximal dose Caution in patients with seizure disorder

assessed frequently with patients and caregivers. These may include cooking safety, driving safety, presence of firearms or other weapons in the home, use of power tools, and wandering.

Behavioral symptoms should also be assessed on a regular basis including aggressive or threatening behaviors; resistance to bathing, changing clothes, or taking medications; hallucinations or delusions; depression or anxiety; and sleep problems. Looking for any patterns associated with behavioral symptoms, for instance hunger, time of day, or specific situations, may help in developing a management plan. Caregiver stress should be assessed and addressed. Caregiver assistance including skills training, education, support groups, and stress management can improve behavioral symptoms and reduce caregiver burden.[17]

Finally, advance care planning, including identifying a health care power of attorney and specifying end-of-life care preferences, should be done early in the disease process before the patient loses the capacity to make these decisions. As dementia progresses to severe or end-stage, aggressive interventions, such as feeding tubes, no longer have potential for benefit and may cause undue harm.[18] Hospice referral may be appropriate in advanced dementia, particularly when other medical complications are present.

Dementia management requires a broad approach that often involves input from an interprofessional team including social worker, speech language pathologist, occupational therapist, and physical therapist. A geriatrician, neurologist, or geriatric psychiatrist may be consulted in the case of atypical disease features, rapid progression, difficult to treat behavioral symptoms, or other clinical challenges.

FALLS
Epidemiology

Falls in older adults pose significant risk for injury, loss of future independent function, and likelihood of recurrent falls. Unfortunately, the burden of falls among this population is not consistently well recognized, in part because falls are often underreported, unsuspected, or simply not asked about. One study estimated that less than half of those who fall report the incident to a medical professional.[19]

According to the Centers for Disease Control and Prevention, falls are the leading cause of fatal and nonfatal injuries among older adults, and accounted for more than 25,000 deaths in 2013.[20] Women are particularly at risk for injuries from falls because of a higher prevalence of osteoporosis. Injuries from falls are most often minor (scrapes and bruises), but pose the potential for more serious outcomes. More than half of older adults who fall are unable to pull themselves up, and many may lie for an extended period of time while waiting for assistance.[21] Perhaps most significant, older adults who fall are more likely to experience a decline in basic and instrumental activities of daily living.[22] Among community-dwelling older adults, falls have been shown to be strong predictors of the need for placement in a supportive living environment.[23]

Screening

The American Geriatrics Society (AGS)/British Geriatrics Society clinical practice guideline for prevention of falls in older persons[24] recommends screening for falls in every patient age 65 and older. Patients should be asked if they have experienced a fall in the past year, and if so, the frequency and circumstances surrounding the fall. Older adult patients should also be questioned about gait problems and balance difficulties. The Centers for Disease Control and Prevention Stopping Elderly Accidents,

Deaths, & Injuries (STEADI) Initiative[25] proposes a third question, "Do you worry about falling?" If patients answer positively to any of these questions, or if they present for evaluation following an acute fall, gait and balance assessment and a multifactorial fall risk assessment should be performed by their health care provider.

Evaluation

Multifactorial fall risk assessment, as outlined by the AGS guidelines,[24] should include a focused history (details surrounding the fall, careful medication review, and relevant comorbidities, such as osteoporosis and urinary incontinence), physical examination, and functional assessment. The components of this assessment align closely with some of the more frequently associated risk factors for falls. These include but are not limited to polypharmacy, visual impairment, orthostatic hypotension, heart rate and rhythm abnormalities, vitamin D deficiency, footwear/feet problems, and unsafe hazardous built environments. Physical examination should include orthostatic vital signs; thorough cardiac and neurologic examination; and assessment of joint stability, gait, and balance. Several tests are widely used to test postural stability. The Get Up and Go test is one of the most well-known, in which the patient rises from a chair, walks a fixed distance, turns around, and returns back to seated position.[26] The time to complete this activity does not correlate precisely with fall risk as shown in a 2013 meta-analysis, but the activity regardless allows for assessment of leg strength, balance, vestibular dysfunction, and gait.[27]

Treatment and Prevention

Management of a patient who has fallen and prevention of future falls should be targeted at a patient's individual conditions and risk factors. Several evidence-based interventions have been shown to lower fall risk. An exercise regimen is recommended for all community-dwelling older adult patients at risk for falls. This regimen should include balance; gait; and strength training, such as tai chi or physical therapy.[24] Medication reduction, particularly discontinuation of psychoactive medications, is recommended. Occupational therapists or similarly qualified health care professionals can perform an in-home environmental assessment and make recommendations to mitigate fall risk and promote safe performance of activities within the home. Both the AGS guidelines and STEADI initiative stress the importance of patient and caregiver education,[24,25] because the risk of falls and their subsequent repercussions carry considerable weight.

POLYPHARMACY
Definition and Epidemiology

Polypharmacy is the concurrent prescription of multiple medications to a patient. Although the exact numerical cutoff varies in literature, it is most often defined as five or more medications.[28–30] An alternate functionally focused definition is based on whether or not drugs are medically indicated, although in practice this may be more difficult to identify. With this definition, polypharmacy is recognized as the presence of one or more drug prescriptions that is inappropriate or potentially unnecessary.[31]

Prevalence in older populations is well established. By one measure up to 50% of Medicare beneficiaries received more than five prescriptions.[32] By other estimates, almost half of older adults take at least one medication that is not medically necessary.[33] The proportion of older adults affected by polypharmacy has been steadily increasing over the past few decades. A recent study found that from 1988 to 2010 the proportion of American adults older than 65 taking more than five medications tripled from 12.8% to 39.0%.[29]

Risks

Geriatric patients are particularly at risk because of a variety of medical and social factors. From a physiologic perspective, older patients have reduced metabolism and clearance of drugs, increasing the risk of overdose or inappropriate dosing.[34] Moreover, older patients tend to have medical comorbidities that require multiple medications to manage, increasing the risk of drug-drug and drug-disease interactions.[35] Older patients are more likely to have barriers to adherence to complex medication regimens because of physical and cognitive limitations, financial, or transportation issues.

The adverse effects of polypharmacy on health outcomes in the geriatric population have been extensively studied. The presence of five or more medications is independently associated with an increased risk of falls,[36,37] whereas potentially inappropriate medications, such as those with anticholinergic side effects, are associated with measurable decreases in cognition.[38] A retrospective study of 300 emergency room visits found that 10.6% of visits were caused by adverse drug events.[39] Finally, a study of more than 5000 patients found a significant association between increasing numbers of discharge medications and prevalence of 30-day hospital readmission.[40]

Evaluation and Management

Several tools have been developed to aid clinicians in avoiding polypharmacy and identifying potentially harmful medications. The Beers Criteria[41] (**Table 3**) is an evidence-based list of potentially inappropriate medications for older adults, most recently updated in 2012. It lists commonly prescribed medications that may be inappropriate or harmful, and categorizes them as "avoid," "potentially inappropriate," and "use with caution." Another tool, the STOPP-START criteria, uses a targeted criteria approach to identify potentially inappropriate prescriptions, while proposing alternative safer medications.[42] Internationally, the 2012 Beers Criteria are suggested to

Table 3
Commonly prescribed potentially inappropriate medications for older adults

Class	Common Examples	Potential Adverse Effects
Benzodiazepines: prescribed for anxiety, insomnia, delirium	Lorazepam Alprazolam Diazepam	Sedation, paradoxic agitation, delirium, falls
Antihistamines: prescribed for allergies (first and second generation)	Diphenhydramine Chlorpheniramine	Anticholinergic side effects (confusion, urinary retention, blurry vision)
Tricyclic antidepressants: prescribed for depression, neuropathic pain	Amitriptyline Imipramine Clomipramine	Anticholinergic side effects Orthostatic hypotension
Antipsychotics: prescribed for delirium, mood stabilizers	Haloperidol risperidone	Decreased cognition; increased risk of falls, stroke, death
Nonsteroidal anti-inflammatory drugs: prescribed for pain	Ibuprofen Naproxen	Increased risk of gastrointestinal bleed, ulcers

Data from American Geriatrics Society 2012 Beers Criteria Update Expert Panel. American Geriatrics Society Updated Beers Criteria for potentially inappropriate medication use in older adults. J Am Geriatr Soc 2012;60(4):616–31.

have superior sensitivity to the STOPP-START criteria for identifying potentially inappropriate medications.[43] However, when applied as an intervention within 72 hours of admission, the STOPP-START criteria was shown to significantly reduce adverse drug events[42] and may detect potential prescribing omissions. In practice, the application of both these tools together has been suggested for complementary benefit.

Naturally, strategies to minimize polypharmacy go beyond the use of the previously mentioned tools. An interdisciplinary approach involving pharmacists, families, patients, and physicians is typically the most successful.[28] Commonly used strategies include detailed medication review, starting with the patient bringing in all of their medications ("brown bag review") or an updated list of all medications if the former is not possible. It is crucial to include over-the-counter medications, including analgesics and cold remedies, which may contain any combination of medications, such as aspirin, acetaminophen, diphenhydramine, dextromethorphan, and ibuprofen,[31] and herbal supplements, because these are known contributors to adverse interactions and almost 75% of older patients endorse taking them.[44] This is also an opportunity to review and discard old prescriptions to prevent confusion with discontinued medications.

There are data suggesting that the number of prescribers is independently associated with patients reporting adverse drug events[45]; thus, by reducing the number of prescribers, the incidence of polypharmacy and potential adverse drug events also could be reduced. For selected patients it may be reasonable to consider having all or most medications prescribed through the patient's primary care physician rather than having multiple subspecialists prescribing medications. Whenever possible, reducing medications should be considered, particularly for medications that lack benefit and can be safely withdrawn with minimal side effects.[28] Finally, when in doubt, referral to a specialized team of geriatricians and/or pharmacists may be beneficial in reducing total number of medications and the risk of adverse drug events.

Polypharmacy is a complex issue affecting many older adults, placing them at higher risk for adverse drug events and negative health outcomes. To some extent the prescription of multiple medications is unavoidable in an era of increasingly complex chronic medical problems. However, by approaching medication prescribing with a thoughtful, structured, and multidisciplinary approach, medication regimens can be tailored to be simple and safe while maintaining effectiveness.

LATE LIFE AND END-OF-LIFE PLANNING AND CARE
Care Planning for Multimorbid Patients

Multimorbidity, the presence of multiple coexisting chronic conditions, affects about 75% of the older adult population.[46] Care planning that incorporates patients' goals and preferences, is feasible for the patient, and involves consideration of potential harms and benefits is important for all patients, but particularly complex, multimorbid older adults. For this population, a care planning approach that uses strict adherence to all individual disease-based clinical practice guidelines has potential for harm because of polypharmacy, drug interactions, and lack of feasibility.[47] Rather, a prioritized approach incorporating specific care principles is recommended by AGS expert consensus (**Table 4**).[48]

Delivering Bad News

Delivering bad news, such as severe or terminal diagnoses, is a common occurrence in primary care, particularly in an older patient population. Delivering bad news requires complex communication skills and is often stressful for provider and patient.

Table 4
Guiding principles for the care of older adults with multimorbidity

Principle	Example
1. Elicit and incorporate patient preferences	Does the patient value quality vs quantity of life? What outcomes are important to the patient?
2. Interpret and apply medical literature; recognize limitations of evidence base	Does the patient population studied represent my patient? Were patient-important outcomes reported?
3. Frame care plan in context of prognosis	Is the care plan likely to achieve expected outcomes within the time frame of the patient's estimated prognosis?
4. Consider treatment complexity and feasibility	Can the care plan be simplified to minimize polypharmacy and nonadherence?
5. Optimize therapies and care plans	What aspects of the care plan should be prioritized? Can patient education, caregivers, or interprofessional team members help to optimize the care plan?

Data from Guiding principles for the care of older adults with multimorbidity: an approach for clinicians. Guiding principles for the care of older adults with multimorbidity: an approach for clinicians: American Geriatrics Society expert panel on the care of older adults with multimorbidity. J Am Geriatr Soc 2012;60:E1–25.

Having a structure for delivering bad news that incorporates patients' values and wishes around decision-making and involves a strategy for addressing emotional distress and providing support and follow-up is essential. One such framework, the SPIKES six-step protocol[49] (**Table 5**), has been studied as a way to support providers and patients in discussing the patient's knowledge and expectations, provide accurate information to the patient, support the patient, and develop a strategy for treatment or follow-up.

Advance Care Planning

Advance care planning is a process of planning for and documenting patients' wishes for future care in the event that they are unable to make their own health care

Table 5
SPIKES: a six-step protocol for delivering bad news

Step	Considerations
1. S: Setting up the interview	Review plan; arrange for privacy, seating, and so forth; minimize interruptions; involve loved ones per patient preferences
2. P: Perception	Assess patient's understanding of any prior testing, current disease state or treatment plan
3. I: Invitation	Assess whether/how the patient would like to receive information
4. K: Knowledge	Warn the patient that bad news is coming; state bad news clearly without modifiers or jargon; deliver information in small chunks and pause for understanding
5. E: Address emotion with empathy	Allow for silence; use empathic statements ("I wish the news were different"); ask exploratory questions ("Tell me how you're feeling")
6. S: Strategy and summary	Summarize discussion and make a plan for next steps; close follow-up with opportunity for further questions

Data from Baile WF, Buckman R, Lenzi R, et al. SPIKES—a six-step protocol for delivering bad news: application to the patient with cancer. Oncologist 2000;5(4):302–11.

decisions. Because goals and preferences may change over time or with health status, this process is most effective when it is an ongoing conversation between patient and provider.[50] Patients who participate in advance care planning with their providers are more likely to have their end-of-life wishes known and followed.[51] Advance care planning often involves completion of an advance directive, a written document that is ideally portable and readily available to the patient and their medical professional team. An advance directive typically involves two parts: designating a health care proxy (Durable Power of Attorney for Health Care); and expressing goals, values, or wishes for future health care (Living Will). Advance directives are only followed if the patient has lost decisional capacity and can be revoked or changed at any time by a decisional patient. Because living wills may not represent every decision necessary for future care, designation of a health care proxy is essential. Patients should have a conversation with their health care proxy about their values and goals. Regulations for advance directives vary by state. The National Hospice and Palliative Care Organization's Web site, CaringInfo,[52] has available links to each state's advance directives forms.

SUMMARY

Older adults are the fastest growing segment of the US population, and most older adults are women.[1] As patients age, chronologic age is not always reflective of physiologic age, and many 80 and 90 year olds are healthier than their younger counterparts. Because of this, primary care for the older adult patient requires a wide variety of skills, reflecting the complexity and heterogeneity of this patient population. Individualizing care through consideration of patients' goals, medical conditions, and prognosis is paramount. Quality care for the older adult patient requires familiarity with common geriatric syndromes, such as dementia, falls, and polypharmacy. In addition, developing the knowledge and communication skills necessary for complex care and end-of-life care planning is essential. Geriatricians and interprofessional team members, such as social workers, physical and occupational therapists, and geriatric case managers, can provide valuable guidance and support for primary care providers in the care of complex older adult patients.

REFERENCES

1. Werner CA. The older population: 2010, 2010 Census Briefs. Available at: https://www.census.gov/prod/cen2010/briefs/c2010br-09.pdf. Accessed September 15, 2015.
2. Plassman BL, Langa KM, Fisher GG, et al. Prevalence of dementia in the United States: the aging, demographics, and memory study. Neuroepidemiology 2007; 29(1–2):125–32.
3. Alzheimer's Association. 2015 Alzheimer's disease facts and figures. Available at: http://www.alz.org/facts/downloads/facts_figures_2015.pdf. Accessed September 15, 2015.
4. Hebert LE, Beckett LA, Scherr PA, et al. Annual incidence of Alzheimer disease in the United States projected to the years 2000 through 2050. Alzheimer Dis Assoc Disord 2001;15(4):169–73.
5. National Center for Health Statistics. Deaths: final data for 2013. National Vital Statistics Report, vol. 64. Number 2. Hyattsville (MD): 2015. Available at: http://www.cdc.gov/nchs/data/nvsr/nvsr64/nvsr64_02.pdf. Accessed September 15, 2015.

6. Tinetti ME, McAvay GJ, Murphy TE, et al. Contribution of individual diseases to death in older adults with multiple diseases. J Am Geriatr Soc 2012;60(8): 1448–56.

7. Mitchell SL, Teno JM, Miller SC, et al. A national study of the location of death for older persons with dementia. J Am Geriatr Soc 2005;53:299–305.

8. American Psychiatric Association. Diagnostic and statistical manual of mental disorders (DSM-5). 5th edition. Arlington (VA): American Psychiatric Association; 2013.

9. Clarfield AM. The decreasing prevalence of reversible dementias: an updated meta-analysis. Arch Intern Med 2003;163(18):2219–29.

10. Lin JS, O'Connor E, Rossom RC, et al. Screening for cognitive impairment in older adults: a systematic review for the U.S. Preventive Services Task Force. Ann Intern Med 2013;159(9):601–12.

11. Folstein MF, Folstein SE, McHugh PR. "Mini-Mental State". A practical method for grading the cognitive state of patients for the clinician. J Psychiatr Res 1975;12: 189–98.

12. Borson S, Scanlan J, Brush M, et al. The Mini-Cog: a cognitive 'vital signs' measure for dementia screening in multi-lingual elderly. Int J Geriatr Psychiatry 2000; 15:1021–7.

13. Nasreddine Z. Montreal Cognitive Assessment. Greenfield Park, Québec, Canada: Center for Diagnosis & Research on Alzheimer's Disease. 2014. Available at: www.mocatest.org. Accessed September 15, 2015.

14. Knopman DS, DeKosky ST, Cummings JL, et al. Practice parameter: diagnosis of dementia (an evidence-based review). Report of the Quality Standards Subcommittee of the American Academy of Neurology. Neurology 2001;56:1143.

15. McKhann GM, Knopman DS, Chertkow H, et al. The diagnosis of dementia due to Alzheimer's disease: recommendations from the National Institute on Aging-Alzheimer's Association workgroups on diagnostic guidelines for Alzheimer's disease. Alzheimers Dement 2011;7(3):263–9.

16. Xie J, Brayne C, Matthews F, Medical Research Council Cognitive Function and Ageing Study Collaborators. Survival times in people with dementia: analysis from population based cohort study with 14 year follow-up. BMJ 2008;336:258.

17. Brodaty H, Arasaratnam C. Meta-analysis of nonpharmacological interventions for neuropsychiatric symptoms of dementia. Am J Psychiatry 2012;169:946–53.

18. Mitchell SL, Kiely DK, Lipsitz LA. The risk factors and impact on survival of feeding tube placement in nursing home residents with severe cognitive impairment. Arch Intern Med 1997;157:327–32.

19. Stevens JA, Ballesteros MF, Mack KA, et al. Gender differences in seeking care for falls in the aged Medicare Population. Am J Prev Med 2012;43:59–62.

20. Centers for Disease Control and Prevention, National Center for Injury Prevention and Control. Web–based Injury Statistics Query and Reporting System (WISQARS). Available at: http://www.cdc.gov/injury/wisqars/. Accessed September 15, 2015.

21. Tinetti ME, Liu WL, Claus EB. Predictors and prognosis of inability to get up after falls among elderly persons. JAMA 1993;269(1):65.

22. Tinetti ME, Williams CS. The effect of falls and fall injuries on functioning in community-dwelling older persons. J Gerontol A Biol Sci Med Sci 1998;53(2): M112.

23. Tinetti MF, Williams CS. Falls, injuries due to falls, and the risk of admission to a nursing home. N Engl J Med 1997;337(18):1279.

24. Panel on Prevention of Falls in Older Persons, American Geriatrics Society and British Geriatrics Society. Summary of the Updated American Geriatrics Society/British Geriatrics Society clinical practice guideline for prevention of falls in older persons. J Am Geriatr Soc 2011;59(1):148–57.
25. Stevens JA, Phelan EA. Development of STEADI: a fall prevention resource for health care providers. Health Promot Pract 2013;14(5):706–14.
26. Fleming KC, Evand JM, Weber DC, et al. Practical functional assessment of elderly persons: a primary-care approach. Mayo Clin Proc 1995;70(9):890–910.
27. Schoene D, Wu SM, Mikolaizak AS, et al. Discriminative ability and predictive validity of the timed up and go test in identifying older people who fall: systematic review and meta-analysis. J Am Geriatr Soc 2013;61(2):202–8.
28. Scott IA, Hilmer SN, Reeve E, et al. Reducing inappropriate polypharmacy: the process of deprescribing. JAMA Intern Med 2015;175(5):827–34.
29. Charlesworth CJ, Smit E, Lee DS, et al. Polypharmacy among adults aged 65 years and older in the United States: 1988-2010. J Gerontol A Biol Sci Med Sci 2015;70(8):989–95.
30. Skinner M. A literature review: polypharmacy protocol for primary care. Geriatr Nurs 2015;36(5):367–71.e4.
31. Shah BM, Hajjar ER. Polypharmacy, adverse drug reactions, and geriatric syndromes. Clin Geriatr Med 2012;28(2):173–86.
32. Tinetti ME, Bogardus ST, Agostini JV. Potential pitfalls of disease-specific guidelines for patients with multiple conditions. N Engl J Med 2004;351(27):2870–4.
33. Hajjar E, Hanlon J, Maher R. Clinical consequences of polypharmacy in elderly. Expert Opin Drug Saf 2014;13(1):57–65.
34. Mallet L, Spinewine A, Huang A. The challenge of managing drug interactions in elderly people. Lancet 2007;370(9582):185–91.
35. Spinewine A, Schmader KE, Barber N, et al. Appropriate prescribing in elderly people: how well can it be measured and optimised? Lancet 2007;370(9582):173–84.
36. Bennett A, Gnjidic D, Gillett M, et al. Prevalence and impact of fall-risk-increasing drugs, polypharmacy, and drug-drug interactions in robust versus frail hospitalised falls patients: a prospective cohort study. Drugs Aging 2014;31(3):225–32.
37. Kojima T, Akishita M, Nakamura T, et al. Polypharmacy as a risk for fall occurrence in geriatric outpatients. Geriatr Gerontol Int 2012;12(3):425–30.
38. Fox C, Richardson K, Maidment ID, et al. Anticholinergic medication use and cognitive impairment in the older population: the medical research council cognitive function and ageing study. J Am Geriatr Soc 2011;59(8):1477–83.
39. Hohl CM, Dankoff J, Colacone A, et al. Polypharmacy, adverse drug-related events, and potential adverse drug interactions in elderly patients presenting to an emergency department. Ann Emerg Med 2001;38(6):666–71.
40. Picker D, Heard K, Bailey TC, et al. The number of discharge medications predicts thirty-day hospital readmission: a cohort study. BMC Health Serv Res 2015;15:282.
41. American Geriatrics Society 2012 Beers Criteria Update Expert Panel. American Geriatrics Society Updated Beers Criteria for potentially inappropriate medication use in older adults. J Am Geriatr Soc 2012;60(4):616–31.
42. O'Mahony D, O'Sullivan D, Byrne S, et al. STOPP/START criteria for potentially inappropriate prescribing in older people: version 2. Age Ageing 2015;44(2):213–8.
43. Blanco-Reina E, Ariza-Zafra G, Ocaña-Riola R, et al. 2012 American Geriatrics Society Beers Criteria: Enhanced applicability for detecting potentially

inappropriate medications in European older adults? A comparison with the screening tool of older person's potentially inappropriate prescriptions. J Am Geriatr Soc 2014;62(7):1217–23.

44. Nahin RL, Pecha M, Welmerink DB, et al. Concomitant use of prescription drugs and dietary supplements in ambulatory elderly people. J Am Geriatr Soc 2009; 57(7):1197–205.

45. Green JL, Hawley JN, Rask KJ. Is the number of prescribing physicians an independent risk factor for adverse drug events in an elderly outpatient population? Am J Geriatr Pharmacother 2007;5(1):31–9.

46. Anderson G. Chronic care: making the case for ongoing care. Robert Wood Johnson Foundation; 2010. Available at: http://www.rwjf.org/en/library/research/2010/01/chronic-care.html. Accessed September 15, 2015.

47. Boyd CM, Darer JD, Boult C, et al. Clinical practice guidelines and quality of care for older patients with multiple comorbid diseases: implications for pay for performance. JAMA 2005;294:716–24.

48. Guiding principles for the care of older adults with multimorbidity: an approach for clinicians. Guiding principles for the care of older adults with multimorbidity: an approach for clinicians: American geriatrics society expert panel on the care of older adults with multimorbidity. J Am Geriatr Soc 2012;60:E1–25.

49. Baile WF, Buckman R, Lenzi R, et al. SPIKES—a six-step protocol for delivering bad news: application to the patient with cancer. Oncologist 2000;5(4):302–11.

50. Ramsaroop SD, Reid MC, Adelman RD. Completing an advance directive in the primary care setting: what do we need for success? J Am Geriatr Soc 2007;55: 277–83.

51. Detering KM, Hancock AD, Reade MC, et al. The impact of advance care planning on end of life care in elderly patients: randomised controlled trial. BMJ 2010; 340:c1345.

52. National hospice and palliative care organization caring info. Available at: http://www.caringinfo.org/i4a/pages/index.cfm?pageid=3289. Accessed September 15, 2015.

Index

Note: Page numbers of article titles are in **boldface** type.

A

Abuse
  alcohol
    macrocytic anemia due to, 249
Acne, 187–189
  diagnosis of, 187–188
  epidemiology of, 187
  presentation of, 187
  prognosis, 188–189
  treatment of, 188
Adiposity
  excess
    obesity in women related to
      biological basis of, 204–205
Advance care planning, 375–376
Age
  as factor in CVD in women, 266
Alcohol abuse
  macrocytic anemia due to, 249
Alcohol use
  CVD in women related to, 271
Alopecia, 189–192
  diagnosis of, 190–191
  epidemiology of, 189
  presentation of, 189–190
  prognosis, 191
  treatment of, 191, 192
Amenorrhea
  functional hypothalamic
    CVD related to, 275
Anemia, **247–264**
  described, 247–248
  evaluation of, **247–264** (*See also types of anemia, e.g., Macrocytic anemia*)
    hemolytic anemia, 256–262
    macrocytic anemia, 248–251
    microcytic anemia, 251–255
    normocytic anemia, 255–256
  general considerations in, 247–248
  hemolytic, 256–262
  of inflammation, 254–255

Obstet Gynecol Clin N Am 43 (2016) 381–395
http://dx.doi.org/10.1016/S0889-8545(16)30017-1
0889-8545/16/$ – see front matter

Printed and bound by CPI Group (UK) Ltd, Croydon, CR0 4YY

03/10/2024

01040394-0006